# THIRD EDITION

# SKELETAL RADIOLOGY
## *The Bare Bones*

## FELIX S. CHEW, M.D., Ed.M., M.B.A.

*Professor of Radiology*
*Director of Musculoskeletal Radiology*
*Vice-Chairman for Radiology Informatics*
*Department of Radiology*
*University of Washington*
*Seattle, Washington*

WITH CONTRIBUTIONS FROM

### LIEM T. BUI-MANSFIELD, M.D.

### CATHERINE C. ROBERTS, M.D.

### MICHAEL L. RICHARDSON, M.D.

Wolters Kluwer | Lippincott Williams & Wilkins
Health

Philadelphia · Baltimore · New York · London
Buenos Aires · Hong Kong · Sydney · Tokyo

*Acquisitions Editor*: Charles W. Mitchell
*Product Manager*: Ryan Shaw
*Vendor Manager*: Alicia Jackson
*Senior Manufacturing Manager*: Benjamin Rivera
*Senior Marketing Manager*: Angela Panetta
*Design Coordinator*: Teresa Mallon
*Production Service*: SPi Technologies

**Library of Congress Cataloging-in-Publication Data**
Chew, Felix S.
  Skeletal radiology : the bare bones / Felix S. Chew ; with contributions from Liem T.
Bui-Mansfield, Catherine C. Roberts, Michael L. Richardson. — 3rd ed.
      p. ; cm.
  Includes bibliographical references and index.
  ISBN 978-1-60831-706-6 (alk. paper)
  1. Human skeleton—Radiography. 2. Bones—Diseases—Diagnosis. 3. Bones—Imaging. I. Title.
  [DNLM: 1. Bone and Bones—radiography. 2. Bone Diseases—radiography. 3. Fractures,
Bone—radiography. WE 200 C526s 2010]
  RC930.5.C48   2010
  616.7'107572—dc22
                                                                                    2009050533

Care has been taken to confirm the accuracy of the information presented and to describe generally accepted practices. However, the authors, editors, and publisher are not responsible for errors or omissions or for any consequences from application of the information in this book and make no warranty, expressed or implied, with respect to the currency, completeness, or accuracy of the contents of the publication. Application of the information in a particular situation remains the professional responsibility of the practitioner.

The authors, editors, and publisher have exerted every effort to ensure that drug selection and dosage set forth in this text are in accordance with current recommendations and practice at the time of publication. However, in view of ongoing research, changes in government regulations, and the constant flow of information relating to drug therapy and drug reactions, the reader is urged to check the package insert for each drug for any change in indications and dosage and for added warnings and precautions. This is particularly important when the recommended agent is a new or infrequently employed drug.

Some drugs and medical devices presented in the publication have Food and Drug Administration (FDA) clearance for limited use in restricted research settings. It is the responsibility of the health care provider to ascertain the FDA status of each drug or device planned for use in their clinical practice.

To purchase additional copies of this book, call our customer service department at (800) 638–3030 or fax orders to (301) 223–2320. International customers should call (301) 223–2300.

Visit Lippincott Williams & Wilkins on the Internet: at LWW.com. Lippincott Williams & Wilkins customer service representatives are available from 8:30 am to 6 pm, EST.

10 9 8 7 6 5 4 3 2 1

RRS1001

# FOREWORD

The initial publication of Felix S. Chew's *Skeletal Radiology: The Bare Bones* filled a long-standing need for a concise, introductory primer to the imaging of musculoskeletal diseases. For this, the third edition, Dr. Chew has the contributions of three outstanding musculoskeletal radiologists; Drs. Liem Bui-Mansfield, Catherine Roberts, and Michael Richardson. Together these authors have thoroughly updated the information available in their new work including considerably more magnetic resonance imaging and CT. Most of the older radiographic images have been replaced with newer digital radiographic images. The text has been revised as necessary, and the sources and readings have been updated. That said, Dr. Chew's basic approach has been maintained throughout; the emphasis remains on explanations and descriptions that are to be understood and applied rather than the now common presentation of lists of facts that tend to be memorized and forgotten.

Medical school curricula do not often include a serious study of afflictions of the bones and joints. Even the most common conditions; trauma, osteoporosis, bone metastases, and degenerative joint disease receive scant attention. As a result, most first year residents come to radiology with a limited knowledge of the musculoskeletal system and its diseases. Therefore, the neophyte resident's introduction to musculoskeletal radiology can be daunting. With this limited background, trainees have thrust upon them a vast array of unfamiliar disease processes, a perplexing variety of normal variants, and the complex radiologic anatomy of several different body regions. What are these new radiology residents to do?

Fortunately, there's *The Bare Bones*. Radiology residents can turn to this excellent text to acquire a firm foundation for musculoskeletal imaging. Dr. Chew provides the uninitiated with a working knowledge of skeletal disease and an awareness of the role and value of imaging in the discovery, analysis, and confirmation of the various skeletal abnormalities.

In stripping skeletal radiology to its essentials, Dr. Chew and his coauthors have actually left considerable flesh on the bones. The information in *The Bare Bones* is hardly bare or even spare. All the essentials are covered. All of the critical aspects of the most common skeletal diseases are described and illustrated. The authors synthesize the current knowledge regarding the clinical, pathologic, and physiologic features of each disease, and then outline the proper approach to the interpretation of radiographs, computed tomography, magnetic resonance imaging, and skeletal scintigrams. The important features of each disorder are demonstrated with exceptional illustrations, augmented, as necessary, by excellent diagrams, and appropriately summarized in tables. This masterful approach is consistently applied with superb results.

The book is divided into four parts. The six chapters of Part I are devoted to trauma, properly reflecting the frequency with which skeletal injuries are encountered and the overriding importance of imaging in the diagnosis and management of fractures and dislocations. The first chapter gives an excellent background to the clinical and biomechanical considerations. The next three chapters address injuries of the upper extremity; spine, thoracic cage, and pelvis; and lower extremity, respectively. Chapter 5 describes the distinctive nature of skeletal trauma in children, and Chapter 6 describes imaging of fracture treatment and healing.

Part II begins with a discussion of the clinical features and imaging approach to lesions of the bone. These lesions are then enumerated individually and described in separate chapters on malignant and benign lesions. The final chapter is justifiably devoted to the frequently encountered clinical problem of metastatic disease to the skeleton, and emphasizes the primary role of imaging techniques in detection and management.

Part III covers joint disease, beginning with a description of basic clinical and pathologic features. An overall approach to the radiology of arthritis is presented, followed by chapters on inflammatory arthritis and noninflammatory joint disease.

In separate chapters, Part IV describes developmental and congenital conditions; metabolic, endocrine, and nutritional conditions; and infections of the bones, joints, and soft tissues. There follows a chapter on postsurgical imaging that includes a thorough discussion of the use of imaging in joint replacement, a topic of particular interest to Dr. Chew.

It is all here. I recommend this book to all residents in diagnostic radiology, indeed to all students of skeletal disease. Medical students with an interest in diagnostic radiology, orthopedic surgery, or rheumatology would certainly benefit from its contents. Experienced radiologists will find it a great refresher and undoubtedly gain new insights into musculoskeletal diseases and pick up several useful pointers on musculoskeletal imaging along the way. Teachers of skeletal radiology will discover that the approaches developed and the excellent tables and figures can be of considerable value in preparing their own presentations.

Dr. Chew's first two editions of *The Bare Bones* were outstanding. This third edition is even better. If you would like to improve your musculoskeletal imaging skills – read on!

*Lee F. Rogers, M.D.*
*Clinical Professor*
*Department of Radiology*
*University of Arizona*
*Tucson, AZ*

# PREFACE

The ranges of pathology and individual variation in the skeleton are too vast for sheer memorization and pattern recognition. One is better able to appreciate abnormalities on images when one understands how the radiologic findings mirror the underlying conditions. For trauma, this requires some familiarity with biomechanics; for oncology, an appreciation of radiologic-pathologic correlation; and for developmental conditions, an understanding of skeletal growth, maturation, and functional adaptation. In the 20 years since the publication of the first edition of *The Bare Bones*, the wider application and further refinement of MRI and CT have continued to reduce the role of radiography in musculoskeletal imaging. Inferential diagnosis on the basis of radiologic signs has lost ground to the deliberate demonstration of specific anatomic and pathophysiologic features of disease. The choice and specific performance of examinations have become particularly dependent on clinical context. It is no longer sufficient to react to an image with a list of differential diagnoses; rather, one must consider the clinically relevant possibilities and devise strategies for distinguishing among them with certainty.

*Skeletal Radiology: The Bare Bones*, Third Edition, is a single unified textbook that teaches general principles of skeletal radiology that are applicable regardless of imaging modality. Organized into four parts, this book presents the core knowledge base in musculoskeletal imaging necessary for a radiology resident. Part I covers musculoskeletal trauma, beginning with an approach to trauma and concluding with separate chapters describing trauma to the upper and lower extremities in adults, trauma to the adult spine, trauma in children, and fracture healing and treatment. Part II covers tumors and tumorlike lesions, beginning with an approach to bone lesions and concluding with separate chapters on malignant and aggressive tumors, benign lesions, and metastatic tumors. Part III covers joint disease, beginning with an approach to joint disease and concluding with separate chapters on inflammatory arthritis and noninflammatory joint disease. Part IV covers miscellaneous topics, including chapters on developmental and congenital conditions, metabolic, endocrine, and nutritional conditions, infection and marrow disease, and postsurgical musculoskeletal imaging. The final chapter covers interventional procedures in musculoskeletal radiology. Although this book is intended specifically for radiologists and radiologists-in-training, it is also suitable for practitioners and trainees in all fields who deal with the diagnosis and management of musculoskeletal disease.

# ACKNOWLEDGMENTS

The images in this textbook were selected from the teaching files and clinical case material at Upstate Medical Center in Syracuse, New York; the Massachusetts General Hospital in Boston, Massachusetts; Wake Forest University Baptist Medical Center in Winston-Salem, North Carolina; Keller Army Community Hospital in West Point, New York; the Cleveland Clinic Foundation in Cleveland, Ohio; the University of Washington Medical Center in Seattle, Washington; Harborview Medical Center in Seattle, Washington; the Mayo Clinic Arizona in Scottsdale, Arizona; and Brooke Army Medical Center, San Antonio, Texas. Friends and colleagues who have graciously provided additional case material include Drs. Carol Boles, William Enneking, Joel Gross, Martin Gunn, Heather Hardie, Terry Hudson, Linda Hughes, John Hunter, Mitchell Kline, Wendy Jones, Susan Kattapuram, Michelle Kraut, Susan Leffler, Leon Lenchik, Mark Levinsohn, Gwilym Lodwick, Catherine Maldjian, Liem Bui-Mansfield, Henry Mankin, Kevin McEnery, Michael Mulligan, Robert Novelline, William Palmer, Michael Richardson, Catherine Roberts, Lee Rogers, Daniel Rosenthal, Dempsey Springfield, and others whom I may have unintentionally overlooked at the moment of this writing. The line illustrations were drawn by Crisianee Berry.

*—Felix S. Chew*

# ABBREVIATIONS AND ACRONYMS

| | |
|---|---|
| ACL | anterior cruciate ligament |
| AIDS | acquired immunodeficiency syndrome |
| ALPSA | anterior labrum periosteal sleeve avulsion |
| ANA | antinuclear antibodies |
| AP | anteroposterior |
| BHAGL | bony humeral avulsion of the inferior glenohumeral ligament |
| BMD | bone mineral density, bone mineral densitometry |
| C1, C2, C3, etc. | first cervical vertebra (atlas), second cervical vertebra (axis), etc. |
| CMC joint | carpometacarpal joint |
| CPPD | calcium pyrophosphate dihydrate |
| CT | computed tomography |
| DDH | developmental dysplasia of the hip |
| DEXA | dual energy x-ray absorptiometry |
| DIP joint | distal interphalangeal joint |
| DISH | diffuse idiopathic skeletal hyperostosis |
| DISI | dorsal intercalated segment instability (dorsiflexion instability) |
| DPA | dual photon absorptiometry |
| DXA | dual x-ray absorptiometry |
| FS | fat suppression |
| Gd | gadolinium |
| GLAD | glenolabral articular disruption |
| GRE | gradient recalled echo |
| HAGL | humeral avulsion of the inferior glenohumeral ligament |
| HIV | human immunodeficiency virus |
| HLA | human leukocyte antigen |
| HU | Hounsfield unit (unit of x-ray attenuation on a CT scan) |
| IM rod | intramedullary rod |
| IP joint | interphalangeal joint |
| K-wire | Kirschner wire |

| | |
|---|---|
| L1, L2, L3, etc. | first lumbar vertebra, second lumbar vertebra, etc. |
| LCL | lateral collateral ligament (of the knee) |
| MCL | medial collateral ligament (of the knee) |
| MCP joint | metacarpophalangeal joint |
| MFH | malignant fibrous histiocytoma |
| MR | magnetic resonance |
| MRI | magnetic resonance imaging |
| MTP joint | metatarsophalangeal joint |
| OCD | osteochondral defect, osteochondritis dissecans |
| ORIF | open reduction internal fixation |
| PA | posteroanterior |
| PCL | posterior cruciate ligament |
| PET | positron emission tomography |
| PIP joint | proximal interphalangeal joint |
| PMNs | polymorphonuclear leukocytes |
| PVNS | pigmented villonodular synovitis |
| QCT | quantitative computed tomography |
| RF | rheumatoid factor |
| S1, S2, S3, etc. | first sacral vertebra, second sacral vertebra, etc. |
| SCFE | slipped capital femoral epiphysis |
| SI joint | sacroiliac joint |
| SLAP tear | superior labrum anterior to posterior tear |
| SLE | systemic lupus erythematosus |
| STIR | short tau inversion recovery |
| T1, T2, T3, etc. | first thoracic vertebra, second thoracic vertebra, etc. |
| TFCC | triangular fibrocartilage complex |
| THR | total hip replacement |
| TKR | total knee replacement |
| TMT joint | tarsometararsal joint |
| VISI | volar intercalated segment instability (volar flexion instability) |
| WBC | white blood cell |

# FIGURE CREDITS

**FIGURE 8.27 A–C:**  From Ramsdell MG, Chew FS, Keel SB. Myxoid liposarcoma of the thigh. *AJR*. 1998;170:1242.

**FIGURE 16.1 A, B:**  From Chew FS, Schulze ES, Mattia AR. Osteomyelitis. *AJR*. 1994;162:942.

**FIGURE 17.27 A, B:**  From Chew FS, Ramsdell MG, Keel SB. Metallosis after total knee replacement. *AJR*. 1998;170:1556.

**FIGURES 1.1–8.26**, **FIGURES 8.28–15.41**, **FIGURES 16.2–17.26**, and **FIGURES 17.28–17.51:**  Used with permission from the following sources: Chew FS. *Skeletal Radiology: The Bare Bones*. Rockville, MD: Aspen Publishers; 1989; Chew FS. *Skeletal Radiology: The Bare Bones Teaching Collection*. St. Paul, MN: Image PSL; 1991; Chew FS. *Skeletal Radiology: The Bare Bones*. 2nd Ed., Baltimore, MD: Williams & Wilkins; 1997; Chew FS. *Skeletal Radiology Interactive*. Baltimore, MD: Williams & Wilkins; 1998; Chew FS, Maldjian C, Leffler SG. *Musculoskeletal Imaging: A Teaching File*. Philadelphia, PA: Lippincott Williams & Wilkins; 1999; Chew FS, Kline MJ, Whitman GJ, eds. *iRAD: Interactive Radiology Review and Assessment*. Philadelphia, PA: Lippincott Williams & Wilkins; 2000; Chew FS. *Skeletal Radiology Interactive 2.0*. Winston-Salem, NC: Bubbasoft of North Carolina; 2002; Chew FS. *Skeletal Radiology Interactive 3.0*, Bainbridge Island, WA: Northwest Bubbasoft; 2009; Chew FS, Maldjian C. *Broken Bones: The X-Ray Atlas of Fractures*. Seattle, WA: BareBonesBooks.com; 2009.

# CONTENTS

# PART I

# Trauma

# Approach to Trauma

T rauma to the human frame may cause deformation and breakage. The radiology of musculoskeletal trauma is more than a search for broken bones; it is an analysis of the effect of traumatic forces on a particular patient. It requires an understanding of the ways in which various forces affect the body: how they are applied, where they concentrate, and how they disrupt structural integrity. Fractures are but one manifestation of trauma; injuries to the soft tissues and other organ systems may be present.

## EPIDEMIOLOGY

Fractures are not isolated phenomena; rather, they occur in the context of individual patients. Characteristics that affect the frequency, severity, location, and type of fracture include age, gender, activity, and health of the musculoskeletal system. The incidence of fractures of the extremities has a bimodal distribution with respect to age. In men, there is a first peak, between 10 and 20 years of age, which is related to immaturity of the skeleton, and a second peak, beginning at approximately 70 years of age, which is related to involutional osteoporosis. In women, there is a first peak at 10 years of age, again related to immaturity of the skeleton, and a second peak, beginning at approximately 50 years of age, that is related to postmenopausal osteoporosis. The skeleton is weak when it is growing, gains strength as it matures, and weakens again as it ages. Under 50 years of age, fractures are more common in males than in females because of greater exposure to trauma, but over 50 years of age, fractures in women become more common because of osteoporosis.

In adolescents and young adults, the most common sites of fractures in the extremities are the phalanges and metacarpals of the hand, the distal humerus, the shaft of the tibia, the clavicle, the distal radius, and the phalanges of the foot. In adults older than 50 years of age, the most common sites of fractures in the extremities are the proximal femur, the proximal humerus, the distal radius, and the pelvis.

## BONE BIOMECHANICS

Bone responds to trauma in predictable ways. From knowledge of the anatomic site involved and the forces applied, one can often predict the fractures that result. Conversely, knowing the site and morphology of a particular fracture frequently allows one to infer the forces that caused it. Such knowledge has practical applications to diagnosis and management.

## Force And Deformation

Application of external force to the bone is called *loading*. Bone is physically deformed (i.e., undergoes strain) when it is placed under a load (Fig. 1.1). At physiologic levels of loading, the bone undergoes elastic deformation as it absorbs and stores the energy imparted by the loading. When the load is removed, the stored energy is dissipated by elastic recoil, the bone recovers its preloaded shape, and no damage is sustained. Loading has a linear relationship to elastic deformation called *stiffness*. The stiffer the material, the less it deforms under a given load. When the severity of loading exceeds the level at which elastic recoil is possible, the bone sustains plastic (also called *ductile*) deformation. The absorbed energy from loading is expended in the work of permanently deforming the bone. The *ductility* of a material describes the degree to which it can sustain plastic deformation without breaking. At even greater levels of loading, the bone fails completely, and the imparted energy is expended in fracturing the bone and displacing the fragments. If loading continues, other body parts may sustain injury. Excessive loading results in injury; in general, the greater the amount of loading and the more rapidly it is applied, the more severe the injury.

The external force of loading involves three fundamental components: compressive, tensile, and shear. The compressive component acts inwardly and squashes the bone together, the tensile component acts outwardly and pulls the bone apart, and the shear component acts parallel to the direction of force and sends different points in the bone past each other. The bone subjected to tensile loading tends to elongate; mechanical failure occurs when cement lines debond and the osteons are pulled apart. The bone subjected to compressive loading tends to shorten; mechanical failure occurs when individual osteons sustain oblique cracking. The bone subjected to shear loading undergoes angular deformity. Both tensile and compressive loadings have shear as a component because angular deformity occurs as the bone elongates or shortens.

Bone is a diphasic material comprised of a rigid calcium hydroxyapatite crystalline structure that is resistant to compressive forces and a collagenous matrix of flexible fibrils and ground

**FIGURE 1.2.** Low-velocity gunshot wound causing comminuted fractures of the ulnar shaft.

**FIGURE 1.1.** Various modes of loading.

substance that is resistant to tensile forces. In compact bone (also referred to as *lamellar bone* or *cortical bone*), the material of bone is organized into concentric layers around the neurovascular supply to form osteons (haversian systems). Osteons are the basic functional and structural unit of compact bone. In cancellous bone (trabecular bone), the material of bone is organized into a three-dimensional latticelike system of plates and columns (trabeculae), with the neurovascular supply passing between trabeculae. Compact bone is stiffer than cancellous bone, but cancellous bone is more ductile. The functional architecture of mature bone reflects a continuing process of remodeling to accommodate the type, magnitude, and direction of physiologic loading. In general, bone resists compression better than tension and tension better than shear.

## Loading And Fractures

Loading can be direct or indirect. Direct loading causes injuries at the site of loading. The morphology of fractures caused by direct loading—although related to the site, direction, and amount of force applied—tends to be unpredictable. Such injuries may be classified as crushing, penetrating, or tapping. A crushing injury results from the application of a large force over a large area, for example, a building collapsing on an individual. Crushing force results in comminuted or transverse fractures and extensive soft-tissue damage. A penetrating injury results from a large force being applied to a small area, for example, a gunshot wound. Penetrating force usually results in comminuted fractures; the degree of comminution depends on the energy of the penetrating projectile (Fig. 1.2). A tapping injury results from

a small force being applied to a small area, for example, a blow to the forearm from a nightstick. Tapping force results in a transverse or stellate fracture at the site of impact (Fig. 1.3). Bones without much soft-tissue coverage, such as the ulna or tibia, are more vulnerable to direct trauma than bones such as the humerus or femur.

Indirect loading causes injuries at a distance from the site of loading. The morphology of fractures caused by indirect loading tends to be predictable. Loading under tension (pulling apart), compression (squashing together), torsion (twisting), angulation (bending), and certain combinations of these produce fractures

**FIGURE 1.3.** Tapping fracture of the ulnar shaft (nightstick fracture).

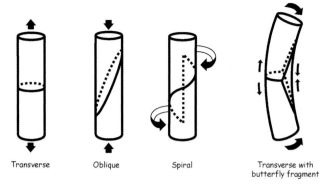

**FIGURE 1.4.** Types of loading correlated with direction of fracture lines.

with predictable shapes that often occur at specific sites (Fig. 1.4). Soft tissues may modify indirect loading—for example, muscles can reduce tensile loads on bones by contracting and supplying an opposing compressive force.

Traction or tension fractures occur as a result of traction on a bone by a tendon or ligament. The bone is pulled apart, or avulsed, and the fracture line is transverse to the direction of force as the bone fibers fail under tension. At the fingers, for example, fragments of bone may be avulsed at the insertions of tendons or ligaments (Fig. 1.5). The size of the avulsed fragment may range from large to tiny (Fig. 1.6). A large fragment may comprise a full-thickness piece of the bone; a small fragment may represent a mere fraction of the cortex. Tension fractures are most common in cancellous bone.

When a long bone is angulated, the convex side is placed under tension, and the concave side is placed under compression. Because the bone fails first under tension, a transverse fracture propagates across the bone from the convex side. On the concave side, the bone may fail under compressive and shearing forces and splinter. Alternatively, a triangular fragment may shear off at an angle to the main fracture line. This results in comminution with a butterfly fragment on the concave side of the bend (Fig. 1.7).

**FIGURE 1.6.** Tiny avulsion fragment at the volar plate attachment at the middle phalanx (*arrow*).

Longitudinal compressive loading of the shaft of a long bone results in an oblique fracture caused by osteons being forced past each other and shearing off (Fig. 1.8). Compressive loading of a whole bone often results in T- or Y-shaped fractures as the hard cortical bone of the shaft is driven into the softer cancellous metaphysis. Such fractures are common at the ends of the humerus or femur and in the hands and toes.

Rotational loading (torsion or twisting) causes horizontal shearing with compressive and tensile components at an angle to the long axis of the shaft (Fig. 1.9). These stresses lead to a spiral fracture that curves around the circumference of the bone, representing a failure

**FIGURE 1.5.** Avulsion fragment at the extensor insertion at the distal phalanx (*arrow*).

**FIGURE 1.7.** Transverse fracture of the tibia with butterfly fragment.

**FIGURE 1.8.** Oblique fracture of the proximal phalanx of the middle finger.

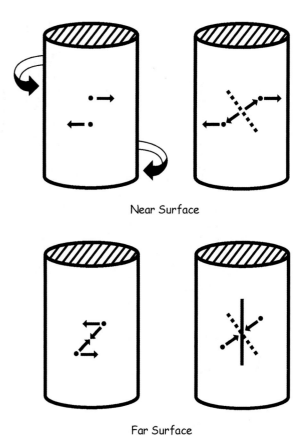

**FIGURE 1.9.** Diagrammatic representation of spiral fracture. On the near cortex of the bone, under torsion, horizontal shear stress forces points in the bone past each other. Tensile stress is present because these points are at the same time pulled apart, leading to an obliquely oriented tension fracture around the circumference of the bone. On the far cortex of the bone, compressive forces are present, leading to a vertical fracture that joins the spiral fracture lines.

in tension, as the bone is pulled apart. The fracture line makes one complete rotation around the circumference of the bone and has sharp pointed ends joined by a vertical component (Fig. 1.10). The vertical fracture acts as a hinge, with the fracture fragments separating on the opposite side along the curved component.

Many fractures are produced by a combination of forces. Angulation with axial compression results in a curved fracture line with oblique and transverse components and sometimes a butterfly fragment. Angulation with rotation results in an oblique fracture with short, blunted ends.

## Bone Bruises

Bone bruises are traumatic injuries to cancellous bone in which hemorrhage and edema displace the normal marrow. These injuries, which involve microfractures of individual trabeculae and disruption of small vessels, are evident on MRI as regions of localized edema with intact overlying articular cartilage and subcortical bone. The mechanism of injury is typically compression, either from direct impact or from indirect loading, with the impact transmitted through an adjacent bone. When the mechanism is direct impact, the bone bruise is usually isolated. When the mechanism is through indirect, transmitted impact, additional significant injuries may be present elsewhere in the anatomic region (Fig. 1.11). The pattern of bone bruises may help to identify associated injuries and suggest the mechanism of injury. Bone bruises typically revert to normal on follow-up MRI within several months; typically, the radiograph remains normal throughout the episode.

## ■ IMAGING FRACTURES

Although some fractures can be identified on virtually any imaging modality, radiography dominates the imaging evaluation for acute fractures. CT has a supporting role in characterizing complex fractures in preparation for possible surgery and occasionally in identifying fractures when radiographs are equivocal. In the spine, CT is used to screen for fractures in the setting of polytrauma.

MRI may be used for identifying fractures, particularly stress and insufficiency fractures, when radiographs are negative or equivocal. MRI is more commonly used for identifying and characterizing soft-tissue and joint injuries. The radionuclide bone scan may be used for identifying stress fractures. Radiographs are a diagnostic supplement to the history and physical examination; care of the patient should not be secondary to performing the radiographic examination. Splinting an injured limb, for example, can alleviate pain without interfering with subsequent radiologic examinations.

On radiographs, fractures of cortical bone are definitively recognized as focal discontinuities in the structure of bone, particularly when displacement is present. Impacted fractures of cortical bone may be recognized as focal alterations in the contour of the bone, typically an abrupt change in what should otherwise be a smooth contour. Compression fractures in cancellous bone may have a discontinuity in the cortex, a change in shape, a linear region of sclerosis, or any combination of these features. Avulsion fractures occur when tension on the attachment of a tendon, ligament, or capsule pulls off a fragment of bone. These fractures may be recognized as displaced fragments that may range in size from less than 1 mm in thickness to several centimeters.

On CT scans, features of fractures are similar to those seen on radiography, but the ability to display the features is greatly enhanced by axial cross sections and multiplanar reconstructions (Fig. 1.12).

**A**    **B**

**FIGURE 1.10.** Spiral fracture of the tibial shaft. **A:** AP view. **B:** Lateral view.

On MRI, fracture lines are dark on T1-weighted images, with surrounding intermediate signal that may involve the adjacent marrow and soft tissues, corresponding to hemorrhage and edema (Fig. 1.13). On T2-weighted images, the surrounding edema and

**FIGURE 1.11.** Bone bruises caused by hyperextension injury. Sagittal T2-weighted fat-suppressed MRI shows a bone bruise in the anterior aspect of the lateral tibial plateau and a matching impaction fracture of the lateral femoral condyle.

hemorrhage are high in signal intensity, while the fracture line remains dark. In compression fractures of cancellous bone, the fracture line may be absent, but the change in signal will be present if the fracture is acute. Avulsion fracture fragments may be difficult to identify on MRI, as the fragment itself may have the same dark signal on T1- and T2-weighted images as the soft tissue structure that pulled it off. Surrounding edema and hemorrhage should be present with acute fractures. Fractures caused by compressive loading tend to have greater amounts of adjacent marrow edema than fractures caused by tensile loading.

On radionuclide bone scans, fractures are evident as regions of focal accumulation of radioactivity. However, because the accumulation of the radioactive tracer depends on increased bone metabolism, radionuclide bone scans are useful only after the healing process has begun and are not used in imaging acute trauma.

## ◼ SOFT-TISSUE BIOMECHANICS

Similar to bone, the soft-tissue structures of the musculoskeletal system deform when loaded. In addition to recoverable or elastic deformation, the soft tissues may also sustain nonrecoverable or nonelastic deformation. *Creep* is continuous deformation under an applied load, and *stress relaxation* is the decrease in internal load over time at a constant deformation. These *viscous effects* vary with time and the rate of loading, and the structure does not instantaneously recover its original size and shape when the load is removed. When a soft-tissue structure is loaded rapidly, it deforms elastically and perhaps fails if the load is great enough; if the same load is applied more slowly, creep and stress relaxation allow the structure to deform to a greater extent, permitting it to absorb more energy without failing. For these reasons, ligaments

A    B

**FIGURE 1.12.** Subtle hip fracture on CT. **A:** Axial CT scan shows subtle discontinuity in the right femoral cortex anteriorly with slight impaction posteriorly (*arrows*), corresponding to a minimally displaced fracture of the greater trochanter. **B:** Coronal reformatted CT shows the extent of the fracture.

and tendons are stronger under tensile loading when the load is applied slowly rather than rapidly. Where they attach to bone, it is generally the rate of loading and the strength of the soft tissues relative to the bone that determine whether a soft-tissue or a bony injury is sustained. In general, rapid rates of loading cause the soft tissues to fail, whereas slower rates of loading avulse the bone. Injuries of tendons or muscle-tendon units are called *strains*;

injuries of ligaments are called *sprains*. Injuries of either may also be called *tears*. Strains and sprains are classified by severity, with grade 1 being a mild injury and grade 3 being a severe, complete discontinuity (Table 1.1). Injuries to soft tissue alone without associated fractures are common and may be difficult to detect on radiographs. Soft-tissue injuries may be directly imaged by MRI and sonography.

A    B

**FIGURE 1.13.** Minimally displaced lateral tibial plateau fracture. **A:** Coronal T1-weighted MRI shows dark fracture line (*arrow*) with surrounding edema. **B:** Coronal inversion recovery MRI shows dark fracture line (*arrow*) with surrounding edema.

| TABLE 1.1 | Grading of Sprains and Strains | | |
|-----------|-------------------------------|--|--|
| | | Clinical Signs | |
| Grade | Injury | Ligament | Muscle-Tendon |
| 1 | Failure of a few fibers | No laxity | No weakness |
| 2 | Partial failure | Laxity | Weakness |
| 3 | Complete rupture | Frank instability | No muscle action |

Collateral soft-tissue injury always accompanies bony injury. Damage may range from superficial abrasions and minimal contusions at the site of injury to massive devitalization involving major segments of the limbs. Direct trauma may cause abrasion, contusion, or crushing of soft tissues. Subcutaneous avulsion of the cutis, compartment syndrome, and a major vascular injury may be caused by indirect mechanisms. For example, displacing fragments from a fracture caused by high-energy indirect loading may slice through the adjacent neurovascular structures and surrounding soft tissues like a meat grinder. In the forearm and lower leg, hemorrhage and acute inflammation from soft-tissue injuries may lead to a compartment syndrome in which increased hydrostatic pressure within a fascial compartment may compromise the circulation and cause ischemic necrosis. Strains of adjacent musculature are common accompaniments to fractures, and sharp bony fragments may lacerate adjacent muscles. Complete fractures of long bones may result in hematomas and sterile collections when the bone marrow spills into the adjacent soft tissues (Fig. 1.14).

The articular cartilage that covers the ends of bones in joints is usually loaded in compression because the coefficient of friction at the surface is too low to generate significant shearing forces. With compressive loading, usually indirect blunt impact transferred through the bone, the structure of the extracellular matrix may sustain damage. With more severe loading, the chondrocytes may die, and the cartilage may crack apart and become fissured. Fibrocartilage articular structures such as articular disks, menisci, and labra may be injured by a variety of mechanisms.

# ◼ IMAGING SOFT-TISSUE INJURIES

Although radiography is typically the first imaging study used for evaluation of soft-tissue injuries, it is performed principally to look for fractures. CT is sometimes used in the same way, particularly in the spine. MRI is the best imaging modality for identifying and characterizing soft-tissue and joint injuries. The radionuclide bone scan is not useful in recognizing sprains and strains. Sonography is typically not used in the acute setting.

On radiographs, injuries of ligaments and joint capsules (sprains) and of muscle-tendon units (strains) may be recognized indirectly, evident as soft-tissue swelling or the loss of anatomic positioning of bony structures. Stress views or kinematic observation under fluoroscopy may be helpful (Fig. 1.15). For example, when bony structures stabilized by a ligament are displaced from their usual positions, injury to the ligament may be inferred. Soft-tissue swelling, particularly when focal, may also indicate a sprain or a strain.

On CT, the ability to identify soft-tissue structures is improved compared with radiographs. As with radiography, indirect signs such as displacement of bony structures or soft-tissue swelling may allow one to infer the presence of a sprain or strain.

On MRI, sprains and strains may be directly imaged. Complete tears (grade 3 sprains) of ligaments may be evident as absence of the structure, displacement of the structure, discontinuity of the structure, or abnormal signal intensity. When tears are acute, displacement and discontinuity with surrounding hemorrhage and edema allow a definitive diagnosis. Partial tears (grade 1 or 2 sprains) may be evident as focally increased signal on T2-weighted

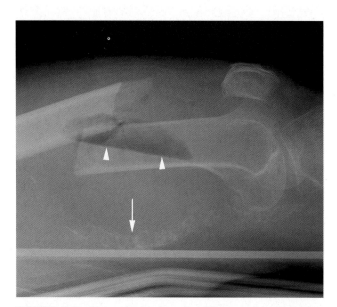

**FIGURE 1.14.** Hematoma and sterile collection of bone marrow spilling into the soft tissues adjacent to a displaced femoral shaft fracture. Note the fat-fluid level (*arrowheads*) on this horizontal beam radiograph and the posterior displacement of the calcified popliteal artery (*arrow*) by the collection.

**FIGURE 1.15.** Ulnar collateral ligament sprain at the first MCP joint. Fluoroscopic image with stress shows widening of the joint on the ulnar side (*arrow*).

**FIGURE 1.16.** Muscle strain accompanying fracture. Axial inversion recovery MRI of the thigh shows high signal in the vastus intermedius muscle (*arrow*) surrounding a femoral shaft fracture.

images with surrounding hemorrhage and edema; at least some portions of the ligament remain in continuity.

Complete tendon tears (grade 3 strains) are usually evident as discontinuity of the tendon with retraction in the direction of the muscle belly. Hemorrhage and edema are typically present in the acute phase but may be absent if the injury is chronic. When tears are partial (grade 1 or 2 strains), focally increased signal on T2-weighted images is present, sometimes with surrounding edema and hemorrhage. Abnormal intrasubstance signal and swelling are generally present in all tendon tears. Fluid within the tendon sheath is also a typical finding in both complete and partial tendon tears. Muscle tears are evident as high signal on T2-weighted images, corresponding to edema and hemorrhage (Fig. 1.16). The abnormal signal is distributed along fascial planes and may be interdigitated within muscle fascicles.

On sonography, the appearance of normal ligaments, tendons, and muscles, because they are structurally organized along the lines of stress, is directionally dependent, a property called anisotropy. Complete tendon tears may be recognized by discontinuity of the tendon with the two ends separated by hypoechoic blood, fluid, or granulation tissue. Sometimes, the structure is simply absent from its expected location. Partial tears may be recognized as focal hypoechoic defects within the substance of the tendon or focal thinning (Fig. 1.17). If a tendon sheath is present, fluid within the tendon sheath will be interposed between the torn fragments of either complete or partial tears.

## ■ OPEN FRACTURES

Open fractures (also called compound fractures) involve a break in the skin. These are distinguished from closed fractures (also called simple fractures), in which the skin remains intact. The presence of a skin wound is often an indication of extensive soft-tissue injury. Traumatized, devitalized soft tissues pose a grave threat of

**A**

**B**

**FIGURE 1.17.** Sonogram of Achilles tear. **A:** Longitudinal scan (feet to left, head to right) shows normal distal tendon fibers (*arrowheads*) and markedly thickened and retracted proximal tendon (*arrow*) with heterogeneous echogenicity (Tibia: posterior tibia). **B:** Sagittal PD MRI of the Achilles tendon with the sonographic field of view indicated by the rectangle. The distal tendon has normal thickness (*arrowheads*) while the retracted proximal tendon is thickened (*arrow*).

infection; exposed bone will not heal. Radiographic signs indicative of an open fracture include a soft-tissue defect, a bone fragment protruding beyond the soft tissues, gas in the soft tissues or within an adjacent joint, the presence of a foreign body, and missing bone fragments.

Open fractures can be classified on the basis of the energy of the injury and consequent extent of soft-tissue devitalization. Type I open fractures are low-energy wounds with a skin wound that is typically 1 cm or less in length. A sharp bone fragment piercing the skin from the inside out usually causes the skin wound, which is generally clean. Muscle and soft-tissue damage are minimal or absent. These injuries are usually debrided and closed. The risk of infection under ideal management is very low. Type II open fractures are usually penetrating wounds with fractures (Fig. 1.18). The extent

**FIGURE 1.18.** Amputation of a fingertip.

of soft-tissue injury is relatively localized, but the skin wound is greater than 1 cm in length. These injuries may be debrided and closed or left open, depending on the circumstance. The infection rate is approximately 2%. Type III open fractures are severe high-energy wounds with gross disruption of skin, soft tissues, and bone. Extensive muscle devitalization and soft tissue disruption or gross contamination are present, and the skin wound is often 10 cm or more in length. The associated fractures are widely displaced, segmental, or badly comminuted, as one would expect with

**FIGURE 1.19.** Comminuted open fracture of the foot from crush injury.

**FIGURE 1.20.** Open, comminuted fracture dislocation of the ankle. Lateral radiograph shows fractures with air within the ankle joint (*arrow*). The joint had been reduced at the scene of the injury before transport.

a high-energy injury (Fig. 1.19). Type III open fractures can be further classified into type III-A, in which there is only limited stripping of the periosteum and soft tissues from the bone; type III-B, in which there is extensive soft tissue loss and gross exposure of bone; and type III-C, in which there is a major vascular disruption. The infection rate is approximately 18% for type III-A open fractures but is more than 50% for types III-B and III-C open fractures. Paradoxically, as techniques of surgical management have improved, the infection rate of open fractures has increased. The explanation lies in the attempted salvage of more severely traumatized limbs that previously would have simply been amputated. The spectrum of infecting organisms has also been changing.

Open fractures that involve a joint often require special care. Gas within a joint that is adjacent to a fracture is an indication that the joint may be contaminated and requires debridement and repair (Fig. 1.20). If the joint was dislocated as well as opened to the environment, contamination may be gross.

## ■ GUNSHOT WOUNDS

Bullets produce open wounds; contaminated material such as clothing and skin is carried deep into the wound. Because insufficient heat is generated during firing and flight, bullets are not bacteriologically sterile. A bullet with a full metal jacket does not fragment in tissue, but partially jacketed or unjacketed bullets tend to expand, deform, and fragment, increasing the volume of the injury. As established by convention, military small arms use fully jacketed ammunition, but civilian small arms may use partially jacketed or unjacketed ammunition. Many police departments use unjacketed, hollow-point bullets in their weapons to reduce the likelihood of a bullet passing through an intended target and striking a bystander.

Low-velocity gunshot wounds are caused by pistols and many small-bore civilian rifles (muzzle velocities of <1,000 ft/second

**FIGURE 1.21.** High-velocity gunshot wound to the lower leg with extensive medial bone and soft-tissue loss. The bullet passed completely through.

or 305 m/second). Tissues are lacerated and crushed as the bullet strikes and passes into the body. The entire energy of the projectile often is absorbed at the site of impact, and the bullet itself frequently comes to rest in the body, its energy spent. Low-velocity gunshot wounds that involve the bone are generally type II open fractures. The extent of soft-tissue injury is restricted to the immediate path of the projectile. The path of the bullet in the body may be erratic, following anatomic tissue planes and other paths of low resistance, sometimes leaving a trail of small metallic fragments. A bullet that comes to rest in a body cavity or lumen may migrate or embolize. The size of a bullet on radiographs depends on its actual size, the radiographic projection, and the degree of magnification. CT may be helpful in localizing the bullet.

High-velocity gunshot wounds are caused by assault rifles and high-powered hunting rifles (muzzle velocities of >2,000 ft/second or 610 m/second). Because kinetic energy increases with the square of the velocity of a projectile, projectiles from high-velocity weapons generally cause severe type III open wounds. On impact, kinetic energy is rapidly transferred from the missile to the tissue. As a high-velocity projectile passes through the body, it compresses the tissues along its path, creating a transient shock wave. Shock waves can cause gas-filled organs to rupture but cause little if any damage to muscle or bone. A temporary vacuum cavity forms behind a high-velocity projectile, similar to the turbulence that forms behind a hand as it is moved rapidly through water. The pressure within the temporary cavity is subatmospheric, causing debris to be sucked into the wound. The cavity oscillates violently and rapidly as it collapses, damaging an extensive volume of tissue. If the projectile strikes the bone, the bone shatters into secondary projectiles. Vascular and neural structures may be extensively damaged, and a volume of tissue extending around the path of the projectile for several centimeters may be devitalized. Even if not hit directly, soft tissue may be pulped, small blood vessels disrupted, and the bone

**FIGURE 1.22.** Shotgun wound to the foot.

shattered. Large vessels may be pushed aside, but intimal damage may lead to thrombosis. The projectile may have enough energy to pass completely through, creating both entrance and exit wounds of highly variable size (Fig. 1.21).

Although shotguns have low muzzle velocity, the aggregate mass of the projectiles may be ten times greater than a single bullet, resulting in proportionally greater wounding power, especially at close range (Fig. 1.22). Multiple projectiles spread over a contiguous area can devitalize a large volume of tissue. Shotgun wounds are considered type III open fractures.

Plastic and rubber bullets from firearms and BBs or small pellets from air guns are inaccurate low-velocity missiles that still have the potential to maim or kill. Blank rounds of ammunition are cartridges with gunpowder but no projectile; however, the explosive force of blank ammunition may kill or injure at close range.

## ■ STRESS INJURIES

Stress fractures may be divided into *fatigue fractures*, in which normal bone fractures in response to abnormal repetitive loads, and *insufficiency fractures*, in which abnormal bone fractures in response to normal repetitive loads. Fractures through focal lesions such as tumors are called *pathologic fractures*.

Fatigue fractures or stress fractures in normal bone are the result of repetitive physical activity, usually occupational or recreational. The individual loads themselves are insufficient to cause fracture, but frequent cyclic loading stimulates remodeling, with the quality and location of the remodeling depending on the magnitude and direction of the loading (Wolff law). The ultimate result is bony hypertrophy. Because cortical bone remodels by a process of resorption and then replacement, there is a vulnerable period during increases in physical activity when the bone has been weakened by resorption but not yet strengthened by replacement. The level and frequency of activity determine the duration of vulnerability. Muscular fatigue is also thought to have a role in the generation of stress fractures. With repetitive exercise to near exhaustion of muscles, decreased stress shielding by muscle action may increase the loads placed on the bones. The site of a stress fracture depends on the type of activity. In runners, for example, common sites include the metatarsal shafts, the tibial shaft, sesamoids of the foot, the medial femoral cortex, and the inferior pubic ramus. Students with heavy book bags and other occupational or recreational backpackers may

**FIGURE 1.23.** Tibial stress fracture (grade 1) with periosteal edema (*arrow*) demonstrated on axial inversion recovery MRI. The marrow is normal.

**FIGURE 1.24.** Calcaneal stress fractures (grade 2). Sagittal inversion recovery MRI shows marrow edema within the cancellous bone of the calcaneus. Retrocalcaneal bursitis is also present (*arrow*).

sustain stress fractures involving the clavicle or upper ribs. Stress fractures are typically identified while they are still incomplete; with rest, the prognosis for healing is excellent.

A similar process of cyclic loading may cause insufficiency fractures, in which abnormally weak bone fractures in response to normal loads. Such fractures may occur, for example, in older, osteoporotic patients who suddenly become more mobile after joint replacement surgery or in patients with metabolic bone disease and decreasing bone strength.

The severity of a stress injury along the spectrum from accelerated stress remodeling to complete structural failure may be graded

on the basis of imaging. The earliest radiologic change is periosteal edema without marrow edema on MRI (Fig. 1.23); the bone scan will be vague, and radiographs will be normal (grade 1). A more advanced injury will show early marrow edema on MRI (inversion recovery only) (Fig. 1.24), a more focally positive bone scan, and normal radiographs (grade 2). The next higher grade injury will show well-established marrow edema on MRI (both inversion recovery and T1) (Fig. 1.25), a focally positive bone scan, and sometimes a fracture line involving part of the cortex on radiographs (grade 3). The highest grade will have a discrete fracture line or cortical signal abnormality on MRI with surrounding edema (Fig. 1.26), an

**A**

**B**

**FIGURE 1.25.** Second metatarsal stress fracture (grade 3). **A:** Axial T1-weighted MRI shows low signal in the marrow of the second metatarsal (*arrow*). **B:** Axial inversion recovery MRI shows marrow edema and surrounding soft-tissue edema (*arrow*).

**FIGURE 1.26.** Tibial shaft stress fracture (grade 4). Coronal T2-weighted MRI with fat suppression shows a focus of marrow edema traversed by a dark fracture line (*arrow*). Surrounding soft-tissue edema is also present.

**FIGURE 1.27.** Tibial stress fracture with graying of the anterior cortex at multiple foci on sagittal CT reformation. Two of the foci are indicated by *arrows*.

intensely positive bone scan, and sometimes a definite fracture line on radiographs. CT may be used to demonstrate fractures or healing (grade 3 or 4). In the absence of a discrete fracture, sometimes the involved cortex may appear less dense on CT, a finding called graying

of the cortex (Fig. 1.27), and corresponding to stress remodeling (grade 1 or 2). Stress fractures may also be oriented longitudinally, along the long axis of the bone (Fig. 1.28). As stress fractures heal, fracture callus with subsequent remodeling is seen (Fig. 1.29).

A

B

**FIGURE 1.28.** Longitudinal stress fracture of the distal tibial shaft. **A:** Axial CT scan shows a vague fracture line in the sagittal plane through the anterior cortex of the distal tibia, with a small amount of periosteal and endosteal fracture callus (*arrows*). **B:** Radionuclide bone scan shows linear activity along the distal tibial shaft.

**FIGURE 1.29.** Healing stress fracture of the second metatarsal (*arrow*).

**FIGURE 1.30.** Soft-tissue ossification at the knee following severe burns. Skin grafting has also been performed.

# ◼ THERMAL TRAUMA

## Burns

Burns cause coagulative tissue necrosis. The depth of the injury is related to the severity and duration of the applied heat. Initially, one may see soft-tissue loss and soft-tissue edema. Osteoporosis and periostitis may occur in the weeks that follow. Periarticular osseous excrescences are common after extensive burns and may be seen 2 to 3 months after injury (Fig. 1.30). The range of motion of involved joints will be limited mechanically. The exact pathogenesis of these ossifications is unknown and seems not to correlate with the severity of the burn.

## Cold Injury

Cold injuries are essentially vascular injuries. In chilblains or immersion foot, prolonged exposure to low but nonfreezing temperatures causes vasoconstriction and hypoxic damage. Leakage of physiologic fluids from damaged small vessels leads to pain and edema. An intense hyperemic and inflammatory response develops; this is usually painful and often lasts for days to weeks. Ultimate recovery is common, but the affected part typically remains more sensitive to cold than before the exposure. Damp cold has a greater effect than cold at low humidity. In freezing injuries or frostbite—to which the digits, nose, and ears are most vulnerable—the formation of ice crystals within the tissues may cause permanent damage. Autoamputation of soft tissue and bone may be the ultimate result. On radiographs, one may see soft-tissue edema, osteoporosis, and periostitis. Soft-tissue and even bone loss from tuftal resorption may occur in the fingers and toes. Cartilage damage may result in secondary degenerative joint disease. Acute evaluation of cold injuries may include arteriography or radionuclide perfusion studies. In children, frostbite may damage the growth plates of fingers or toes, with subsequent growth deformity.

# ◼ DESCRIBING FRACTURES AND DISLOCATIONS

Precise use of language in describing fractures and dislocations is imperative for patient care. The most important fact about a fracture is its site within the skeleton. The location within the involved bone should be precisely noted. In the long bones, it is conventional to divide the shaft into thirds and to indicate which third is involved (proximal, middle, or distal). A fracture site can also be located at the junction of the proximal and middle thirds or the junction of the middle and distal thirds. If anatomic landmarks are present, they may be used for reference; some anatomic regions have specific terminology.

Fractures may be closed or open and complete or incomplete. The morphology of the fracture should be described in terms of the principal fracture line: transverse, spiral, or oblique, and so forth. Simple fractures have one fracture plane and two major fragments. Comminuted fractures have two or more fracture planes and three or more major fragments. Examples of comminuted fractures include transverse fractures with butterfly fragments and segmental fractures (transverse fractures at different levels of a shaft that isolate a segment of the bone) (Fig. 1.31).

*Alignment* refers to the long axis of the fragments; *angulation* is a change from the normal alignment and refers specifically to the angle between the long axes of the major fragments. The direction of angulation of a fracture reflects the direction of loading. By convention, varus or medial angulation of the distal fragment is deviation of the distal part toward the midline of the body; valgus or lateral angulation of the distal fragment is deviation of the distal part away from the midline of the body. Angulation can also be anterior or posterior. An alternative method of reporting fracture angulation is to describe the direction of the apex of the angle formed by the major fragments. A fracture with valgus (lateral) angulation of the distal fragment would be described as apex medial.

**FIGURE 1.31.** Segmental fracture of the femoral shaft with complete displacement.

*Position* refers to the relationship of the fracture fragments to their normal anatomic location. Loss of position is called *displacement*. Fragments that are completely separated from each other are completely displaced. Fragments that maintain partial contact with their anatomic location are partially displaced; partial displacement of cortical fractures is usually described in terms of the proportion of the shaft width. In nondisplaced fractures, the fragments remain in their normal anatomic location. In rotary displacement, the fragments turn away from each other; documentation of rotary displace-

**FIGURE 1.33.** Osteochondral fracture of the patella. The fracture fragment (*arrow*) consists of articular cartilage with an attached segment of subchondral bone.

ment requires a single film that includes both ends of the fractured bone. *Shortening* is the overlap of fragments along the axis of the limb, and *distraction* is separation of fragments along the axis of the limb.

Loss of position by articulating bones is called *dislocation* or *luxation* if there is no remaining contact between the articulating bones and *subluxation* if partial contact has been maintained. Dislocations and subluxations should be described by the location of the distal part relative to the proximal part. For example, in a dorsal proximal interphalangeal (PIP) dislocation, the middle phalanx has dislocated to a position that is dorsal to the proximal phalanx (Fig. 1.32).

The apparent position and alignment of bones and fragments on radiographs can vary with the positioning of the part relative to the X-ray beam. In general, two views obtained 90 degrees to each other is

**FIGURE 1.32.** Dorsal PIP dislocation.

**FIGURE 1.34** Axial T2-weighted fat suppressed MRI shows a cartilage injury of the patella (*arrowhead*) with loose cartilage fragment (*black arrow*) and medial retinacular sprain (*white arrow*). Other loose cartilage fragments and bone bruises were demonstrated on other images.

the minimum necessary to determine the relative position and alignment of fracture fragments in three dimensions. Sequential measurements of fracture position and angulation on films are often not possible unless great care is taken to obtain films in the same projection.

Intra-articular fractures are those at the end of a bone in which the fracture line extends into the articulating portion of the bone, although not necessarily into the articular surface itself. Osteochondral fractures are intra-articular fractures that extend through both the bone and the articular cartilage. On radiographs, the presence of the cartilage fragment may be inferred from the donor site of the bony fragment (Fig. 1.33). Cartilage injuries may be imaged directly by MRI (Fig. 1.34).

Avulsion fractures are traction fractures from tensile loading of tendons or ligaments and range from large transverse fractures to tiny flecks of cortex at the insertion or origin of the involved muscle or tendon. These fractures indicate disruption of the bone-tendon or bone-ligament complex and have great clinical significance. They also imply that the soft-tissue structure—the tendon or ligament that has pulled off the bone fragment—is itself still intact.

# ◼ RADIOLOGIC REPORTING

The ultimate work product of diagnostic radiology is information for clinical decision making. The work is not complete until that information is transferred to those who are attending the patient. The information that the radiologist obtains from the images is documented in the radiologic report and should be sufficient to satisfy the clinical imperative for the radiologic examination. The radiologist's report becomes part of the patient's medical record. It should be composed with care and diligence and rendered in a timely fashion. Direct communication between the radiologist and the attending physician by telephone or in person is often appropriate.

A radiologic report of a fracture should begin with the date (time) of the examination, the type of examination (portable or not), the date of the report, the body part examined, the projections obtained, and the appliances present (e.g., casts or splints). A description of the fracture is the body of the report and should include as a minimum the location, direction, position, and alignment of the fracture. Additional descriptive and diagnostic observations are included as appropriate. In radiologic reports, unless otherwise specified, fractures can be assumed to be acute, complete, not comminuted, not displaced, not angulated, extra-articular, nonpathologic, and closed.

There are many different systems of classification for fractures in most regions of the body, often devised for different purposes by practitioners with different interests. The best classifications are those that provide a conceptual basis for understanding patterns of injuries, facilitate clinical management decisions, or correlate with prognosis. Descriptive and anatomic classifications are useful in radiology, and when both writers and readers of the radiologic report use the same classifications in the same way, precise communication is possible. However, for complex systems of fracture classification, observer variability may be quite high. Rather than guess the classification scheme that the referring clinician may be using, the radiologist should strive to describe the injuries (present and absent) in sufficient detail for any classification system to be applied on the basis of the radiologic report.

## SOURCES AND READINGS

Browner B, Jupiter J, Levine A, Trafton P, Krettek C. *Skeletal Trauma: Fractures, Dislocations, Ligamentous Injuries.* 4th Ed. Philadelphia, PA: Saunders; 2008.

Bucholz RW, Heckman JD, Court-Brown C, Tornetta P. *Rockwood and Green's Fractures in Adults.* 7th Ed. Philadelphia, PA: Lippincott Williams & Wilkins; 2009.

Chew FS, Maldjian C. *Broken Bones: The X-ray Atlas of Fractures.* Seattle: BareBonesBooks.com; 2009.

Einhorn TA, O'Keefe RJ, Buckwalter JA. *Orthopaedic Basic Science: Foundations of Clinical Practice.* 3rd Ed. Rosemont, IL: American Academy of Orthopaedic Surgeons; 2007.

eMedicine. http://emedicine.medscape.com.

Griffin LY. *Essentials of Musculoskeletal Care.* 3rd Ed. Rosemont, IL: American Academy of Orthopedics; 2005.

Helms CA, Major NM, Anderson MW, et al. *Musculoskeletal MRI.* 2nd Ed. Philadelphia, PA: WB Saunders; 2009.

Hoppenfeld S, Zeide MS. *Orthopedic Dictionary.* Philadelphia, PA: Lippincott Williams & Wilkins; 1994

Jacobson JA. *Fundamentals of Musculoskeletal Ultrasound.* Philadelphia, PA: Saunders; 2007.

Nordin M, Frankel VH. *Basic Biomechanics of the Musculoskeletal System.* 3rd Ed. Philadelphia, PA: Lippincott Williams & Wilkins; 2001.

Rogers LF. *Radiology of Skeletal Trauma.* 3rd Ed. New York, NY: Churchill Livingstone; 2002.

Schultz RJ. *The Language of Fractures.* 2nd Ed. Baltimore, MD: Williams & Wilkins; 1990.

Wheeless CR III, ed. *Wheeless' Textbook of Orthopaedics.* http://www.wheelessonline.com.

Wilson AJ. Gunshot Injuries: What Does a Radiologist Need to Know? *Radiographics.* 1999;19:1358–1368.

# Trauma in Adults: Upper Extremity

 his chapter describes the radiology of many common injuries to the upper extremities in adults.

## ◼ HAND

Fractures of the metacarpals and phalanges of the hand are approximately three times more common in men than in women. These injuries have a peak incidence in young men and decrease in incidence with increasing age.

## Fingers

Avulsion injuries of the phalanges involve tensile failure of ligamentous or musculotendinous units. These injuries result when excessive loading occurs while the tendon or ligament is already under tension. The substance of a tendon or ligament may tear, or there may be avulsion of its bony insertion. For example, sudden, forcible flexion of the distal interphalangeal (DIP) joint of an extended finger, as occurs when an outstretched finger is struck by a baseball, may result in tensile failure of the extensor mechanism of the distal phalanx. The injury is called a *baseball finger*, and the resulting clinical deformity is called a *mallet finger*, in which the DIP joint is maintained in flexion and cannot be extended (Fig. 2.1). An avulsion fracture of the dorsal proximal corner of the distal phalanx is present in 25% of cases of baseball finger; thus, most of these injuries are tendinous. An avulsed bone fragment can be retracted by muscle pull. The converse injury occurs with forcible extension of the DIP joint of a flexed finger or with forcible hyperextension at the DIP joint. In this case, the volar plate of the distal phalanx at the flexor digitorum profundus tendon insertion may be avulsed; alternatively, the tendon may tear. Similar injuries may occur at the proximal interphalangeal (PIP) joint.

Purely ligamentous and tendinous injuries are more common than bony avulsions in the fingers, so radiographs may show only soft-tissue swelling or deformities of alignment. Avulsion fractures at the base of a phalanx from the volar edge indicate disruption of the attachment of the volar plate. Avulsions from the lateral edge indicate disruption of the attachments of collateral ligaments

(Fig. 2.2). Avulsions from the dorsal edge indicate disruption of the extensor tendon. The avulsed fragments always contain the tendinous or ligamentous insertion (enthesis) and may range in size from a tiny sliver of cortical bone to a large intra-articular fragment. If the intra-articular fragment involves one third or more of the articular surface, the joint may subluxate and require operative fixation. A bony defect should be present where the fragment originated, and although one portion of the fragment has cortex, one portion does not. In contrast to the situation with fracture fragments, accessory ossicles and sesamoid bones invariably are completely corticated, and no donor site should be present. Deformities of alignment reflect the function of the injured unit. In some cases, stress views may be necessary to demonstrate the loss of function.

The most common dislocation occurs at the PIP joint. Nonmedical personnel often reduce PIP joint dislocations, and many fracture subluxations are actually reduced fracture dislocations. After reduction, if there are no fractures, one may see only soft-tissue swelling. Dorsal dislocations are common, lateral dislocations are less common, and volar dislocations are rare. Fractures involving the phalangeal tufts are the result of direct sharp or blunt trauma.

The most common metacarpal fracture is an impacted fracture of the fifth metacarpal neck with volar angulation (boxer's fracture). It is sustained by bending and axial loading when the closed fist strikes an object (e.g., a wall or chin). In severe cases, the fourth metacarpal neck may also be fractured.

## Thumb

Ligamentous disruption of the ulnar collateral ligament of the thumb's metacarpophalangeal joint, or gamekeeper's thumb, is sustained during downhill skiing when an improperly planted pole places sudden valgus stress on the thumb. Similar mechanisms of injury may also occur in sports such as football, hockey, wrestling, and basketball. Unless there is an avulsion of a fragment of bone, stress views may be necessary to show this injury on radiographs (Fig. 2.3). On MRI, the torn ulnar collateral ligament may be imaged directly. The adductor pollicis aponeurosis is normally superficial to the ulnar collateral ligament. Interposition of the adductor pollicis

**FIGURE 2.1.** Mallet finger resulting from extensor tendon rupture.

aponeurosis between the ruptured ulnar collateral ligament and its distal attachment is called a *Stener lesion* (Fig. 2.4). A Stener lesion will prevent healing of the ligament and result in chronic instability.

The exceptional mobility of the thumb in opposing the other digits is possible in part because of a shallow saddle-shaped

**FIGURE 2.3.** Avulsion fracture (*arrow*) at the proximal phalanx of the thumb by the ulnar collateral ligament (gamekeeper's thumb).

articulation between the first metacarpal and the trapezium. Axial loading of a partially flexed first metacarpal can produce a simple intra-articular fracture. The adductor pollicis and abductor pollicis longus muscles pull the metacarpal base and shaft proximally, but the anterior lip remains attached to the trapezium by its ligaments (Bennett fracture) (Fig. 2.5). These intra-articular fractures usually require operative reduction and fixation. If a T- or Y-shaped comminuted fracture (Rolando fracture) rather than a simple fracture is sustained, anatomic reduction and fixation may become more problematic (Fig. 2.6). In contrast to these injuries, extra-articular fractures of the first metacarpal shaft present few problems in management because muscle origins along the length of the shaft prevent displacement.

**FIGURE 2.2.** Avulsion fracture at the collateral ligament insertion of the middle phalanx (*arrow*). The soft tissues are swollen.

# ■ WRIST

## Biomechanics

The wrist positions the hand in space, transmits power to the hand from muscles in the forearm, and transmits mechanical force between the hand and the forearm. Its range of motion is magnified in flexion and extension and in radial and ulnar deviation by a dual articulation: one between the radius and the lunate and one between the lunate and the capitate. With ulnar and radial deviation of the hand, the distal carpal row rotates as well as turns. The carpus can be envisioned as having a central column that consists

**A**

**B**

**FIGURE 2.4.** Stener lesion. Coronal inversion recovery **(A)** and coronal T1-weighted MRI **(B)** show a torn ulnar collateral ligament with proximal retraction (*arrow*). The adductor pollicis aponeurosis (*arrowhead*) is interposed between the torn ligament and its distal site of attachment.

**FIGURE 2.5.** Intra-articular fracture of the base of the first metacarpal with dislocation (Bennett fracture). The small medial fragment (*arrow*) maintains its attachment to the joint, while the metacarpal has dislocated proximally.

**FIGURE 2.6.** T-shaped fractures (*arrow* and *arrowheads*) at the base of the first metacarpal (Rolando fracture) shown by coronal reformatted CT.

**FIGURE 2.7.** Ligaments of the wrist. The strong ligaments are on the volar aspect of the wrist and form a sling that suspends the carpus from the distal forearm. The space of Poirier exists because there is no strong ligamentous attachment of capitate to lunate. Many indirect injuries of the carpus involve a carpal sling disruption that extends into the space of Poirier.

of the lunate and the capitate. Flexion and extension and the transmission of mechanical force occur through the central column. The capitate, distal carpal row, and hand comprise a single functional unit. The lunate is an intercalated segment between the capitate and the radius that has no direct muscular control (no muscles insert on the lunate). The scaphoid flanks the lunate on one side and functions as a connecting rod alongside the capitate and lunate, providing stability during motion. The triquetrum acts as a pivot for intercarpal rotation through a sloping, helicoid articulation with the hamate.

Ligaments of the wrist limit motion when they become taut at their maximum excursion. The volar carpal ligaments are strong and form a sling that suspends the carpus from the radius and triangular fibrocartilage complex (TFCC) (Fig. 2.7). Dorsal ligaments are weaker. Interosseous ligaments bind adjacent carpal bones to

each other; those of clinical importance are the scapholunate and lunotriquetral ligaments. The scaphoid and triquetrum flank the lunate on either side and have strong ligamentous attachments to the distal carpal row as well as attachments to the lunate and to the distal forearm. Because no strong ligaments connect the capitate and lunate to each other, the stability of that articulation depends on the integrity of the adjacent scaphoid and triquetrum and their ligamentous attachments. The gap in the volar ligamentous sling at the lunate-capitate articulation is called the *space of Poirier*.

Radiographic evaluation of the wrist is based primarily on the appearance of each bone and its relationship with the other bones. The arcs made by the proximal articular surfaces of the proximal carpal row, the distal articular surfaces of the proximal carpal row, and the proximal articular surfaces of the distal carpal row are helpful anatomic landmarks. The positions of the scaphoid fat stripe and the pronator quadratus fat pad are occasionally helpful indirect signs of wrist fracture.

## Scaphoid Fractures

Scaphoid fractures account for approximately 85% of all isolated carpal bone fractures. The scaphoid bridges the lunate-capitate articulation. With extreme, forceful dorsiflexion between the lunate and the capitate and perhaps the impingement of the scaphoid on the dorsal radial rim, the scaphoid starts to bend, and the fracture line begins on its volar aspect under tensile loading, propagating transversely through the narrowest region (the scaphoid waist). Most scaphoid fractures have no comminution (70% of cases). Less common are fractures through the proximal (10%) or distal (20%) poles. The scaphoid may also fracture during perilunate injuries (discussed later in this chapter). Many scaphoid fractures are nondisplaced and difficult to recognize without special scaphoid views (Fig. 2.8). Indirect signs of scaphoid fracture are obscuration or lateral displacement of the scaphoid fat stripe and soft-tissue swelling over the dorsum of the wrist. Sometimes, it is worthwhile for the radiologist to examine the patient directly. MRI or CT may demonstrate radiographically occult fractures of the scaphoid and other carpal bones (Fig. 2.9). Because the blood supply to the proximal pole of the scaphoid enters the

**A**

**B**

**FIGURE 2.8.** Scaphoid waist fracture. **A:** The fracture is not visible on the standard PA radiograph. **B:** Special scaphoid radiograph shows the fracture (*arrow*).

**FIGURE 2.9.** Radiographically occult scaphoid waist fracture (*arrow*) demonstrated on T1-weighted MRI.

**FIGURE 2.10.** Triquetral fracture. Lateral radiograph shows displaced avulsion fragment (*arrow*) with overlying soft-tissue swelling.

distal pole and courses proximally across the waist, posttraumatic osteonecrosis of the proximal pole with nonunion is a common complication seen in up to 30% of cases. Osteonecrosis of the scaphoid may be directly imaged with MRI. The ultimate prognosis of complicated scaphoid fractures after surgical intervention is favorable. Wrist instability is a common sequela of scaphoid nonunion.

## Other Isolated Carpal Fractures

Isolated fractures of carpal bones other than the scaphoid are relatively uncommon. Isolated triquetral fractures usually involve the dorsal surface and are seen best on lateral or slightly oblique radiographs (Fig. 2.10). Isolated lunate fractures usually involve the dorsal or volar surface and are ligamentous avulsions. Pisiform fractures may occur with direct trauma and are best seen on oblique radiographs. Hamate fractures may involve any part, but fractures of the hook of the hamate become displaced by the insertion of the transverse carpal ligament. These may follow falls or direct trauma from the handle of a racquet, golf club, or baseball bat. Complications include nonunion, osteonecrosis, and ulnar or median nerve injury, and most are treated surgically. Dorsal fracture dislocations may also occur at the articulation of the hamate with the bases of the fourth and fifth metacarpals (Fig. 2.11).

**A**

**B**

**FIGURE 2.11.** Fracture dislocation of the hamate. **A:** Radiograph shows dorsal fracture dislocation (*arrow*) involving the articulations of the fourth and fifth metacarpals with the hamate. **B:** Axial CT scan shows the displaced, comminuted hamate fracture (*arrow*).

## Perilunate Injuries

A consistent pattern of injuries is sustained around the lunate when the hand is extended to break a backward fall. On impact, the hand and wrist undergo hyperextension, ulnar deviation, and intercarpal supination (rotary motion between the proximal and distal carpal rows). The ligamentous sling of the carpus is loaded in tension from the radial side, and a sequence of injuries may ensue (Table 2.1). In stage 1, scapholunate dissociation or rotary subluxation, there is rupture of the proximal ligamentous attachments of the scaphoid, opening the space of Poirier on the radial side. The separation of the scaphoid from the middle column leaves scapholunate dissociation. Disruption of the ligaments of the scaphoid allows it to rotate about its short axis in a volar direction (Fig. 2.12). This mechanism of loading may also fracture the scaphoid. In stage 2, perilunate dislocation, the capitate dislocates from the lunate dorsally, taking with it the hand and the scaphoid (Fig. 2.13). The space of Poirier opens on the radial side, often through a scaphoid fracture between the ligamentous attachments to the capitate and lunate, but the triquetral ligaments remain intact. In stage 3, midcarpal dissociation or triquetral dislocation, under continued loading, the

| TABLE 2.1 | Perilunate Injuries of the Wrist |
|-----------|----------------------------------|
| Stage | Injury |
| 1 | Rotary subluxation of the scaphoid (scapholunate dissociation) |
| 2 | Perilunate dislocation |
| 3 | Midcarpal dissociation (triquetral dislocation) |
| 4 | Lunate dislocation |

triquetral ligaments fail by tear or avulsion of insertions, separating the triquetrum from the lunate. Although the lunate remains in place, the rest of the carpus is dislocated dorsally, coming to rest on the dorsal surface of the lunate. The lunate is subluxated and tilted volarly but is not completely dislocated (Fig. 2.14). Lunate dislocation (stage 4) occurs if there is sufficient force to tear the dorsal radiocarpal ligament, allowing the dorsally dislocated carpus to eject the lunate from the radius volarly. The capitate comes to rest in the radial articular surface. The dislocated lunate is also rotated 90 degrees volarly, still held to the radius by its volar ligaments

**A**

**B**

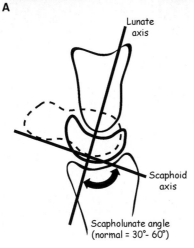

Lunate axis

Scaphoid axis

Scapholunate angle (normal = 30°- 60°)

Lateral Projection

**C**

**FIGURE 2.12.** Rotary subluxation of scaphoid. **A:** Lateral radiograph shows volar rotary subluxation of the scaphoid. The scapholunate angle is nearly 90 degrees. **B:** PA radiograph shows foreshortening of the scaphoid with a cortical ring sign over its distal pole. **C:** Scapholunate angle measurement. Normal SL angle is 30 to 60 degrees.

A

B

**FIGURE 2.13.** Transscaphoid perilunate dislocation. **A:** Lateral radiograph shows complete dorsal dislocation of the capitate with normal location of the lunate. **B:** PA radiograph shows the overlap of the scaphoid and capitate but not the triquetrum. The scaphoid is fractured.

A

B

**FIGURE 2.14.** Midcarpal dislocation. **A:** Lateral radiograph shows complete dorsal dislocation of the capitate and volar subluxation of the lunate. **B:** PA radiograph shows separation of the scaphoid, capitate, and triquetrum from the lunate. Avulsion fractures of the triquetrum and radial styloid are present.

A    B

**FIGURE 2.15.** Lunate dislocation. **A:** Lateral radiograph shows volar dislocation of the lunate with 90 degrees rotary displacement. The capitate occupies the normal position of the lunate. **B:** PA radiograph shows the lunate as an overlapping triangular structure.

(Fig. 2.15). Avulsion fractures instead of ligamentous ruptures may occur, including avulsion and tension fractures of the carpal bones (especially the scaphoid) and of the distal radius and ulna. The radiographic signs of reduced perilunate injuries may be subtle, particularly in the absence of bony involvement.

## Triangular Fibrocartilage Complex and Ulnar-Sided Injuries

The TFCC is a biconcave fibrocartilage disk interposed between the proximal carpal row and the ulna and suspended by dorsal and volar radioulnar ligaments that extend from the medial aspect of the distal radius to the ulnar styloid process. The TFCC extends the articular surface of the distal radius across the distal ulna, separating the radiocarpal compartment of the wrist from the distal radioulnar joint. Tears of the TFCC may be traumatic or degenerative. Most tears occur through the central portion of the disk where it is thinnest, leading to ulnar-sided wrist pain (Fig. 2.16). Tears that involve the radioulnar ligaments may result in instability of the distal radioulnar joint. Disruption of other carpal ligaments on the ulnar side of the wrist may occur with or without injury to the TFCC. The mechanism and classification of these injuries are not well established.

## Carpal Instability

The seriousness of ligamentous injuries of the wrist is often overlooked during the acute clinical presentation, particularly if fractures are absent and dislocations have been reduced. When untreated, patients with "wrist sprains" often return with chronic, disabling wrist symptoms, including instability, pain, decreased grip strength, posttraumatic arthritis, and painful "clicks." Fractures of the distal radius may be associated with more serious carpal dysfunction

that becomes apparent once the radial fractures have healed. When the normal wrist is held in neutral position, the axes of the radius, lunate, and capitate are collinear on lateral radiographs. With flexion or extension, approximately half the motion occurs between the lunate and the radius and half between the capitate and the lunate. In dorsiflexion instability (also called *dorsal intercalated segment instability*, or DISI), the axes of the radius, lunate, and capitate assume a

**FIGURE 2.16.** Central TFCC tear (*arrow*) shown on T1-weighted fat-suppressed MR arthrogram.

**FIGURE 2.17.** Carpal instability patterns on sagittal CT reformations. (*R*, radius; *C*, capitate; *D*, dorsal aspect; *V*, volar aspect). **A:** DISI with capitate subluxation. The lunate (*arrow*) is tilted dorsally. **B:** VISI. The lunate (*arrow*) is tilted volarly.

zigzag configuration with dorsal angulation of the lunate (relative to the radius) and volar angulation of the capitate (relative to the lunate). Dorsiflexion instability may be associated with rotary subluxation of the scaphoid but more often follows an impacted distal radius fracture. In volar flexion instability (also called *volar intercalated segment instability*, or VISI), the zigzag is the reverse, with volar angulation of the lunate (relative to the radius) and dorsal angulation of the capitate (relative to the lunate) (Fig. 2.17). Scapholunate dissociation (rotary subluxation of the scaphoid) may be found following an episode of trauma or in the setting of arthritis. MRI, wrist arthrography, or stress radiographs may be required to document carpal instability or the underlying ligamentous injuries.

# ▩ DISTAL RADIUS AND FOREARM

Fractures of the distal radius usually occur from falls on the outstretched hand (FOOSH). A Colles fracture is a nonarticular transverse fracture of the distal radial metaphysis with dorsal displacement, dorsal angulation, and dorsal impaction (Fig. 2.18). This injury—common in older persons with osteoporosis, particularly women—is sustained during a fall forward onto an outstretched, dorsiflexed hand with the impact force aligned to the long axis of the radius. The fracture results from tensile failure of cancellous metaphyseal bone on the volar side and compressive failure on the dorsal side. The distal radial articular surface and the carpus are spared. In 60% of cases, the ulnar styloid is avulsed by the TFCC. Alternatively, the TFCC may tear, the distal radioulnar joint may dislocate, or the distal ulnar shaft may fracture. Because the radial fracture traverses the spongy bone of the metaphysis, healing is generally prompt with closed treatment, but associated ulnar styloid fractures frequently do not unite. Residual, posttraumatic dorsal tilt of the distal radial articular surface may result in instability of the wrist. A transverse radial metaphyseal fracture that displaces and angulates volarly is called a *reverse Colles fracture* or a *Smith fracture*.

Simple intra-articular fractures of the distal radius that involve either its dorsal or its volar margin are called *Barton fractures*.

Complex intra-articular fractures of the distal radius may be caused by high-energy axial compression forces transmitted through the lunate to the medial half of the radial articular surface. The articular surface usually splits into three major fragments: the radial styloid and two medial fragments, one dorsal and one volar. The medial fragments may be angulated dorsally or volarly, depending on the degree of flexion or extension of the wrist at the time of injury. Additional impaction and comminution may be present depending on the magnitude of the loading. Most patients with these fractures also have intracarpal soft-tissue injuries, including ligament tears and TFCC injuries. The distal radioulnar joint is disrupted, and the ulnar styloid may be fractured. These injuries are typically treated surgically.

Isolated avulsion fractures of the radial styloid may follow avulsions of the radial collateral ligament. Compressive forces transmitted through the scaphoid may cause isolated shear fractures of the radial styloid; these may be associated with avulsion fractures of the ulnar styloid. Simple intra-articular fractures of the distal radius that involve the radial styloid process are sometimes called *Hutchinson* or *chauffeur's fractures*.

Dislocation or subluxation of the distal radioulnar joint may occur in association with other fractures of the radius or in isolation. Because this injury is often overlooked and difficult to document on radiographs, CT may be required for the definitive diagnosis (Fig. 2.19). Often, an unstable distal radioulnar joint reduces in neutral or supination and subluxates in pronation. Therefore, the CT examination should be performed in both pronation and supination. Chronic dislocation or instability of the distal radioulnar joint may result in posttraumatic wrist disability.

Most fractures of the forearm (60%) involve both the radius and the ulna. Less common are isolated fractures of the ulna with or

**FIGURE 2.18.** Transverse fracture of the distal radial metaphysis with dorsal displacement and angulation in an elderly woman (Colles fracture). **A:** Lateral radiograph. **B:** PA radiograph.

**FIGURE 2.19.** Subluxation of the left distal radioulnar joint demonstrated by CT. **A:** In supination, the joint is normally located. **B:** In pronation, the ulna is dorsally subluxated (*arrow*).

**FIGURE 2.20.** Angulated, displaced fracture of the distal radial shaft at the junction of the middle and distal thirds with dislocation of the distal radioulnar joint (Galeazzi fracture).

without radial dislocation (25%), and the least common are isolated fractures of the radius with or without ulnar dislocation (15%). The greater the loading, the more likely it is that both bones are fractured. Raising the forearm to ward off a blow by a blunt instrument such as a nightstick may result in a tapping fracture from direct loading of the ulnar shaft.

A fracture of the radial shaft with dislocation of the distal radioulnar joint is called a *Galeazzi fracture* (Fig. 2.20). An impacted or comminuted fracture of the radial head with dislocation of the distal radioulnar joint is called an *Essex-Lopresti fracture* (Fig.2.21). A fracture of the ulnar shaft with dislocation of the radial head is called a *Monteggia fracture* (Fig. 2.22). Monteggia fractures are described using the Bado classification. The common type of Monteggia fracture is an angulated fracture of the proximal ulnar shaft with the apex anterior along with anterior dislocation of the radial-capitellar joint (Bado type I). Less common types may also occur, including the apex posterior angulation of the ulnar shaft fracture with posterior dislocation of the radial-capitellar joint (Bado type II), the apex lateral angulation of the ulnar shaft fracture with lateral dislocation of the radial-capitellar joint (Bado type III), and fractures of both the proximal ulnar and radial shafts with radial-capitellar dislocation (Bado type IV).

## ◼ ELBOW

The most common elbow fractures in adults involve the radial head or neck. Radial head and neck fractures are sustained during falls onto an outstretched hand, impacting the radial head against the capitellum. One of two types of fractures is typically sustained: a linear shear fracture through the radial head (Fig. 2.23) or an impaction fracture of the radial neck (proximal radial metaphysis) (Fig. 2.24). Because

**A**

**B**

**FIGURE 2.21.** Essex-Lopresti fracture. **A:** PA view of wrist shows dislocation of the distal radioulnar joint and a perilunate injury. **B:** AP view of elbow shows comminuted radial head fracture (*arrow*).

**FIGURE 2.22.** Apex anterior fracture of the ulnar shaft with anterior dislocation of the radial capitellar joint (Monteggia fracture, Bado type 1).

they are intra-articular, a fat pad sign is often present. Approximately half of these fractures are nondisplaced and may require oblique views for demonstration. More severe fractures have displacement and comminution and may also involve the capitellum.

An intra-articular olecranon process fracture may be caused by a fall onto an outstretched hand with the elbow in flexion. The combination of axial compression with tension from contraction of the triceps produces oblique or transverse fractures through the semilunar notch (Fig. 2.25). Fractures may also be caused by direct falls onto the flexed elbow.

Most acute dislocations of the elbow result from falls or sports-related mishaps. Typically, the ulna dislocates posteriorly relative to the humerus, taking the radius with it. In many cases, there are no

**FIGURE 2.24.** Impacted radial neck fracture (*arrow*) with anterior and posterior fat-pad signs (*arrowheads*).

associated fractures. When there are fractures associated with elbow dislocations, the fragments are most commonly avulsions from the coronoid process of the ulna (Fig. 2.26). Although posterior elbow dislocations are the most common, dislocation in other directions may occur. Elbow dislocations are more common in children than in adults.

Intercondylar fractures of the distal humerus involve impaction of the ulna into the trochlear groove, where it splits the

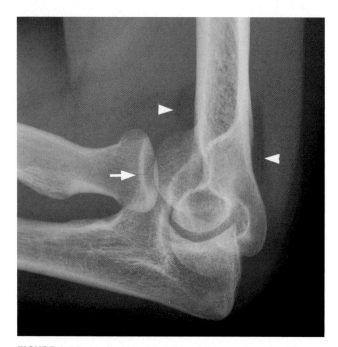

**FIGURE 2.23.** Nondisplaced radial head fracture (*arrow*) with anterior and posterior fat-pad signs (*arrowheads*).

**FIGURE 2.25.** Intra-articular fracture of the olecranon process (*arrow*).

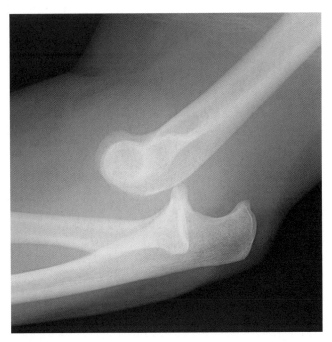

**FIGURE 2.26.** Posterior elbow dislocation.

**FIGURE 2.28.** Ulnar collateral ligament tear. Coronal T2-weighted MRI shows high signal and disruption of the ulnar collateral ligament (*arrow*). Note that the flexor muscle origin is intact.

distal humerus like a wedge, often separating the medial and lateral fragments with a T- or Y-shaped fracture line. Comminution and displacement are common. These fractures are treated with open reduction and internal fixation.

Soft-tissue injuries of the elbow in adults may occur on the lateral (radial), medial (ulnar), anterior, or posterior aspects. Lateral epicondylitis is a stress injury of the origin of the common extensor tendon at the lateral epicondyle that can be caused by a discrete injury or by repetitive stress. Also called *tennis elbow* because of its association with the backhand stroke in tennis, the condition may be demonstrated on MRI as high signal on T2-weighted images

and thickening of the extensor carpi radialis brevis muscle origin (Fig. 2.27). The lateral ligamentous complex may be injured acutely or chronically and consists of tears of the radial collateral ligament and the extensor-pronator muscle group origin. On the medial aspect of the elbow, tears of the ulnar collateral ligament may accompany activities such as baseball pitching. These injuries are best demonstrated on MRI (Fig. 2.28); MR arthrography often increases the conspicuity of the abnormality. At the anterior aspect of the elbow, tears of the biceps tendon from its insertion at the bicipital tuberosity of the radius may occur. On radiographs, a complete tear is manifested by proximal retraction of the muscle belly. On clinical examination, weakness in elbow flexion when the hand is supinated is present, along with the bulging biceps muscle belly. MRI demonstrates complete as well as partial tears of the distal biceps tendon (Fig. 2.29). At the posterior aspect of the elbow, tears of the triceps tendon may occur but are relatively rare compared with the soft-tissue injuries on the other aspects of the elbow.

# ■ SHOULDER AND ARM
## Humerus

Fractures of the proximal humerus usually occur through the shaft at the surgical neck (Fig. 2.30). The rotator cuff abducts and rotates the proximal fragment. The greater or lesser tuberosities may also be fractured, and in very severe injuries, the anatomic head may be dislocated. Anatomic neck fractures are rare and have a poor prognosis because the blood supply to the humeral head is disrupted. Fractures of the humeral shaft are laterally and posteriorly angulated when the fracture separates the insertions of the pectoralis major and the deltoid, allowing the pectoralis major to adduct the proximal fragment. A fracture below the deltoid insertion allows it to abduct the proximal fragment, resulting in medial angulation.

**FIGURE 2.27.** Lateral epicondylitis. Coronal inversion recovery MRI shows thickening and high signal at the extensor musculature origin at the lateral epicondyle (*arrow*).

**FIGURE 2.29.** Biceps tendon tear. **A:** Lateral radiograph of the arm shows a focal bulge of the biceps muscle (*arrow*). **B:** Sagittal T1-weighted MRI shows the retracted biceps tendon (*arrow*).

Most simple humeral shaft fractures are treated by closed means; occasionally, screws, plates, or rods are used.

Isolated fractures of the greater tuberosity may occur in falls or other trauma. Because the supraspinatus and infraspinatus tendons of the rotator cuff have their insertion on the greater tuberosity, patients may present with signs and symptoms of rotator cuff tears. MRI is the preferred method for identifying radiographically occult greater tuberosity fractures (Fig. 2.31) as well as identifying rotator cuff tears and other causes of shoulder pain.

**FIGURE 2.30.** Surgical neck fracture (*arrows*) of the proximal humerus. **A:** External rotation radiograph. **B:** Internal rotation radiograph.

**FIGURE 2.31.** Greater tuberosity fracture and SLAP tear. Oblique coronal T2-weighted fat-suppressed MR arthrogram shows high signal in the greater tuberosity (*arrow*) with a nondisplaced fracture line. Fluid entering the superior labrum indicates a SLAP tear (*arrowhead*). The rotator cuff is intact.

## Glenohumeral Joint Anatomy

The glenohumeral joint is highly mobile and is the most common site of subluxation or dislocation. The glenoid fossa is the shallow depression in the articular surface of the glenoid process, made deeper and larger by a circular rim of fibrocartilage, the glenoid labrum. The rotator cuff tendons surround the glenohumeral joint and represent the major dynamic stabilizers of the joint. The supraspinatus and infraspinatus tendons cover the superior aspect of the joint and insert along the greater tuberosity of the humerus. The subscapularis tendon covers the anterior aspect of the joint and inserts on the lesser tuberosity of the humerus. The teres minor tendon covers the posterior aspect. The rotator cuff interval is a gap between the supraspinatus and subscapularis tendons, through which the long head of the biceps tendon passes to insert along the superior aspect of the glenoid labrum. The superior glenohumeral and the middle glenohumeral ligaments extend from the humerus to the superior and anterior aspects of the glenoid labrum, respectively. The inferior glenohumeral ligament, a primary static stabilizer of the shoulder joint, passes from the medial aspect of the proximal humeral shaft in the anterior and posterior bands to attach to the inferior glenoid labrum anteriorly and posteriorly. The presence, size, and attachments of the glenohumeral ligaments are variable from patient to patient. The shoulder has a strong joint capsule. In the acute setting, radiographs and CT are the primary means of imaging the shoulder; in the subacute and chronic setting, MRI (with or without arthrography) is the primary means. Because the articular surface of the glenoid is oriented obliquely, the radiographic examination should always include a lateral view (axillary, transscapular, or transthoracic) when shoulder dislocation is suspected.

## Glenohumeral Joint Dislocations

In approximately 95% of cases of glenohumeral dislocation, the humeral head dislocates anteriorly and ends up anterior, inferior, and medial to the glenoid process in a subcoracoid location

**A**                    **B**

**FIGURE 2.32.** Anterior shoulder dislocation. **A:** AP radiograph shows the humeral head dislocated medially and inferiorly. **B:** Axillary radiograph shows the humeral head dislocated anteriorly.

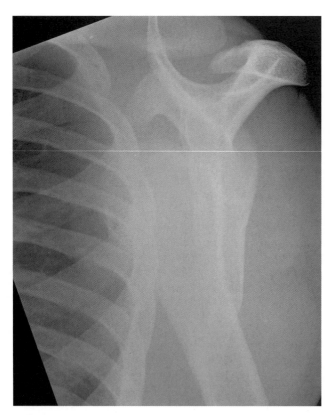

**FIGURE 2.33.** Anterior shoulder dislocation demonstrated on transscapular radiograph ("Y-view").

(Figs. 2.32 and 2.33). Abduction and external rotation of the arm cause the acromion to come in contact with the surgical neck of the humerus, and the humeral head can be levered out of the glenoid fossa. A direct blow to the back of the shoulder can eject the humeral head, and traction on the limb can pull it out. Impaction of the anterior-inferior surface of the glenoid labrum on the posterolateral aspect of the humeral head after it dislocates may cause a depressed humeral head fracture called the *Hill-Sachs lesion* (Fig. 2.34). Less dramatic but perhaps more important than the dislocation itself is the concomitant detachment of the labrum and capsule from the anterior glenoid process (Bankart lesion) sometimes associated with an avulsion fracture (Fig. 2.35). These injuries often result in posttraumatic anterior shoulder instability or recurrent dislocations. In approximately 5% of shoulder dislocations, the humeral head comes to rest posterior to the glenoid process, and the dislocation may be difficult to recognize on standard AP views (Fig. 2.36). An impaction fracture of the anterior aspect of the humeral head may be present, *reverse Hill-Sachs lesion* (Fig. 2.37). Posterior shoulder dislocations may occur in the setting of tonic-clonic seizures. Other types of shoulder dislocations are rare. Acute dislocations are treated with closed reduction; associated soft-tissue or glenoid rim injuries may require surgical repair.

## Rotator Cuff Injuries

The tendons of the rotator cuff may tear as a result of acute or repetitive trauma, mechanical impingement, degeneration, focal ischemia, or some combination of these. Rotator cuff tears may also be associated with rheumatoid arthritis. More than 90% of rotator cuff tears present with chronic weakness and pain. A minority of rotator

**A**

**B**

**FIGURE 2.34.** Hill-Sachs lesion. **A:** Internally rotated AP radiograph of the shoulder shows impaction fracture (*arrow*) of the humeral head was sustained during previous anterior dislocation. **B:** Axial T2-weighted fat-suppressed MRI shows high signal (*arrow*) at the site of impaction.

**FIGURE 2.35.** Avulsion fracture of the glenoid rim (osseous Bankart injury) following anterior shoulder dislocation. Axial T2-weighted fat-suppressed MRI shows a displaced fragment of bone (*arrow*) from the anterior glenoid process with attached labrum and capsule.

cuff tears presents after a discrete episode of trauma; however, many patients with chronic presentations have a history of glenohumeral dislocation or other shoulder trauma. Full-thickness rotator cuff tears result in a discontinuity that may fill with fluid or granulation tissue; the involved muscle belly may retract. Partial-thickness tears may involve either the inferior or the superior surfaces of the cuff or may be entirely within the substance of the tendons. The most common rotator cuff tear is an isolated tear of the supraspinatus tendon at its insertion at the greater tuberosity (Fig. 2.38). When the infraspinatus tendon is torn, it is typically in combination with a tear of the supraspinatus tendon, allowing the humeral head to subluxate superiorly underneath the acromion process (Fig. 2.39). Partial-thickness tears are more common than full-thickness tears, and partial-thickness tears involving the articular surface of the cuff are more common than those involving the bursal side. Rotator cuff tears are much more common among older patients.

On radiographs, superior subluxation of the humeral head with loss of the normal radiographic space between the inferior aspect of the acromion process and the superior aspect of the humeral head is indicative of rotator cuff tear or atrophy. When the inferior surface of the acromion has remodeled to accommodate the humeral head, it is an indication that the supraspinatus and infraspinatus tendons are massively torn and retracted. These findings are often incidentally made on chest radiographs of elderly patients.

On arthrography, contrast medium or contrast medium and air are injected into the shoulder capsule. A full-thickness rotator cuff tear is indicated by leakage of contrast medium or air through the tear into the subdeltoid-subacromial bursa. The size of the tear is often difficult to establish using this technique. Partial tears involving the articular surface may be sometimes demonstrated on air contrast arthrography but generally not with single contrast arthrography. Arthrography may be combined with CT or MRI for greater accuracy.

On MRI, the shoulder should be examined in axial, oblique coronal, and oblique sagittal planes. The normal rotator cuff tendons have generally low signal on all sequences, similar to that of

**FIGURE 2.36.** Posterior shoulder dislocation. **A:** AP radiograph shows internal rotation of the humeral head. **B:** Y-view shows posterior position of the humeral head relative to the glenoid fossa.

**FIGURE 2.37.** Posterior shoulder dislocation with impaction fracture of anterior humeral head (reverse Hill-Sachs lesion).

tendons in other parts of the body. Many normal supraspinatus tendons have gray zones within the substance of the tendon that may reflect imaging artifact (magic angle phenomenon) or anatomic variation. Rotator cuff tears on MRI may be confidently recognized if there is a discontinuity of the tendon, retraction of the involved muscle belly, and fluid interposed between the fragments of the tendon. If a full-thickness tear does not involve the entire width of the tendon, and the gap is filled with granulation tissue rather than fluid, one may only see increased signal in the tendon without retraction of the muscle belly. Secondary signs of rotator cuff tears include fluid in the subdeltoid-subacromial bursa, fluid in the subcoracoid bursa, fluid in the glenohumeral joint, loss of the peribursal fat plane around the subdeltoid-subacromial bursa, and muscle atrophy. None of the secondary signs is diagnostic of a tear when occurring in isolation.

Partial-thickness tears of the rotator cuff are evident as focal regions of high signal on T2-weighted images. Secondary signs of rotator cuff tear may be present. MRI is less accurate in identifying partial-thickness tears of the rotator cuff than full-thickness tears.

Rotator cuff tendinopathy is evident on MRI as thickening of the tendon with increased signal on T2-weighted images. Tendinopathy is commonly found in the supraspinatus tendon (Fig. 2.40) and may progress to partial or complete tear.

**FIGURE 2.38.** Full-thickness partial-width supraspinatus tendon tear (*arrows*) on T1-weighted MR arthrogram. Gadolinium-based contrast medium that was injected into the glenohumeral joint has flowed through the tear into the subdeltoid-subacromial bursa. **A:** Oblique coronal. **B:** Oblique sagittal. **C:** Axial.

**A**　　　　　　　　　　　　　　　　　　　　**B**

**FIGURE 2.39.** Full-thickness tears of the supraspinatus and infraspinatus tendons. **A:** Oblique coronal T2-weighted fat-suppressed MRI shows retraction of the supraspinatus tendon (*arrow*) and superior subluxation of the humeral head. **B:** Oblique sagittal T2-weighted fat-suppressed MRI shows absence of the supraspinatus and infraspinatus tendons (*arrows*) due to retraction.

Tears of the subscapularis tendon are uncommon, and tears of the teres minor tendon are even less common. Isolated tears of the subscapularis tendon may occur with anterior dislocation. Dislocations of the long head of the biceps tendon from the bicipital groove of the proximal humerus may accompany a subscapularis tendon tear, and sometimes the long head of the biceps tendon may dislocate into the glenohumeral joint.

Rotator cuff tears are repaired surgically if conservative methods do not improve symptoms. Imaging after a surgical repair can

**FIGURE 2.40.** Rotator cuff tendinopathy. Oblique coronal T2-weighted MRI shows high signal (*arrow*) and thickening of the supraspinatus tendon, without discontinuity.

be difficult because of imaging artifacts from the surgery and the variable correlation between imaging findings of recurrent tear and patient symptoms.

## Glenoid Labral and Glenohumeral Ligament Injuries

Injuries of the labrum and associated capsular structures are often related to sports activities. Most occur in one of two locations: the anterior-inferior labrum or the superior labrum (Table 2.2). A detachment of the anterior-inferior labrum during avulsion of the inferior glenohumeral ligament results in anterior shoulder instability. The superior labral anterior to posterior tear, in which the labral-capsular-bicipital tendon complex is detached from the superior aspect of the glenoid process by traction on the long head of the biceps tendon during sudden arm abduction, does not result in instability (see Fig. 2.31). MRI signs of SLAP tear include "Cheerio sign," "double Oreo cookie sign," linear high signal intensity in the posterior half of the superior labrum curving laterally away from the glenoid resulting in a "V" or "Y" appearance of the superior labrum, increased width of high signal between the superior labrum and glenoid, and paralabral cyst. A detachment of the anterior-inferior labrum by tension on the inferior glenohumeral ligament is a Bankart lesion, with its variants the Perthes lesion and the ALPSA lesion (anterior labroligamentous periosteal sleeve avulsion lesion) (Fig. 2.41). Labral and capsular injuries are shown best by MR arthrography or CT arthrography. Normal variants in the anterosuperior aspect of the glenoid may mimic labral pathology (Table 2.3). These variants include the sublabral sulcus (Fig. 2.42), the sublabral foramen (Fig. 2.43), and the Buford complex (Fig. 2.44).

Posterior labral tears at the attachment of the posterior cord of the inferior glenohumeral ligament may result in the POLPSA lesion (posterior labroligamentous periosteal sleeve avulsion lesion) (Fig. 2.45), which may be associated with paralabral cysts. These cysts are thought to arise from the chronic leakage of synovial fluid through the tear into the periarticular soft tissues, perhaps with a

| TABLE 2.2 | Injuries of the Glenoid Labrum |
|---|---|
| Name of Lesion | Salient Feature |
| SLAP | Superior labrum-anterior-posterior lesion |
| Bankart | Detachment of the anterior-inferior labrum and inferior glenohumeral ligament from the glenoid process. The tear is between the labrum and the bone |
| Perthes | Incomplete avulsion of the anterior-inferior labrum with intact scapular periosteum. The labrum is displaced minimally or not at all |
| ALPSA | Anterior labrum periosteal sleeve avulsion. The tear of the anterior-inferior labrum is between the bone and the periosteum |
| POLPSA | Posterior labrum periosteal sleeve avulsion. The tear of the posterior labrum is between the bone and the periosteum |
| GLAD | Glenolabral articular disruption |
| OCD | Osteochondritis dissecans or osteochondral defect of the glenoid has a high incidence of associated labral tear |
| GLOM | Glenoid labrum ovoid mass is the appearance of a labral tear |
| Bennett | Extra-articular posterior ossification associated with posterior labral injury and undersurface rotator cuff damage |
| HAGL | Humeral avulsion of the inferior glenohumeral ligament |
| BHAGL | Bony humeral avulsion of the inferior glenohumeral ligament |
| FAIGHL | Floating anterior-inferior glenohumeral ligament. Anterior HAGL lesion with an associated labral tear |
| FPIGHL | Floating posterior-inferior glenohumeral ligament. Posterior HAGL lesion with an associated labral tear |

one-way valve effect. The presence of such cysts is associated with a posterior labral tear in the majority of cases (Fig. 2.46), although an actual communication between the cyst and the joint is often difficult to demonstrate. When large, such cysts may cause entrapment neuropathy of the suprascapular nerve in the suprascapular notch or spinoglenoid notch, resulting in denervation atrophy changes in the supraspinatus muscle, supraspinatus and infraspinatus muscles, or infraspinatus muscle, respectively. Early denervation may be recognized on MRI as a slight increase in muscle signal on T2-weighted images; late denervation may be recognized by loss of bulk and the presence of intramuscular fat on T1-weighted images. Cysts are not generally associated with labral tears at other locations, because it is only posteriorly where the joint capsule is immediately apposed to the labrum. Posterior labral tears are commonly found in association with ossification adjacent to the posteroinferior aspect of the glenoid rim (Bennett lesion). Bennett lesions are found commonly in throwing athletes and often have associated posterior undersurface rotator cuff damage.

Injuries of the inferior glenohumeral ligament include tears through the mid-substance as well as avulsions from its humeral attachment. Mid-substance tears are best demonstrated by MR arthrography and are associated with tears of the shoulder capsule

**FIGURE 2.41.** ALPSA lesion. Axial GRE MRI shows displacement of the anterior labrum (*black arrow*) and stripping of the periosteum anteriorly (*white arrow*).

| TABLE 2.3 | Anterosuperior Labral Variants of the Shoulder |
|---|---|

Sublabral recess or sulcus: potential space or recess between superior labrum and glenoid

Sublabral foramen or hole: hole located anterior to glenoid providing communication of glenohumeral joint with subscapular recess

Buford complex: cord-like or thickened middle glenohumeral ligament with absent or diminutive anterosuperior labrum

and consequent leakage of contrast (Fig. 2.47). *HAGL* (humeral avulsion of the inferior glenohumeral ligament) injuries occur when the ligament is torn from its humeral insertion (Fig. 2.48), and BHAGL (bony humeral avulsion of the inferior glenohumeral ligament) injuries occur when there is an associated fragment from the humerus (Fig. 2.49). HAGL lesions may involve the anterior or posterior band (Fig. 2.50), with or without bony avulsion and with or without associated labral tear. When there is an associated labral tear with a HAGL, the lesion is called *floating anterior* (Fig. 2.51) or *posterior-inferior glenohumeral ligament*. The majority of patients with HAGL lesions have associated injuries. The most commonly associated injuries are labral tears, Hill-Sachs lesions, and rotator cuff tears.

GLAD (glenolabral articular disruption) is a nondisplaced superficial anteroinferior labral tear associated with an adjacent chondral injury (Fig. 2.52). This mechanism of injury is forced adduction to the shoulder from an abducted and external rotated position. It has many similarities to osteochondral lesions of the glenoid fossa (Fig. 2.53). History of dislocation, instability on physical examination, mechanism of injury, and radiologic findings distinguish osteochondral lesion of the glenoid from the GLAD lesion.

**FIGURE 2.43.** Sublabral foramen. Axial GRE MRI shows high signal (*arrow*) between the anterosuperior labrum and the glenoid.

# CLAVICLE

Fractures of the clavicle usually occur in the middle third, medial to the coracoclavicular ligaments. The sternocleidomastoid muscle displaces the proximal fragment superiorly, and the shoulder, acting through the coracoclavicular ligament, displaces the distal fragment inferiorly. With immobilization, healing is usually prompt.

**FIGURE 2.42.** Sublabral sulcus. Oblique coronal T2-weighted fat-suppressed MRI shows high signal (*arrow*) between the superior labrum and the glenoid curving medially toward the glenoid.

**FIGURE 2.44.** Buford complex. Axial GRE MRI shows a thickened middle glenohumeral ligament (*arrow*) and an absent anterosuperior labrum.

**FIGURE 2.45.** POLPSA lesion. Axial GRE MRI shows displacement of the posterior labrum and stripping of the periosteum posteriorly (*arrow*).

**FIGURE 2.47.** Tear of the anterior band of the inferior glenohumeral ligament (*arrow*) with leakage of contrast (*arrowheads*) shown on coronal T1-weighted fat-suppressed MR arthrogram.

**FIGURE 2.46.** Posterior labral tear with labral cyst. Axial GRE MRI shows a paralabral cyst (C) associated with a posterior labral tear (*arrow*).

**FIGURE 2.48.** HAGL lesion. Axial GRE MRI shows detachment of the anterior band of the inferior glenohumeral ligament (*arrow*) with extravasation of joint fluid across the torn humeral attachment.

**FIGURE 2.49.** BHAGL lesion. Coronal CT reformation of the right shoulder shows a linear bone fragment (*arrow*) medial to the proximal humerus.

**FIGURE 2.50.** Posterior HAGL lesion. Axial PD fat-suppressed MRI shows that the posterior band of the inferior glenohumeral ligament (*arrow*) is avulsed from the proximal humerus with extravasation of the joint fluid across the torn humeral attachment.

A

B

**FIGURE 2.51.** Floating anterior inferior glenohumeral ligament **A:** Oblique coronal T2-weighted fat-suppressed MRI shows a J-shaped anterior band of the inferior glenohumeral ligament with extravasation of the joint fluid across the torn humeral attachment (*arrow*). **B:** Axial GRE MRI shows a glenoid labrum ovoid mass (*arrow*) consistent with anterior labral tear.

**FIGURE 2.52.** GLAD lesion. Axial T2-weighted fat-suppressed MR arthrogram shows a chondral flap tear (*arrow*) of the glenoid.

Clavicular fractures distal to the coracoclavicular ligaments may be complicated by tears of the coracoclavicular ligaments or avulsion of the coracoid process.

Acromioclavicular injuries involve the disruption of the acromioclavicular and coracoclavicular ligaments (shoulder separation). The inferior surfaces of the acromion process and the distal clavicle are normally at the same level on AP radiographs.

In a type I injury, the acromioclavicular ligaments are stretched but not disrupted, and radiographs are normal or show a slight increase in the joint space. When the acromioclavicular ligaments are completely torn (type II), the distal clavicle subluxates superiorly. If the coracoclavicular ligaments are also torn (type III), the clavicle dislocates and the space between the clavicle and the coracoid process widens (Fig. 2.54). Other types of acromioclavicular injuries are rare.

Dislocations of the sternoclavicular joint are usually sustained in high-speed motor vehicle collisions. Although radiographs may demonstrate superior dislocation (Fig. 2.55), CT may be required to demonstrate a posterior dislocation. Anterior dislocations of the sternoclavicular joint are more common than posterior dislocations, but the latter have more serious complications.

**FIGURE 2.53.** Osteochondral lesion of glenoid. Axial GRE MRI shows a multiloculated cyst (*black arrow*) in the posterior aspect of the glenoid and a loose body (*white arrow*) anterior to the glenoid.

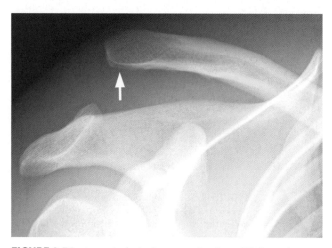

**FIGURE 2.54.** Acromioclavicular separation (type III) (*arrow*).

**FIGURE 2.55.** Posterior-superior dislocation of the right sternoclavicular joint. **A:** Radiograph shows medial position of the right clavicular head (*arrow*). **B:** Axial CT scan shows posterior dislocation (*arrow*). **C:** Coronal CT reformation shows superior dislocation (*arrow*).

## SOURCES AND READINGS

Berquist TH. *MRI of the Musculoskeletal System*. 5th Ed. Philadelphia, PA: Lippincott Williams & Wilkins; 2005.

Browner B, Jupiter J, Levine A, Trafton P, Krettek C. *Skeletal Trauma: Fractures, Dislocations, Ligamentous Injuries*. 4th Ed. Philadelphia, PA: Saunders; 2008.

Bucholz RW, Heckman JD, Court-Brown C, Tornetta P. *Rockwood and Green's Fractures in Adults*. 7th Ed. Philadelphia, PA: Lippincott Williams & Wilkins; 2009.

Chew FS, Maldjian C. *Broken Bones: The X-ray Atlas of Fractures*. Seattle, WA: BareBonesBooks.com; 2009

eMedicine. http://emedicine.medscape.com.

Gilula LA, ed. *The Traumatized Hand and Wrist: Radiographic and Anatomic Correlation*. Philadelphia, PA: WB Saunders; 1998.

Griffin LY. *Essentials of Musculoskeletal Care*. 3rd Ed. Rosemont, IL: American Academy of Orthopedics; 2005.

Helms CA, Major NM, Anderson MW, et al. *Musculoskeletal MRI*. 2nd Ed. Philadelphia, PA: WB Saunders; 2009.

Hilbrook TL, Grazier K, Kelsey JL, et al. *The Frequency of Occurrence, Impact, and Cost of Selected Musculoskeletal Conditions in the United States*. Chicago, IL: American Academy of Orthopedic Surgeons; 1984.

Lichtman DM, Alexander AH. *The Wrist and its Disorders*. 2nd Ed. Philadelphia, PA: WB Saunders; 1997.

Mayfield JK. Patterns of injury to carpal ligaments. A spectrum. *Clin Orthop*. 1984;187:36–42.

Pedowitz R, Resnick D, Chung CB. *Magnetic Resonance Imaging in Orthopedic Sports Medicine*. Berlin: Springer; 2008.

Rockwood CA Jr, Matsen FA, Wirth M. *The Shoulder*. 3rd Ed. Philadelphia, PA: WB Saunders; 2004.

Rogers LF. *Radiology of Skeletal Trauma*. 3rd Ed. New York, NY: Churchill-Livingstone; 2002.

Steinbach LS, Chung CB. *MRI of Upper Extremity: Shoulder, Elbow, Wrist, and Hand*. Philadelphia, PA: Lippincott Williams & Wilkins; 2009.

Stoller DW. *Magnetic Resonance Imaging in Orthopaedics and Sports Medicine*. 3rd Ed. Philadelphia, PA: Lippincott Williams & Wilkins; 2006.

Wheeless CR III, ed. *Wheeless' Textbook of Orthopaedics*. http://www.wheelessonline.com.

# 3 Trauma in Adults: Axial Skeleton

**T**his chapter describes the radiology of common injuries to the spine, thoracic cage, and pelvis in adults.

## ■ GENERAL PRINCIPLES

Injuries to the spine often occur in the setting of severe trauma. Approximately 45% of spine injuries are sustained in motor vehicle collisions, 20% in falls, 15% in recreational or sports-related accidents, 15% from intentional acts of violence, and 5% from other causes. There is a 4:1 male predominance. Although spinal cord injuries often accompany spine trauma, neurologic damage is not an invariable concomitant (Table 3.1). Precautions against causing or worsening a neurologic injury should be scrupulously observed at all levels of care. There are clinical criteria for predicting whether an injury is present or not; the simplest of these are the NEXUS criteria (Table 3.2). It is generally not the role of the radiologist to determine whether imaging is indicated or not, but rather to provide the radiologic care that is necessary for the clinical situation. In the setting of suspected spine trauma, if any imaging is deemed necessary, CT with multiplanar reformations should be obtained. A single lateral radiograph is also typically obtained as part of the initial survey in multiple trauma patients. Abnormality of the soft tissues or the spinal cord may be imaged directly by MRI.

The vertebral bodies and intervertebral disks usually bear compressive loads, and the posterior elements and associated ligaments usually bear distractive (tensile) loads. The three-column concept is used widely to assess fracture stability (Fig. 3.1). The anterior

### TABLE 3.1 Neurologic Damage in Spine Trauma

| Level of Injury | Percentage with Neurologic Damage |
| --- | --- |
| Cervical spine | 39 |
| Thoracic spine | 10 |
| Thoracolumbar junction (T11–L1) | 4 |
| Lumbar spine | 3 |
| Overall | 14 |

*Source*: Riggins RS, Kraus JF. The risk of neurologic damage with fractures of the vertebrae. *J Trauma*. 1977;17:126–133.

### TABLE 3.2 NEXUS Criteria Indicating Low Risk of Spinal Injury (All Criteria Must be Met)

No midline cervical tenderness
No focal neurologic deficits
No intoxication or indication of brain injury
No painful distracting injuries
Normal alertness

*Source*: Hoffman JR, Mower WR, Wolfson AB, Todd KH, Zucker MI. Validity of a set of clinical criteria to rule out injury to the cervical spine in patients with blunt trauma. National Emergency X-Radiography Utilization Study Group. *N Engl J Med*. 2000;343:94–99.

column consists of the anterior part of the vertebral bodies, the anterior part of the intervertebral disks, and the anterior longitudinal ligament. The middle column consists of the posterior annulus of the intervertebral disk, the posterior wall of the vertebral body, and the posterior longitudinal ligament. The posterior column consists of the posterior elements, the facet joints, and the posterior ligament complex. An injury that disrupts the middle and at least one other column is considered unstable. Most injuries can be described by the mechanisms of flexion, extension, shearing, and rotation (Table 3.3 and Fig. 3.2). These mechanisms may be combined with axial compression or axial distraction (tension). Flexion is by far the most common mechanism of injury and may occur throughout the spine. Flexion injuries result in compression of the anterior column and distraction of the posterior column. They have the radiologic features of vertebral body fractures and narrowing of the disk space anteriorly and widening of the interspinous space posteriorly. Severe injuries may disrupt the middle column, resulting in anterolisthesis and dislocated facets. Extension injuries are common only in the cervical region. They result from distraction of the anterior column and compression of the posterior column. They have the radiologic features of avulsion fractures of the anterior aspect of the vertebral end plate and widening of the disk space anteriorly and fractures of the neural arch posteriorly. Severe injuries may disrupt the middle column, resulting in retrolisthesis. Shearing injuries are common in the thoracic and lumbar regions and result from disruption of ligaments. Lateral distraction, lateral dislocation, avulsion fractures of the vertebral end plates, and transverse process fractures may

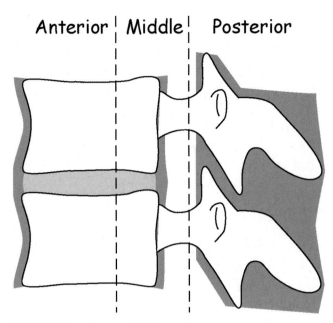

**FIGURE 3.1.** Diagram of the three-column concept.

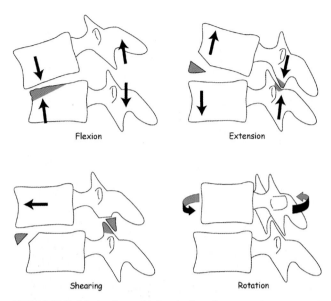

**FIGURE 3.2.** Mechanisms of injury in the spine.

be seen. Rotational injuries may occur throughout the spine and may be evident by rotational misalignment, dislocation, avulsion fractures of the vertebral end plates, and facet or pillar fractures. Axial compression may result in compression injuries in all three columns, whereas axial distraction may result in tension injuries.

The normal alignment of the spine is lordotic in the cervical region, kyphotic in the thoracic region, and lordotic in the lumbar region. Arcs drawn along any of the bony margins of the vertebrae on any view should be straight or should curve smoothly.

| TABLE 3.3 | **Radiologic Features of Vertebral Injuries** |
|---|---|
| Mechanism | Key Radiologic Features |
| Flexion | Vertebral body fracture |
| | Narrow disk space |
| | Wide interspinous space |
| | Facet dislocation |
| | Anterolisthesis |
| Extension | End-plate avulsion fracture |
| | Wide disk space |
| | Neural arch fracture |
| | Retrolisthesis |
| Shearing | Lateral distraction |
| | Lateral dislocation |
| | End-plate avulsion fracture |
| | Transverse process fracture |
| Rotational | Rotational misalignment |
| | Dislocation |
| | End-plate avulsion fracture |
| | Facet or pillar fracture |

*Source*: Adapted from Daffner RH, Deeb ZL, Rothfus WE. "Fingerprints" of vertebral trauma-a unifying concept based on mechanisms. *Skeletal Radiol.* 1986;15:518–525.

The various joints throughout the spine should be congruent. The paraspinal soft tissues may be seen in the cervical region anteriorly and in the thoracic region laterally. As a general guideline, above the esophagus, the prevertebral soft tissues should measure 5 mm or less; at the level of the upper esophagus, usually C6, they should measure 22 mm or less. In the thoracic region, the lateral soft tissues should follow the bony margins closely; they are more prominent in the presence of osteophytes. Asymmetry of the soft tissues may indicate injury. Discontinuity of any cortical margin may indicate a fracture. Some injuries that may be difficult to identify in the axial plane are often better seen in the sagittal or coronal planes.

Because of differences in anatomy, biomechanics, and exposure to loading, spine trauma is considered in four regions: upper cervical (Occiput-C1–2), lower cervical (C3–T1), upper thoracic (T2–10), and thoracolumbar (T11–L5). Spinal column injuries are most common in the lower cervical spine and in the thoracolumbar region. A significant minority of patients have fractures at multiple noncontiguous levels. The most dangerous of these situations is a C2 fracture combined with a C7–T1 injury.

# ■ UPPER CERVICAL SPINE (OCCIPUT-C1–2)

The cervical spine occupies a vulnerable position as the mobile linkage between the head and the thorax. The internal stresses on the spine and the injuries that result depend primarily on the positions of the head, spine, and body at the time of injury, and the sequence, direction, magnitude, and rate of loading. When structural failure occurs, it is most often restricted to a single intervertebral or vertebral level, but as many as 10% of patients with upper cervical spine injuries also have lower cervical spine injuries. In clinical practice, two types of events account for most cervical spine injuries: (a) axial loading on the head that is transmitted into the spine and (b) acceleration or deceleration of the head and body relative to each other. Axial loading occurs when the moving head strikes a stationary object and may be combined with loading in flexion or extension. Acceleration and deceleration loading may occur because of the substantial difference in mass between the head and body. Forward or backward translation of the head relative to the body during

**FIGURE 3.3.** Craniocervical junction injury. **A:** Lateral radiograph shows prevertebral soft-tissue swelling between the endotracheal tube and vertebral column. **B, C:** Sagittal CT reformation shows forward subluxation (*arrows*) of the left and right occipital condyles (C) relative to C1. **D:** Coronal CT reformation shows a displaced avulsion fragment from the left occipital condyle (*arrow*).

acceleration or deceleration results in complex, changing forces on the cervical spine. In addition to the hyperflexion or hyperextension loading that occurs when the cervical spine reaches its limit of mobility, there are additional distractive forces in the axial direction. The predominant mode of loading is tensile in either flexion or extension. The injuries that occur depend on how the spine is loaded as well as individual variations in the mechanics and anatomy.

High energy is required to injure the craniocervical junction, typically through distractive hyperflexion or hyperextension forces with or without associated rotation. Most survivable injuries are subluxations of the atlanto-occipital joints or fractures of the occipital condyles. The subluxations are typically anterior subluxations of the occipital condyles over C1, seen best on sagittal reformatted CT or sagittal MRI. Fractures of the condyles may be impactions,

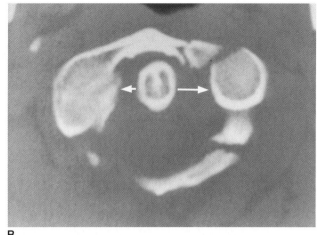

**A**

**B**

**FIGURE 3.4.** Axial compression fracture of C1 suffered in a diving accident. **A:** Lateral radiograph shows soft-tissue swelling and displaced fractures of the posterior arch (*arrows*). **B:** CT scan shows comminuted fractures involving the left lateral and the posterior portions of the ring of C1. The fragments have displaced asymmetrically from the odontoid process (*arrows*).

extensions from fractures of the base of the skull, or avulsions (Fig. 3.3). Patients occasionally survive atlanto-occipital dislocation.

Fractures of the ring of C1 are sustained during axial loading. An axial load applied to the top of the head with the cervical spine in neutral position spreads apart the ring of C1 between the sloped articular surfaces of the occiput and C2. This results in multiple, displaced fractures of C1 (Jefferson fracture). More commonly, the axial load is applied obliquely, or the cervical spine does not remain straight, and the fractures of the ring of C1 are more posterior or lateral (Fig. 3.4). Neurologic damage is often absent because the

spinal canal is relatively capacious at this level, and the fragments are displaced away from the cord.

In traumatic spondylolisthesis of C2 (hangman's fracture), there are bilateral pars interarticularis fractures with forward sub-luxation of C2 over C3. The *pars interarticularis* is the bridge of bone that occupies the position in the articular mass between the superior and inferior articular facets. An individual subjected to judicial hanging drops feet first through a trap door with a rope secured around the neck and the hangman's knot located under the chin. When he or she reaches the end of the rope, the upper

**FIGURE 3.5.** Traumatic spondylolisthesis (hangman's fracture) in a traffic accident victim. Horizontal fractures through the pars interarticularis (*arrow*).

**FIGURE 3.6.** CT scan of C2 hangman's fracture (*arrows*).

**FIGURE 3.7.** Odontoid fracture (type II) shown on sagittal CT reformation (*arrows*).

cervical spine is pulled violently into hyperextension and simultaneously subjected to massive distractive forces from the downward inertia of the body. The ligaments of the anterior column tear at the C2–3 level, and the posterior elements are fractured at the pars interarticularis. Similar fractures of the C2 posterior elements may also occur when an axial load (compressive rather than distractive) is applied with the neck hyperextended (Figs. 3.5 and 3.6). This may occur in a motor vehicle collision in which the passenger slides forward and strikes the forehead, forcing the neck into hyperextension.

In young adults, most fractures of the odontoid process of C2 (dens) occur transversely across the base, probably as a result of hyperextension or hyperflexion. The fracture is accompanied by ligament tears at the same level separating the odontoid process and C1 from the remainder of C2 as a single, mechanically unstable unit (Fig. 3.7). The odontoid is composed primarily of cortical bone, so an odontoid fracture heals less well than the fractures through portions of the vertebrae that are primarily cancellous.

In elderly adults, the most common odontoid fracture is through the base of the dens with extension into the body of C2 (Fig. 3.8). When the fracture is caused by flexion, a tension fracture begins at the posterior base of the dens and propagates anteriorly and inferiorly into the body of C2 where compression and impaction occur, resulting in an anteriorly angulated dens. When the fracture is caused by extension, a tension fracture begins at the anterior base of the dens and propagates posteriorly where compression and impaction occur, resulting in a posteriorly angulated dens.

Fractures of the dens can be classified according to Anderson and D'Alonzo. A type I fracture involves the tip of the dens and is rare. A type II fracture extends transversely across the base of the dens and is the most common type. A type III fracture involves the body of C2. A fracture of the base of the odontoid process, through the substance of the body of C2 rather than through the odontoid process itself, also represents a mechanically unstable fracture. Because the fracture is through cancellous bone, healing is usually prompt and nonunion is unlikely. These fractures are much less common than fractures through the odontoid process. Odontoid fractures are the most common cervical spine fractures in patients older than 70 years of age.

Isolated fractures of the anterior-inferior margin of the body of C2 are the most common type of hyperextension teardrop fracture (Fig. 3.9), so called because the mechanism of injury is hyperextension and the fracture fragment resembles a teardrop. The hyperextension teardrop fracture represents an avulsion fracture with tension mediated through the anterior longitudinal ligament. The hyperextension teardrop fracture occurs less commonly at C3—and even less commonly at other levels—but may be associated with a hangman's fracture.

Dislocations of C1 over C2 require severe ligamentous disruption, are rare, and are usually fatal. Subluxation at the C1–2 level typically requires disruption of the transverse ligament of C1 that maintains the normal anatomic position of the odontoid process.

**A**      **B**

**FIGURE 3.8.** Odontoid fracture (type III) (*arrows*) shown on coronal (**A**) and sagittal (**B**) CT reconstructions. Note the subluxation of C1 relative to C2 (*arrowheads*).

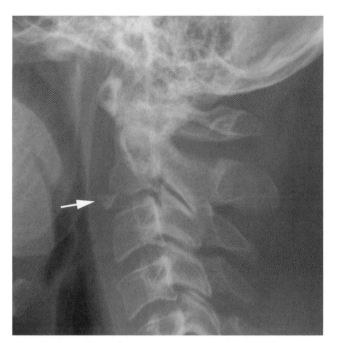

**FIGURE 3.9.** C2 hyperextension teardrop fracture (*arrow*).

**FIGURE 3.10.** Posterior ligament tear between C5 and C6 without fracture (hyperflexion sprain). The anterior disk space is narrowed (*arrow*) while the posterior elements are splayed apart (*arrowhead*).

Nontraumatic laxity of the transverse ligament is associated with Down syndrome, rheumatoid arthritis, and mucopolysaccharidosis.

# ■ LOWER CERVICAL SPINE (C3–T1)

Axial loading of the head occurs in events such as a fall from a height in which the individual lands on the head or a motor vehicle collision in which he or she is thrown forward and strikes the head. The attitude of the cervical spine and the location and direction of impact relative to the spine determine the stresses that result. Moderately severe axial loading with the cervical spine in neutral position causes vertebral body failure with central depression of the subjacent superior end plate, most often at C5. With massive axial loads, the intervertebral disk herniates through the end plate of the subjacent vertebral body and causes the body to explode from within, dispersing the fragments (burst fracture). Retropulsed fragments frequently damage the spinal cord. If the neck is flexed or if the location and direction of impact force the neck into flexion, the cervical spine is distracted posteriorly and compressed anteriorly. If the forces are relatively small, the injury may consist of a posterior ligament sprain (hyperflexion sprain) and possibly a compression fracture of the vertebral body. Disruption of the posterior ligament complex may be evident on radiographs as a focal kyphosis localized to the level of the sprain, often with subluxation of the facet joints and fanning of the spinous processes (Figs. 3.10 and 3.11). The abnormalities are accentuated with flexion and reduced with extension. The anterior compression fracture may be evident as loss of height, buckling of the anterior cortex, disruption of the end plate, and wedging of the disk space. Because the middle column is intact, this injury tends to be stable. Prevertebral soft-tissue swelling tends to be minimal and focal, reflecting the integrity of the anterior longitudinal ligament. If the direction of force is slightly to one side, the injuries may be eccentric. Delayed or failed ligament healing is a common complication.

If axial compression with hyperflexion is caused by large forces, a fracture dislocation may result (hyperflexion teardrop injury). This grievous injury is usually accompanied by quadriplegia from contusion of the anterior portion of the spinal cord. Massive posterior distractive forces disrupt the posterior ligament complex and dislocate the facet joints. The anterior and middle columns

**FIGURE 3.11.** Hyperflexion sprain. Sagittal inversion recovery MRI shows edema within the spinal cord (*arrow*) and interspinous ligaments (*arrowheads*).

**FIGURE 3.12.** Hyperflexion teardrop fracture. **A:** Lateral radiograph shows C6 fractures (*arrow*) with anterior soft-tissue swelling. **B:** Midline sagittal CT reformation shows retropulsion of the body of C6 (*arrowhead*).

are disrupted with tears of the longitudinal ligaments and the intervertebral disk. A triangular fragment (teardrop fragment) is sheared off the anterior-inferior corner of the dislocating vertebral body. The result is complete disruption of the cervical spine, with the superior portion displaced posteriorly and angulated anteriorly. The injury is recognized radiographically by focal kyphosis, posterior dislocation, distraction of the posterior elements, and the teardrop fragment of the anterior-inferior corner of the superior body (Figs. 3.12 and 3.13). Diffuse, marked anterior prevertebral soft-tissue swelling is always present.

The major injury vector in bilateral facet dislocation is hyperflexion of large magnitude without axial compression. Bilateral facet dislocation is a tension injury that propagates from posterior to anterior. Complete disruption of the ligaments and forward displacement of one involved vertebra over another allow the inferior articular facets of the superjacent vertebra to dislocate into the intervertebral foramen. The superior vertebra is anteriorly displaced by approximately 50% of the width of its body (Fig. 3.14). Sometimes the facets are subluxated (perched) but not dislocated. There may be accompanying fractures of the articular processes of the subjacent vertebra. The spine is unstable.

Axial loading with hyperextension places the anterior column under tension and the posterior column under compression. Structures of the spine fail in sequence, depending on the magnitude of the loading: tear of the anterior longitudinal ligament, disruption of the intervertebral disk, and tear of the posterior longitudinal ligament. A tension fracture of the vertebral body rather than disk disruption may occur; if the fracture involves only the anterior-inferior corner, a triangular (teardrop) fragment is present (hyperextension teardrop fracture). Compression fractures of the posterior elements are common, including fractures of the lamina and lateral masses. One or both facet joints may become dislocated. If only ligaments are disrupted and the spine relocates on the rebound, radiographs

may show a nearly normally aligned spine without fracture in an acutely quadriplegic patient (hyperextension sprain) (Fig. 3.15). Marked prespinal soft-tissue swelling should be present.

Large forces causing hyperextension and distraction, as might occur with a massive blow to the face or forehead, result in an injury similar to hyperextension with axial compression.

**FIGURE 3.13.** Hyperflexion fracture dislocation at C5–6. Sagittal T2-weighted MRI shows transection of the spinal cord (*arrow*).

**FIGURE 3.14.** Bilateral facet dislocation at C6–7. **A:** Radiograph shows anterior dislocation of C6 relative to C7 (*short arrow*). Gross prespinal soft-tissue swelling is present. The facet joints are locked (*long arrow*). There are fractures of the spinous processes (*arrowheads*). **B:** Axial CT scan shows bilateral locked facets (*arrows*).

The injury consists of tension injuries of the anterior and middle columns with transient posterior dislocation. Sometimes the disruption includes a tension fracture of the vertebral body, occasionally isolating a triangular fragment. Compressive injury to the posterior column is absent. Some degree of acute cervical cord syndrome is present, even though the cervical vertebrae on the lateral view may appear normally aligned after spontaneous reduction of the dislocation.

**FIGURE 3.15.** Hyperextension injury at C5–6. **A:** Lateral radiograph and **B:** sagittal reformatted CT scan show widened anterior intervertebral space at C5–6 with retrolisthesis. A small avulsion fragment of the anterior inferior corner of C5 is present (*arrows*).

**FIGURE 3.16.** Unilateral facet dislocation at C3–4. **A:** Lateral radiograph shows forward subluxation of C3 (*arrows*). **B:** Axial CT scan shows dislocation of the right facet (*arrow*), but not the left.

Unilateral facet dislocation occurs with hyperflexion, lateral bending, and rotation. Axial rotation and lateral bending are normally coupled in the middle and lower cervical spine because of the angle of the facet joints. With lateral bending, the facet joint on the concave side of the bend is compressed and essentially fixed; the contralateral articular mass rides forward and up and dislocates into the intervertebral foramen. The superior portion of the inferior facet is frequently fractured, presumably from impaction. Unilateral facet dislocation is recognized by forward subluxation and rotary misalignment (Fig. 3.16). The ligaments are disrupted on the side of the dislocation.

Lateral fracture dislocations of the cervical spine are very uncommon (Fig. 3.17). In this circumstance, the lateral radiograph

**FIGURE 3.17.** Lateral cervical spine fracture dislocation. **A:** Coronal reformatted CT scan shows lateral translation of C6 over C7 with rotatory displacement. **B:** Sagittal T2-weighted MRI shows abnormal high signal (*arrow*) between the spinous processes of C6–7 indicative of ligamentous disruption. Spinal cord contusion is also present.

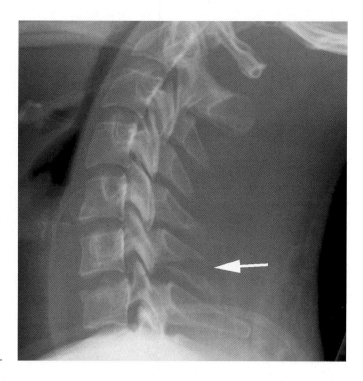

**FIGURE 3.18.** Clay shoveler's fracture at C6 (*arrow*).

may be misleading in demonstrating normal or nearly normal alignment. Secondary signs, such as soft-tissue swelling, should be present, and a cervical spinal cord injury may be clinically apparent. The mechanism of injury is likely to be lateral shearing.

Whiplash injuries occur in motor vehicle collisions when the individual's car is struck from behind, accelerating the body forward relative to the head. After the head bounces off the back of the car seat, the neck rebounds into flexion. The usual whiplash injury is a strain of the paravertebral and other neck muscles, often the *longus colli* group. In more severe injuries, the anterior longitudinal ligament and the anterior attachment of the intervertebral disk may be sprained. Bony fractures and dislocations are distinctly uncommon. Properly positioned headrests may prevent these injuries.

A clay shoveler's fracture is a horizontal tension fracture of a spinous process, most often at C7 and less commonly C6 or T1 (Fig. 3.18). Workers digging drainage ditches in southwestern Australia, in 1933, sustained these fractures when clay stuck to their shovels as they tried to throw the clay, suddenly increasing the stress on the neck musculature and its insertions. Similar injuries are sustained in motor vehicle collisions.

## ■ THORACIC REGION (T2–10)

The thoracic spine is supported by the rib cage and therefore is not very mobile. Fractures are uncommon and require major trauma. Acute traumatic compression fractures are most common

**FIGURE 3.19.** Hyperextension fracture distraction at T4–5. Sagittal reformatted CT scan shows posterior translation of T4 over T5 with widening of the intervertebral disk space and posterior distraction of the facet joints (*arrows*). **A:** Left; **B:** Midline; **C:** Right.

**FIGURE 3.20.** Hyperflexion fracture distraction at T9–10 shown by sagittal reformatted CT scans. **A:** On the left, there is an anterior superior corner fragment of T10 (*short arrow*) attached to T9, which is anteriorly translated. The superior T10 facet is fractured and the inferior T9 facet is dislocated anteriorly (*long arrow*). **B:** In the midline, the disk space is obliterated and the spinous processes are splayed (*arrowhead*). The anterior superior corner fragment of T10 is present (*short arrow*). There is a bone fragment in the spinal canal (*long arrow*). **C:** On the right, the superior T10 and inferior T9 facets are fractured (*arrowhead*). The anterior superior corner fragment of T10 is present (*short arrow*).

at the T6–7 levels. Most are anterior wedge fractures; the rest are lateral wedge fractures. Patients complain of localized pain and may have increased kyphosis. On imaging, paraspinal swelling, disruption of the cortical surface, and loss of height are present. Severe trauma may cause burst fractures, but these are much more common in the thoracolumbar region (discussed later in this chapter).

Although the upper thoracic spine is protected from bending forces by the rib cage, it is nonetheless vulnerable to torsional or shearing forces. Fracture dislocations are severe injuries that are probably the result of torsional or shearing forces, presumably combined with hyperflexion or axial compression (Fig. 3.19). The posterior ligaments are torn, there is fracture or dislocation of the facet joints, and the vertebral body may have a rotary shear fracture just below the subjacent end plate. Horizontal shearing forces may be sustained in a direct blow that translates the upper portion of the spine over the lower portion at the level of injury. Typically, the blow is from behind and causes an anterior fracture dislocation. The posterior column usually sustains traumatic spondylolisthesis with ligament tears, and the anterior and middle columns may have shear fractures of the vertebral body or soft-tissue injuries of the intervertebral disk (Fig. 3.20). There is a high incidence of spinal cord injury; 60% to 70% of patients with thoracic fracture dislocation have a neurologic deficit. Thoracic fracture dislocations are often reduced or partially reduced when patients are placed on backboards for extrication or transport. A massive injury may then be present with only subtle signs on the obligatory AP radiograph of the chest. Misalignment of the spinous processes, misalignment of the lateral margins of the vertebral bodies, focal angulation, widening of the interspinous distance, and paraspinal hematoma should be carefully sought. Sometimes, the paraspinal hematoma dissects into the mediastinum and over the apex of the left lung, simulating transection of the thoracic aorta. The presence of any of these findings necessitates further investigation, usually by CT.

# ◼ THORACOLUMBAR REGION (T11–L5)

Most injuries to the thoracolumbar region occur at the thoracolumbar junction (T11–L2), where the greatest degree of mobility is present. This region is particularly vulnerable to hyperflexion injuries.

**FIGURE 3.21.** Hyperflexion fracture distraction at T11–12. Sagittal T2 MRI shows disruption of the posterior longitudinal ligament and ligamentum flavum, with distraction of the posterior elements and extensive hemorrhage in the posterior soft tissues (*arrowheads*). There is focal kyphosis at T11–12 with narrowing of the anterior aspect of the intervertebral disk space (*arrow*) and anterior translation of the T11 body.

**FIGURE 3.22.** Lumbar burst fracture at L2. **A:** Axial CT shows comminuted vertebral body fractures that allow the pedicles to separate. **B:** Sagittal CT reformation shows flattening of L2 with retropulsion of fragments into the spinal canal. The posterior elements remain aligned.

During hyperflexion, compression fractures with anterior wedging of the vertebral body may be sustained, but the tensile loads are not great enough to disrupt the posterior ligaments (Fig. 3.21). Pure axial loading of the spine causes axial compression fractures that appear indistinguishable from hyperflexion injuries. With moderate loading, a simple compression fracture of the superior end plate is typical. If the loads are asymmetric, the fractures may be eccentric. Lateral bending may cause tension fractures of the transverse processes. With massive loading, a burst fracture may occur

(Fig. 3.22), with the involvement of the posterior elements and possible injury to the spinal cord. Simple compression fractures are stable because the middle and posterior columns remain intact; they may be treated with a brace or body cast. Burst fractures involving anterior and middle columns may require internal fixation.

Seat belt injuries are sustained in hyperflexion when the body is thrown forward against a restraining lap belt during sudden deceleration. Unlike the usual flexion injury, in which the axis of rotation is through the vertebral body, the axis of rotation in seat

**FIGURE 3.23.** Tension fracture of the entire L2 vertebra in a motor vehicle accident victim (Chance fracture). **A:** Lateral view shows sharp kyphotic angulation at the fracture level. The fractures extend through the vertebra from the posterior elements (*arrow*) to the body. **B:** AP radiograph shows the fractures through the body, posterior elements, and transverse processes (*arrows*).

**FIGURE 3.24.** Multiple left rib fractures sustained in a high-speed automobile crash.

belt injuries is at the anterior abdominal wall. Tensile forces disrupt the spine from posterior to anterior, usually at the L2 or L3 level. The resulting injury may consist of a tension fracture that extends horizontally through the vertebral body and neural arch (Chance fracture), intervertebral ligament disruption, or a combination of both (Fig. 3.23). A shoulder harness or air bag may prevent these injuries. Fractures or dislocations are uncommon at L3 or L4 and are rare at L5. Injuries to L3–5 are seen most often in patients with multiple traumas.

**A**

**B**

**FIGURE 3.25.** Manubrial fracture. Lateral radiograph (**A**) and sagittal reformatted CT (**B**) show nondisplaced fracture (*arrows*) of the manubrium.

**FIGURE 3.26.** Sternal body fracture. Axial CT shows nondisplaced fracture (*arrow*) through the body of the sternum.

# ■ THORACIC CAGE

Blunt chest trauma sustained in motor vehicle collisions may crush the bony thorax on direct impact. Pulmonary contusion, pneumothorax, myocardial contusion, diaphragmatic rupture, and abdominal injuries may result. The sudden deceleration that accompanies direct impact may cause transection of the thoracic aorta.

Rib fractures may occur from direct blows or crush injuries (Fig. 3.24). Oblique views of the chest are often necessary to demonstrate fractures of the ribs because of their arcuate course. Rib fractures may be difficult to see initially but are more obvious later as they become displaced by constant respiratory motion. Knowing the sites of maximal pain and point tenderness is helpful. Rib fractures may be multiple, in which case they involve adjacent ribs in a linear array. A flail chest occurs when there are multiple rib fractures that isolate a segment of the chest wall and cause paradoxic motion with respiration. Complications and associated conditions include pulmonary contusion, pneumothorax, hemopneumothorax, hemothorax, tracheal or bronchial tear, and interstitial emphysema. Fractures of the first three ribs usually follow severe trauma. The most common rib fractures are of the posterior or lateral aspects of the fourth through ninth ribs. Fractures of the lower ribs may be associated with visceral injuries. A rib may fracture with violent coughing or sneezing, usually at the anterior aspect along the diaphragmatic insertion. Stress fractures may also occur at the insertions of the serratus anterior muscles (first through ninth ribs) or scalene muscles (first and second ribs). Rib fractures that occur without trauma or with minimal trauma raise suspicion for a pathologic fracture.

The sternum fractures only with severe trauma as might be sustained with direct impact on the chest, for example, hitting the steering wheel during a motor vehicle collision. Most sternal fractures are transverse through the body of the sternum or the

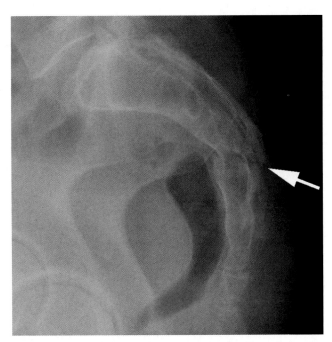

**FIGURE 3.27.** Fracture of the sacrum. Lateral radiograph shows a transverse fracture (*arrow*) through the sacrum at the S3 level.

sternomanubrial junction (Figs. 3.25 and 3.26). Hyperflexion of the thoracic cage is another mechanism of sternal fracture.

# ■ PELVIC RING

The pelvic ring comprises the sacrum and the two innominate bones. These three rigid components have resilient articulations where small degrees of motion are possible: the sacroiliac (SI) joints and the pubic symphysis. Thus, the pelvic ring is not a single rigid structure. Biomechanically, the sacrum can be considered the keystone of a femoral-sacral arch that supports the spine over the legs. The upper portion of the SI joint is a fibrous articulation with an extremely strong interosseous ligament; the lower portion of the SI joint is synovial and does not contribute mechanical strength to the joint. Anterior and posterior sets of SI ligaments attach the upper sacrum to the ilium, and sacrotuberous and sacrospinous ligaments attach the lower sacrum to the ischium. The functional stability of the pelvic ring depends on these ligaments. The pubic rami act as a stabilizing strut anteriorly, but their role is not crucial, provided that the posterior structures remain intact. Fractures of the pelvis can be divided into those that do not disrupt the integrity of the weight-bearing femoral-sacral arch (stable fractures) and those that do (unstable fractures).

## Stable Fractures

Stable fractures account for approximately two thirds of all pelvic fractures. These injuries include isolated fractures of the sacrum and pubic rami, avulsion fractures around the periphery of the pelvis, and simple acetabular fractures (see Chapter 4). Many stable fractures of the pelvis, especially isolated fractures around the obturator foramen, are sustained by elderly osteoporotic adults who fall. Although the bony margins of the obturator foramen form a rigid ring, the arrangement of its components is such that when the ring is loaded, one portion may be subjected to shearing forces, whereas another may be subjected to compressive forces. Bone resists shearing forces less well than compressive forces, so the bones may fail under shear but not under compression, leaving a single fracture of the ring. The most common pelvic fracture is an isolated fracture of an ischial ramus sustained in a fall. An isolated fracture of an iliac wing is called a *Duverney fracture*. It is frequently sustained in blunt trauma, such as motor vehicle crashes.

Isolated fractures of the sacrum are caused by direct trauma or a fall. These fractures tend to be transversely oriented, below the

**FIGURE 3.28.** Fracture of the sacrum. Oblique coronal T1-weighted MRI shows dark signal (*arrow*) extending vertically along the left sacral ala, indicating the fracture line and adjacent hemorrhage and edema.

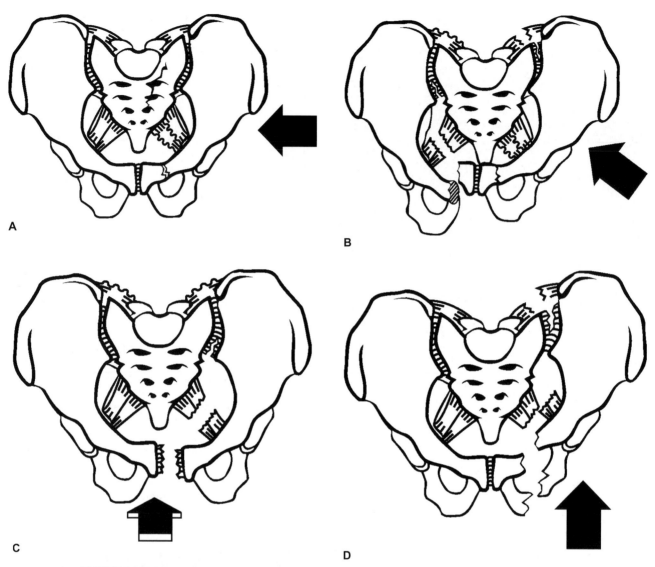

**A**

**B**

**C**

**D**

**FIGURE 3.29.** Diagram of pelvic ring fractures. **A:** Lateral compression (type I). SI joint compression and pubic ramus fracture. The hemipelvis on the side of impact rotates inward. **B:** Lateral compression (type II). The SI joint is opened posteriorly as the hemipelvis continues to rotate inward. **C:** AP compression fracture (type II). Diastasis of the symphysis with opening of the SI joint anteriorly. **D:** Vertical fracture dislocation of a hemipelvis.

**FIGURE 3.30.** Lateral compression fracture. CT scan shows a buckle fracture of the right sacral ala (*arrow*).

level of the SI joints, and anteriorly displaced or anteriorly angulated (Figs. 3.27 and 3.28). They are best demonstrated on the lateral radiograph or by CT images reformatted in the sagittal plane. Fractures of the sacrum that occur with pelvic ring fractures are typically vertical in orientation.

Stress fractures of the pubic rami may occur in runners. The clinical presentation is groin pain that is much worse with activity. As with stress fractures elsewhere, a radionuclide bone scan may be necessary to identify the injury.

## Unstable Injuries

Unstable injuries of the pelvic ring are the result of severe trauma, usually motor vehicle collisions involving either pedestrians or car occupants. Because these injuries are common in the setting of multiple trauma, an AP radiograph of the pelvis should be part of the initial evaluation of all multiple trauma patients. Patients with

**FIGURE 3.31.** Lateral compression fracture with complex acetabular fractures. **A:** AP radiograph shows fractures of the inferior pubic ramus (*arrowhead*), complex fractures of the acetabulum (*short arrows*), fracture of the iliac wing (*long arrow*), and very subtle fractures of the sacral ala, all on the right side. **B:** CT scan at the level of the sacral ala shows a shear fracture of the iliac wing (*short arrow*) and compression fracture of the sacrum (*long arrow*). **C:** CT scan at the level of the hips shows fractures of both the anterior (*arrow*) and posterior (*arrowhead*) columns of the acetabulum.

pelvic fractures may have serious vascular injury, exsanguinate, and die. Because reduction and stabilization of pelvic fractures usually control bleeding, early discovery and evaluation of these injuries have significant practical importance for the orthopedist. Urologic injuries are commonly associated with severe pelvic fractures. Fractures that involve the vagina or rectum are open fractures and carry a grave risk of sepsis. Three distinct patterns of injury can be recognized (Fig. 3.29).

The most common mechanism of unstable pelvic ring injury is lateral compression. Lateral compression may occur when a pedestrian or a vehicle occupant is struck from the side. The pelvis is crushed as the hemipelvis on the side of impact is rotated inward by the force, sustaining a shear fracture of the pubis and a compression fracture of the ipsilateral sacral ala; ligamentous injury is minimal (Fig. 3.30). With a force of greater magnitude, continued inward rotation causes either disruption of the posterior SI ligaments or fracture of the ilium. The opposite hemipelvis may be rotated outward, opening the SI joint anteriorly. Central hip dislocation may be associated with lateral pelvic compression injuries (Fig. 3.31). The severity of the injury depends on the precise direction and magnitude of the forces.

When force is applied anteriorly to the pelvis, the pelvis is flattened open. The anterior arch is first pulled apart and sustains a

**FIGURE 3.32.** AP compression fracture. **A:** The symphysis pubis is diastatic (*arrow*). **B:** The left SI joint has opened anteriorly (*arrow*).

**FIGURE 3.33.** Straddle fractures of the pelvis, involving the right and left superior and inferior pubic rami (*arrows*).

**FIGURE 3.35.** Posterior wall acetabular fractures (*arrow*).

tension injury, usually a vertically oriented tension fracture of the pubic ramus or, less often, soft-tissue disruption of the symphysis. If the force is of sufficient magnitude, one hemipelvis rotates outward, opening the pelvis like a book (Fig. 3.32). The sacrotuberous and sacrospinous ligaments are disrupted in turn and followed by the anterior, interosseous, and posterior SI ligaments. An even

more severe injury is total SI joint disruption that leaves a floating, unsupported hemipelvis. AP compression fractures are associated with massive vascular damage and high mortality rates. A posterior column acetabular fracture may be an associated injury.

A variant of the anterior compression fracture is the *straddle fracture*, which refers not to the mechanism of injury but to the morphology of the fractures. In this situation, there are bilateral vertical fractures of the superior and inferior pubic rami, with an intact pubis (Fig. 3.33).

Vertical shear forces typically occur in falls from a height onto an extended leg. The usual pattern of injury is a vertical fracture of the anterior ring and fracture dislocation of the ipsilateral SI joint with vertical displacement (Malgaigne fracture) (Fig. 3.34). The vertical fractures of the anterior ring may be ipsilateral or contralateral to the SI joint lesion. Because there is total disruption of the posterior ligaments combined with anterior fractures, this relatively uncommon injury is grossly unstable. Occasionally, both SI joints are dislocated as the sacrum drops through the femoral-sacral arch.

Complex patterns of pelvic ring fractures occur with the application of forces from two or more directions, either together or sequentially. The most common combination is lateral compression and AP compression. The injuries have features of both types of injury. One helpful clue in the analysis of pelvic ring fractures is the direction of displacement of the acetabulum. In lateral compression injuries, the acetabulum moves medially; in AP compression, it moves laterally; and in vertical shear, it moves superiorly. The configuration of pubic rami fractures is another helpful clue. Pubic rami fractures oriented in the horizontal or coronal planes are sustained under lateral compression; fractures oriented in the vertical plane are sustained under AP compression or vertical shear.

**FIGURE 3.34.** Vertical shear fractures sustained in fall. Vertical fractures extend from the left pubic rami through the iliac wing (*arrows*).

**A**    **B**

**FIGURE 3.36.** Complex right acetabular fracture involving both columns (*arrows*). **A, B:** Judet views reconstructed from multidetector CT scan.

## ■ ACETABULUM
### Acetabular Fractures

The acetabulum is nestled at the confluence of the ilium, pubis, and ischium under an arch formed by two columns: the iliopubic (anterior) and ilioischial (posterior). The posterior column, the

**FIGURE 3.37.** Partially reduced posterior fracture dislocation of the right hip. Fractures of the rim and wall of the posterior column of the acetabulum are present. Because of the intra-articular fragment, the dislocation is not fully reducible. A fat-fluid level and gas bubble (*arrow*) are present.

thicker of the two, includes the major portion of the acetabular roof. The *acetabular roof*, or dome, is the articular and weight-bearing surface of the hip socket and includes portions of both columns. The quadrilateral plate forms the medial wall of the acetabulum and does not bear weight. The anterior column forms the iliopectineal line on AP radiographs; the posterior column forms the ilioischial line. Each column has a wall and a rim. Acetabular fractures result from indirect forces transmitted through the femoral head, most often in high-energy motor vehicle collisions or falls. Approximately 20% of pelvic ring fractures in adults involve the acetabulum. The morphology of the fracture depends on the position of the femur at the moment of impact, the magnitude and direction of the force, and the strength of the bone. Acetabular fractures can be simple or complex. Complex fractures can be described as combinations of fractures of the anterior and posterior columns, the anterior and posterior rims, and the acetabular roof. A transverse fracture separates the innominate bone into a superior iliac fragment and an inferior ilioischial fragment, and a T-shaped fracture combines a transverse fracture with a vertical separation of the anterior and posterior columns. The most common fracture of the acetabulum is a simple fracture of the posterior wall or rim (Fig. 3.35), sometimes associated with posterior hip dislocation (discussed in the next section). The other common fractures are simple transverse fractures and complex fractures that involve the posterior column. With complex fractures, the orthopedist is often most concerned about whether both anterior and posterior columns are involved or separated from each other, the severity of acetabular dome involvement, and the concomitant presence of pelvic ring injuries, especially ipsilateral iliac wing fractures or SI joint disruption. CT is often necessary for full delineation of the sites of fracture and configuration of the fragments. Acetabular fractures can also be demonstrated by three-dimensional reconstructions or radiographs of the pelvis in 45-degree oblique projections (Judet views) that show the anterior and posterior columns (Fig. 3.36). CT is often helpful for identifying intra-articular fragments following reduction of a fracture dislocation of the acetabulum (Fig. 3.37).

A                                                                    B

**FIGURE 3.38.** Posterior fracture dislocation of the right hip. **A:** Radiograph shows the femoral head lateral and superior to the acetabulum. The femoral shaft is adducted. **B:** CT shows the femoral head posterior to the empty acetabulum.

A                                                                    B

**FIGURE 3.39.** Anterior dislocation of the left hip (different patients). **A:** Radiograph shows the femoral head is inferior to the acetabulum. The femoral shaft is abducted. **B:** CT shows the femoral head anterior to the obturator ring.

**FIGURE 3.40.** Posterior fracture dislocation of the femoral head with a fragment remaining in the acetabulum. A fat-fluid level (*arrowheads*) and gas bubble (*arrow*) are present in the joint.

## Hip Dislocation

Hip dislocations result from severe trauma such as motor vehicle collisions. Posterior dislocations with or without acetabular fractures (Fig. 3.38) account for 85% to 90% of cases. The mechanism of posterior dislocation is a blow along the axis of the femoral shaft with the hip flexed (as in hitting the dashboard with the knee in a motor vehicle collision). The posterior wall or column of the acetabulum is often fractured, and the femoral shaft or knee may also be injured. Sciatic nerve injury, sometimes transient, is present in approximately 10% of cases. Anterior dislocations may occur in motor vehicle collisions or falls from heights when the hip is abducted (Fig. 3.39). CT can identify intra-articular fragments and confirm relocation of the hip after reduction. The presence of a gas bubble within the hip capsule is indicative of previous dislocation. Complications of hip dislocation include avascular necrosis of the femoral head, transient or permanent sciatic nerve palsy, myositis ossificans, and posttraumatic degenerative joint disease. A fragment of the femoral head may shear off as the hip is dislocated (Fig. 3.40).

## Acetabular Labrum

Patients with acetabular labral abnormalities may present with intractable, mechanical hip pain or snapping hip syndrome. The *acetabular labrum* is a fibrocartilaginous structure that is apposed to the bony acetabular rim. Similar to the glenoid labrum, it serves to deepen the hip socket. The labrum covers the anterior, superior,

A

B

**FIGURE 3.41.** Tear of the anterior acetabular labrum. **A:** Coronal T2-weighted MRI with fat suppression shows a small cyst (*arrow*) at the anterior-inferior margin of the labrum. **B:** Axial T2-weighted MRI with fat suppression shows the tear (*arrow*) filled with fluid that tracks into the cyst.

and posterior portions of the acetabular rim; the deficient inferior portion is connected by a transverse ligament and is the site of insertion of the ligamentum teres. The labrum has a triangular cross section and normally has uniformly dark signal on T1-weighted, PD, and T2-weighted MRI, similar to the glenoid labrum or the menisci of the knee. Abnormalities of the labrum can be identified noninvasively with MRI or MR arthrography. As with the glenoid labrum, there is considerable variability in the appearance of the acetabular labrum, but tears can be identified by discontinuities in the fibrocartilage that are filled with fluid or contrast, in the case of MR arthrography. Disruptions of the peripheral attachment of the labrum to the bony acetabulum may also occur. The presence of a paralabral cyst is highly associated with labral tear (Fig. 3.41).

## SOURCES AND READINGS

Browner B, Jupiter J, Levine A, Trafton P, Krettek C. *Skeletal Trauma: Fractures, Dislocations, Ligamentous Injuries.* 4th Ed. Philadelphia, PA: Saunders; 2008.

Bucholz RW, Heckman JD, Court-Brown C, Tornetta P. *Rockwood and Green's Fractures in Adults.* 7th Ed. Philadelphia, PA: Lippincott Williams & Wilkins; 2009.

Chew FS, Maldjian C. *Broken Bones: The X-ray Atlas of Fractures.* Seattle, WA: BareBonesBooks.com; 2009

Daffner RH, Brown RR, Goldberg AL. A new classification for cervical vertebral injuries: Influence of CT. *Skeletal Radiol.* 2000;29:125–132.

Daffner RH, Deeb ZL, Rothfus WE. "Fingerprints" of vertebral trauma—a unifying concept based on mechanisms. *Skeletal Radiol.* 1985;15:518–525.

Daffner RH, Hackney DB. ACR appropriateness criteria on suspected spine trauma. *J Am Coll Radiol.* 2007;4:762–775

Delignanis AV, Baxter AB, Hanson JA, et al. Radiologic spectrum of craniocervical distraction injuries. *Radiographics.* 2000;20:S237–S250

Demetriades D, Charalambides K, Chahwan S, et al. Nonskeletal cervical spine injuries: Epidemiology and diagnostic pitfalls. *J Trauma.* 2000;48:724–727.

eMedicine. http://emedicine.medscape.com.

Griffin LY. *Essentials of Musculoskeletal Care.* 3rd Ed. Rosemont, IL: American Academy of Orthopedics; 2005.

Holmes JF, Miller PQ, Panacek EA. Epidemiology of thoracolumbar spine injury in blunt trauma. *Acad Emerg Med.* 2001;8:866–872.

Lowery DW, Wald MM, Browne BJ, et al. Epidemiology of cervical spine injury victims. *Ann Emerg Med.* 2001;38:12–16.

Olson SA, Burgess A. Classification and initial management of patients with unstable pelvic ring injuries. *Instr Course Lect.* 2005;54:383–393.

Rao SK, Wasyliw C, Nunez DB Jr. Spectrum of imaging findings in hyperextension injuries of the neck. *Radiographics.* 2005;25:1239–1254

Resnick D. *Diagnosis of Bone and Joint Disorders.* 4th Ed. Philadelphia, PA: WB Saunders; 2002.

Riggins RS, Kraus JF. The risk of neurologic damage with fractures of the vertebrae. *J Trauma.* 1977;17:126–133.

Rogers LF. *Radiology of Skeletal Trauma.* 3rd Ed. New York, NY: Churchill-Livingstone; 2002.

Ryan MD, Henderson JJ. The epidemiology of fractures and fracture-dislocations of the cervical spine. *Injury.* 1992;23:38–40.

Tile M, Helfet DL, Kellam J. *Fractures of the Pelvis and Acetabulum.* 3rd Ed. Philadelphia, PA: Lippincott Williams & Wilkins; 2003.

Wasnich RD. Vertebral fracture epidemiology. *Bone.* 1996;18:79S–183S.

Wheeless CR III, ed. *Wheeless' Textbook of Orthopaedics.* http://www.wheelessonline.com.

White AA, Panjabi MM. *Clinical Biomechanics of the Spine.* 2nd Ed. Philadelphia, PA: Lippincott Williams & Wilkins; 1990.

# Trauma in Adults: Lower Extremity

his chapter describes the radiology of many common injuries to the lower extremities in adults.

## ■ PROXIMAL FEMUR

Fractures of the proximal femur are common only in the elderly because of osteoporosis (see Chapter 15); more than 95% of these fractures occur in patients older than 50 years, and the incidence is increasing as the population ages. The eventual mortality rate associated with hip fractures approaches 20%, and many survivors lose their independence of movement. Ninety-nine percent of fractures of the proximal femur are caused by simple falls. Even osteoporotic femurs are resistant to the compressive and tensile forces that occur during normal weight bearing, but there is great vulnerability to torsional or shearing stress. The roles of preexisting insufficiency microfractures in osteoporotic bone and decreased muscle tone as they relate to proximal femur fractures are unclear. Patients present with a painful, shortened, externally rotated limb that is unable to bear weight. Femoral fractures in persons younger than 40 years result from high-energy trauma and usually have associated injuries. Fractures of the proximal femur can be classified as intracapsular in 37% of cases, intertrochanteric in 49%, and subtrochanteric in 14%. Women sustain three to six times as many intracapsular fractures as men, but the incidence of intertrochanteric fractures is equal between the sexes. The initial evaluation in a suspected fracture should begin with radiographs. If a fracture is not identified and there is high clinical suspicion of a fracture, MRI should be obtained. If MRI is not available, CT or radionuclide bone scan should be used, although they are slightly less accurate than MRI. In the elderly population, fractures may not show radionuclide uptake until several days after the injury. A patient who was ambulatory before the fall but is unable to bear weight afterward should be presumed to have a fracture until proved otherwise.

### Intracapsular Fractures

The capsule of the hip joint encloses the head and most of the neck of the femur, extending from the acetabulum to the intertrochanteric line anteriorly and to the midneck posteriorly. Most femoral neck fractures are intracapsular and therefore heal less rapidly (synovial fluid lyses clot) than intertrochanteric and subtrochanteric fractures. In addition, the vascular supply to the head is largely disrupted. Subcapital femoral neck fractures extend transversely across the neck, just below the femoral head. Intracapsular fractures can be classified as either nondisplaced (Fig. 4.1) or displaced (Fig. 4.2). Fractures through the base of the neck are similar to two-part intertrochanteric fractures in mechanism and treatment (discussed in the next section). The greater the displacement, the greater the likelihood of subsequent femoral head osteonecrosis. With displaced fractures, the incidence of osteonecrosis and nonunion is approximately 25%. Patients with impacted fractures are usually ambulatory with an antalgic limp and pain that is referred to the groin or the medial knee. Nondisplaced fractures have no inherent stability and may displace with continued ambulation. Femoral neck fractures heal by endosteal callus formation. Nondisplaced fractures are usually fixed with multiple pins placed in parallel; displaced fractures may be reduced and fixed with a variety of methods, including multiple pins, a telescoping hip screw, or some combination thereof. When the risk of femoral head osteonecrosis is high or the quality of trabecular bone is too poor for internal fixation, femoral endoprosthesis or total hip replacement may be used as primary treatment.

### Intertrochanteric Fractures

The major fracture line of intertrochanteric fractures extends diagonally from superolateral (greater trochanter) to inferomedial (lesser trochanter). Most intertrochanteric fractures are comminuted, with the greater and lesser trochanters sometimes present as separate fragments (Fig. 4.3). In describing these fractures, the major fragments and the fracture lines should be enumerated in relation to the trochanters, the neck, and the shaft. The degree of displacement and comminution and the presence or absence of subtrochanteric extension along the femoral shaft affect the orthopedic treatment plan and prognosis. Open reduction and internal fixation with a dynamic hip screw are usual. Unlike intracapsular femoral neck fractures, these injuries tend to heal promptly and

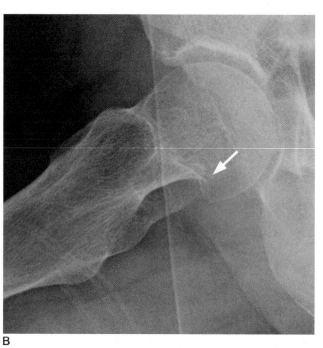

A

B

**FIGURE 4.1.** Impacted subcapital femoral neck fracture in an elderly woman. **A:** AP radiograph shows subtle contour abnormality of the lateral cortex at the head-neck junction (*arrow*) with linear density traversing the neck (*arrowhead*). **B:** Frog lateral radiograph shows buckled posterior cortex (*arrow*).

without complication. The incidence of avascular necrosis of the femoral head is approximately 1%. Incomplete intertrochanteric fractures may occur in elderly adults as a result of falls. Radiographs in this circumstance may be normal, but MRI will demonstrate the fracture (Fig. 4.4). Isolated fractures of the greater trochanter occur in elderly adults as a result of direct trauma sustained in falls. Isolated fractures of the lesser trochanter in adults are

pathologic and usually indicate an underlying osseous metastasis (see Chapter 10).

## Subtrochanteric Fractures

Subtrochanteric fractures in the elderly may represent extensions of intertrochanteric fractures into the shaft. In other age groups,

A

B

**FIGURE 4.2.** Displaced subcapital femoral neck fracture (*arrows*). **A:** AP radiograph. **B:** True lateral radiograph.

**FIGURE 4.3.** Four-part intertrochanteric fracture with greater and lesser trochanters as separate fragments.

**FIGURE 4.5.** Osteoporotic supracondylar femur fracture. Lateral radiograph shows fat-fluid level (*arrow*).

subtrochanteric fractures are sustained in high-energy trauma such as motor vehicle collisions. The opposing pull of the gluteal and ili-opsoas muscles and the thigh adductor muscles distracts and angulates the major fracture fragments. The cantilevered configuration of the femoral shaft and neck creates large stresses on the medial femoral cortex that complicate orthopedic management. A possibility of a pathologic or insufficiency fracture must be considered in subtrochanteric fractures that occur in the absence of significant trauma.

# SHAFT AND DISTAL FEMUR

Fractures of the femoral shaft occur typically in young adults as a result of major blunt force trauma, such as motor vehicle crashes. Because the femur is the largest and strongest bone in the human body and is protected by the largest and strongest muscle groups, considerable force is necessary to fracture it. Blood loss of two or

**FIGURE 4.4.** Incomplete intertrochanteric fracture (*arrows*) on coronal T1-weighted MRI.

more units typically accompanies an acute femoral shaft fracture. When the femoral shaft fractures with minimal trauma in an adult, an underlying pathologic lesion should be sought. Femoral fractures can also occur when there is advanced bony demineralization (Fig. 4.5). Insufficiency fractures in the elderly with osteoporosis sometimes may only be identified with MRI.

# KNEE

Radiographs are frequently obtained in the initial evaluation of knee injuries. Radiographs may show fractures, joint effusion, and dislocation or subluxation. Small avulsion fractures, particularly of the fibular head, medial femoral condyle, lateral tibial margin, or tibial spines, may indicate major ligamentous disruptions. When the mechanism of injury or the clinical examination suggests a ligament, cartilage, or other soft-tissue injury, MRI is the imaging method of choice.

## Extensor Mechanism

The extensor mechanism of the knee is composed of the quadriceps muscles and tendons, the patella, and the infrapatellar tendon. The *patella* is a large sesamoid bone. The quadriceps and infrapatellar tendons are continuous with each other across the patella; the medial and lateral retinacula are tendinous extensions that pass beside the patella. Injuries to the extensor mechanism may result from forced flexion during strong quadriceps contraction. With complete disruption of the extensor mechanism, voluntary knee extension is lost; a partial disruption results in weakness of extension. In the adult, the extensor tendons are thinnest where they pass over the patella. Tear of the tendon coupled with a fracture of the patella from tensile loading results in a transverse patellar fracture with the fragments distracted by the quadriceps muscle (Fig. 4.6). The quadriceps and infrapatellar tendons are also subject to injury.

**FIGURE 4.6.** Avulsion fracture of the inferior pole of the patella (*arrow*).

**FIGURE 4.8.** Infrapatellar tendon sprain (grade 3). Proximal retraction of the patella by the quadriceps muscles. Note the high position of the patella (patella alta).

Quadriceps tears usually occur at the musculotendinous junction in patients who have degenerative changes in their tendons, resulting in a low-lying patella (patella baja). Quadriceps tendon injuries are best demonstrated by MRI (Fig. 4.7). Infrapatellar tendon tears are seen most often in young adult athletes. In complete tears, superior retraction of the patella by unopposed pull of the quadriceps results in a high-riding patella (patella alta) (Fig. 4.8). Partial tears of the infrapatellar tendon are seen as increased T2-weighted signal within the tendon on MRI (Fig. 4.9). Stellate fractures of the patella may be caused by direct trauma. The extensor mechanism remains intact, and the fragments are not distracted. Hemarthrosis in the knee capsule is invariably present (Fig. 4.10).

**FIGURE 4.7.** Quadriceps tendon tear. Sagittal proton density MRI shows discontinuity of the tendon (*arrow*) at the superior pole of the patella.

**FIGURE 4.9.** Infrapatellar tendon sprain (grade 2). Sagittal PD MRI shows partial tear of the infrapatellar tendon (*arrow*) at its insertion on the anterior tibial tubercle. The patella has not retracted proximally because the tear is incomplete.

**FIGURE 4.10.** Minimally displaced comminuted patellar fracture (*long arrow*). Lateral radiograph with horizontal X-ray beam demonstrates a fat-fluid level, (*short arrow*) indicative of intra-articular fracture.

**FIGURE 4.12.** Medial retinaculum tear postpatellar dislocation. Axial T2-weighted fast spin echo MRI of the knee shows tear of the medial retinaculum (*arrow*).

Patellar dislocations are typically lateral and may occur with flexion and internal rotation of the femur on a fixed tibia. Impaction injuries of the medial patella and lateral femoral condyle are characteristic of patellar dislocation (Fig 4.11), and associated tears of the medial patellar retinaculum (Fig. 4.12), MCL, and ACL may be found. Chondral or osteochondral fractures may involve either the patella or the femoral trochlea, sometimes with displaced fragments (Fig. 4.13; see also Fig. 1.34).

**FIGURE 4.11.** Lateral patellar dislocation. Axial inversion recovery MRI shows reduced lateral patellar dislocation with bone bruises of the medial patellar facet (*short arrow*) and lateral femoral condyle (*long arrow*). There is a sprain of the medial patellar retinaculum (*arrowhead*) and a large joint effusion.

**FIGURE 4.13.** Axial T2-weighted fat-suppressed MRI shows reduced lateral patellar dislocation with medial retinacular separation (*arrowhead*) and osteochondral injuries of the patella (*short arrow*) and lateral femoral trochlea (*long arrow*).

## Complex Knee Injuries

Similar to the spine, the knee may be thought of as an articulated column stabilized by surrounding soft-tissue structures. The joint capsule invests the entire knee and supports it on all sides. The medial side is also supported by the MCL and medial retinaculum; the lateral side by the LCL complex (iliotibial band, LCL itself, biceps femoris tendon) and lateral retinaculum; the anterior aspect by the structures of the quadriceps mechanism; and the posterior aspect by the gastrocnemius muscles. The posterolateral corner has the popliteus muscle and tendon and arcuate ligament; the posteromedial corner has the semimembranosus tendon and posterior oblique ligament. The ACL and PCL occupy the central portion of the knee, with the ACL lateral to the PCL. The medial and lateral menisci deepen the articular surface of the tibial plateaus.

When the extended knee is loaded by bending forces, the structures on the concave side of the bend are compressed, and the structures on the convex side are distracted. Compressive injuries include bone bruises and impaction fractures; distractive injuries include tears of ligaments, tendons, muscles, and capsule, or avulsions of their bony attachments. Under *valgus* loading, an MCL injury is combined with lateral compartment bone bruises or impaction fractures. If the loading is severe enough, the ACL and PCL also tear under tension (Fig. 4.14). Under *varus* loading, the LCL complex tears under

A

B

C

FIGURE 4.14. Valgus knee injury in a pedestrian struck by a car. **A:** Coronal T2-weighted fat-suppressed MRI shows torn MCL (*black arrow*) and lateral condyle bone bruise (*white arrow*). **B:** Sagittal proton density MRI shows torn ACL (*arrow*). **C:** Sagittal proton density MRI shows torn PCL (*arrow*).

**FIGURE 4.15.** Varus knee injury in pedestrian struck by car. **A:** Coronal inversion recovery MRI shows tears of the LCL complex, including an avulsion of the iliotibial tract (*black arrow*). There is a compression injury on the medial side with tibial bone bruise (*white arrow*) and medial meniscal tear. **B:** Sagittal PD fat-suppressed MRI shows ACL tear (*arrow*). **C:** Sagittal PD fat-suppressed MRI shows PCL tear (*arrow*).

tension, and the medial compartment sustains the compressive injury; with severe loading, the ACL and PCL also tear (Fig. 4.15). With *hyperextension*, the compressive injury involves the contiguous anterior aspects of the femur and tibia (see Fig. 1.11), and the tensile injury involves the posterior capsule and gastrocnemius muscles; if there is accompanying anterior or posterior translation of the tibia, the ACL or PCL may tear, respectively. With *hyperextension-valgus* loading, the compressive injury is anterolateral, and the distractive injury involves the posteromedial corner, the MCL, and the PCL. With *hyperextension-varus* loading, the compressive injury is anteromedial, and the distractive injury involves the posterolateral corner and ACL (Fig. 4.16).

**FIGURE 4.16.** Hyperextension-varus injury. Axial inversion recovery MRI shows anteromedial bone bruise (*short arrow*) in the distal femur and posterolateral corner injury (*long arrow*).

When the flexed and externally rotated knee sustains valgus stress, the ACL and the MCL are loaded under tension. If the ACL tears, the tibia is able to translate anteriorly beneath the femur and impact the lateral condyle, resulting in the pivot-shift bone bruise pattern that is highly correlated with ACL tears (Fig. 4.17). The medial and lateral menisci, which act as buttresses against translation of the knee, may also be torn. With weight-bearing or axial compression, meniscal tears are more likely. The combination of tears of the ACL, the MCL, and a meniscus (usually lateral) is called the unhappy triad; if both menisci are torn, it is an unhappy tetrad. Much less commonly, varus stress on the internally rotated and flexed knee may result in tears of the ACL, lateral, and posterolateral structures; the Segond fracture may be part of this injury complex (Fig. 4.18).

Isolated PCL tears may occur with dashboard injuries or falls on the flexed knee, in which the tibia is translated posteriorly. A bone bruise may occur at the anterior aspect of the tibia (Fig. 4.19).

The specific pattern of bone bruises seen on MRI may suggest the mechanism of injury and associated injuries: Kissing contusions (contiguous bruises or impaction fractures) indicate a bending injury to the extended knee; the opposite side will typically sustain distraction injuries. The pivot shift pattern (bruises or impaction fractures of the lateral femoral condyle and posterolateral tibia) occurs with ACL tears; MCL and lateral meniscal tears are commonly associated. Isolated bruise of the anterior aspect of the tibia may indicate a dashboard injury with PCL tear. Bruises of the medial facet of the patella and lateral femoral condyle may indicate previous lateral patellar dislocation.

## Meniscal Tears

The menisci are C-shaped fibrocartilaginous structures that rest on the medial and lateral plateaus, deepening the articular surfaces into shallow bowls that receive the femoral condyles. Collagen fibers provide structural support: circumferential fibers provide hoop strength, and radial fibers provide attachment to the surrounding capsule. Acute traumatic meniscal tears may occur when the meniscus is crushed or sheared between the femoral condyle and tibial plateau, producing vertical or radial tears. Vertical longitudinal tears run between the circumferential fibers and across the radial fibers. Radial tears run across the circumferential fibers and between the radial fibers. Parrot-beak tears are longitudinal with a radial component that exits the inner edge of the meniscus. Bucket-handle tears are longitudinal tears in which the inner fragment separates from the peripheral fragment and displaces, usually into the intercondylar notch. Tears not easy to categorize are considered complex. In older individuals, meniscal tears are horizontal or oblique in morphology and in menisci weakened by chondrocyte death and myxoid degeneration.

On MRI, the normal menisci are visualized as sharp, well-defined low-signal structures, with a triangular cross section. Meniscal tears are evident as higher signal regions that extend to an articular margin (Figs. 4.20 and 4.21). Gross distortions of meniscal shape or intrameniscal fluid collections indicate meniscal tears with displaced fragments (Fig. 4.22). Parameniscal cysts are highly associated with meniscal tears (Fig. 4.23).

## ■ TIBIA

### Tibial Plateau

Most tibial plateau fractures are sustained in motor vehicle collisions, but fractures of the tibial plateau may also occur in older individuals during twisting falls (Figs. 4.24 and 4.25; see also Fig. 1.13). Isolated lateral tibial plateau fractures are the most common (55% to 70%); the rest involve the medial plateau alone or both plateaus. These injuries consist of compression fractures of the subchondral cancellous bone with depressions of the articular surface, vertical splits (shear fractures) of the joint margin, or a combination of depression and vertical split. A knee effusion is invariably present. Conventional tomography can establish the depth of the depression and the number and location of depressed fragments; CT with coronal and sagittal reconstructions serves the same purpose. Associated injuries include lateral meniscal tears (50% of cases), lateral femoral condylar fractures, cruciate ligament tears, and fibular head fractures. These injuries may be treated surgically, depending on the amount of depression and displacement. Posttraumatic degenerative joint disease occurs in 20% of cases.

### Tibial Shaft

Transverse and segmental tibial shaft fractures commonly occur in high-energy motor vehicle collisions, particularly in pedestrians and motorcyclists. Because the soft tissues covering the tibia anteriorly are thin, many of these fractures are open. The complications of infection and osteonecrosis of large cortical fragments are common. Even if uncomplicated, these high-energy fractures tend to heal slowly and may take as long as 2 years to unite completely. The combination of transverse fractures of the femoral shaft and tibial shaft isolates the knee joint and is called a *floating knee*. Twisting injuries may result in spiral fractures of the tibia (see Fig. 1.10); bending injuries may result in transverse fractures with butterfly fragment (see Fig. 1.7).

A

B

C

**FIGURE 4.17.** Flexion-external rotation-valgus injury (unhappy triad). **A:** Sagittal T2 fat-suppressed MRI through the lateral compartment shows impaction fracture of the anterior aspect of the lateral femoral condyle (*long arrow*) and bone bruise in posterolateral tibia (*short arrow*) (pivot shift pattern). **B:** Sagittal T2 fat-suppressed MRI through the intercondular notch shows ACL tear (*arrow*). **C:** Coronal inversion recovery MRI shows MCL sprain, grade 2 (*arrow*). A lateral meniscal tear was also present (not shown).

# ◼ ANKLE
## Ankle Mortise

The leg articulates with the foot at the talus. The *talus* is a hard, slippery bone with much of its surface covered by articular cartilage. Because the talus has no direct muscular control, its movements follow the push and pull of adjacent bones and ligaments. The talus is maintained in the ankle mortise (tibiofibular socket) by geometric fit and with ligaments. The articular surfaces of the ankle mortise are the tibial plafond superiorly and the medial (tibial) and lateral (fibular) malleoli on either side. The mortise is wider anteriorly than posteriorly. The posterior lip of the tibia is designated as the *posterior malleolus*. At the distal tibiofibular syndesmosis, anterior

and posterior tibiofibular ligaments bind the fibula to the tibia. The tibial and fibular shafts are also joined along their length by an interosseous membrane. The lateral malleolus is attached to the foot by anterior and posterior talofibular ligaments and a calcaneofibular ligament. The medial malleolus has a superficial deltoid ligament that inserts on the talus, calcaneus, and navicular and a deep deltoid ligament that inserts on the talus. The mortise, ligaments, and calcaneus form a ring in the coronal plane with the talus in the center (Fig. 4.26). Most ankle injuries are sustained by indirect loading when the leg angulates or rotates around a malpositioned and stationary foot. Forced movement of the talus breaks open the mortise. Most ankle injuries are reduced or partially reduced by the time they are radiographed, so the direction and magnitude

**FIGURE 4.18.** Segond fracture of the lateral tibial margin (*arrow*).

of loading must be inferred from the pattern of injury. The most useful classification of ankle injuries is the AO-Weber classification (Table 4.1). Ankle injuries may also be described by the location and morphology of the fractures. A practical mechanistic classification of indirect ankle injuries has four types: adduction, external rotation, abduction, and axial compression.

Adduction or inversion of the foot is inward rotation along the foot's long axis. With forcible inversion, the lateral malleolus and its ligaments are loaded. The first injury is a sprain of the anterior talofibular ligament, which may be followed by a sprain of the calcaneofibular ligament. The appearance on radiographs is lateral soft-tissue swelling; the talus may be tilted but will not be displaced. This lateral ankle sprain is the most common ankle injury in adults (Fig. 4.27). Less commonly, a tension fracture of the lateral malleolus occurs rather than a ligamentous sprain. With continued loading, the talus impinges against the medial malleolus and moves medially, causing an oblique or vertical shear fracture of the medial malleolus as the talus subluxates.

External rotation of the foot loads the anterior portion of the lateral malleolus and the posterior portion of the medial malleolus as the talus moves within the mortise like a lever. The first injury is disruption of the anterior tibiofibular ligament of the syndesmosis. Loading then transfers to the lateral malleolus, resulting in a short oblique fracture that runs anteroinferior to posterosuperior (Fig. 4.28). With continued loading, the talus displaces the lateral malleolar fragment, causing the posterior malleolus to be avulsed by the strong posterior tibiofibular ligaments; the lateral and posterior malleoli remain attached to the talus and each other. Finally, with loss of the lateral and posterior supports of the ankle, the medial side is loaded as the talus dislocates laterally and posteriorly, and either the medial malleolus fractures or the deltoid ligament tears (Fig. 4.29). In an isolated lateral malleolar external rotation injury, the talus is subluxated; in a trimalleolar injury, it may be completely dislocated. If the posterior malleolar fragment includes 25% or more of the articular surface, an associated component of axial compression can be inferred. Sometimes, CT is necessary to establish the proportion

**A**    **B**

**FIGURE 4.19.** Dashboard injury during a motor vehicle crash on sagittal PD fat-suppressed MRI. **A:** Image at the intercondylar notch shows tears of the PCL (*short arrow*) and the posterior knee capsule (*long arrow*). There is extensive posterior edema. **B:** Image at the lateral compartment shows an anterior tibial bone bruise from impact with the dashboard (*short arrow*). There is a popliteus muscle strain (*arrowhead*) and a tear of the posterior knee capsule (*long arrows*), indicative of posterolateral corner injury.

**FIGURE 4.20.** Sagittal PD-weighted MRI shows horizontal tear (*arrow*) of the posterior horn of the medial meniscus extending into the inferior articulating surface.

**FIGURE 4.21.** Sagittal PD-weighted MRI shows vertical tear (*arrow*) in the anterior horn of the lateral meniscus.

A

B

C

**FIGURE 4.22.** Bucket-handle tear of the medial meniscus. **A:** Axial T2 fat-suppressed MRI through the knee joint shows a tear of the entire medial meniscus with displacement of the central portion of the meniscus (*arrows*) into the intercondylar region. **B:** Coronal proton density MRI shows the displaced meniscal fragment (*short arrow*) inferior to the PCL (*long arrow*). **C:** Sagittal proton density MRI shows the displaced meniscal fragment (*short arrows*) parallel to the PCL (*long arrow*), the "double PCL" sign. There has been previous ACL reconstruction.

**FIGURE 4.23.** Lateral meniscus tear with meniscal cyst. Sagittal T2-weighted MRI with fat suppression shows horizontal tear in the anterior horn of the lateral meniscus associated with a meniscal cyst (*arrow*).

**FIGURE 4.24.** Severely comminuted lateral tibial plateau fracture with extension to the medial plateau and shaft.

**A**   **B**

**FIGURE 4.25.** Lateral tibial plateau fracture (*arrows*). **A:** Radiograph. **B:** Axial CT.

**FIGURE 4.26.** Ligaments of the ankle. Lateral aspect shows the lateral collateral ligaments. Medial aspect shows the deltoid ligament. Coronal section shows how the structures of the ankle joint form a ring with the talus in the center. Axial section shows how the distal fibula is attached to the tibia by the syndesmosis.

of articular surface involvement. The most common ankle fracture in adults is an isolated lateral malleolar fracture from external rotation.

Abduction or eversion of the foot relative to the ankle causes a tension fracture of the medial malleolus more often than a tear of the deltoid ligament. With continued loading in abduction, the talus impinges against the lateral malleolus and displaces it laterally, disrupting the syndesmotic ligaments or avulsing their bony attachments. As the talus dislocates laterally, taking the fibula with it, the interosseous ligament tears until the fibular shaft fractures. The fibular fracture may occur anywhere along the shaft and typically runs inferomedial to superolateral. A proximal fracture of the fibula may be missed on routine films of the ankle.

Three fracture eponyms may be encountered in clinical consultation. The *Maisonneuve fracture* is an abduction injury in which the fibular fracture is quite proximal (Fig. 4.30). The *Tillaux fracture* is an abduction injury with an avulsion fracture of the anterior tibial tubercle by the anterior tibiofibular ligament (Fig. 4.31). The *Wagstaffe-LeFort fracture* is an avulsion fracture of the anterior

medial portion of the distal fibula by the anterior tibiofibular ligament.

Ankle injuries usually require anatomic restoration of the mortise; otherwise, excessive motion and instability lead to early degenerative joint disease. Simple ankle sprains are treated conservatively with casting and bracing. Most heal over a period of several weeks, but a few have chronic pain and recurrent instability. MRI in this circumstance may reveal a chronic anterior talofibular ligament tear (Fig. 4.32) or other pathology. If satisfactory restoration of the mortise is not achieved by closed means, open reduction and internal fixation are performed. Displacements of 1 to 2 mm are acceptable for the medial joint space; displacements of 3 to 4 mm are acceptable for the posterior malleolus. Medial malleolar fractures are usually fixed by lag screws. Lateral malleolar fractures may be fixed by various methods such as cortical plates, screws, pins, or combinations of these appliances.

Axial compression (vertical loading) fractures (also called *pilon fractures*) are sustained in falls from a height or in automobile collisions in which the talus is driven into the tibial plafond. These injuries are characterized by severe distal tibial shaft comminution, intra-articular fractures through the tibial plafond, and talar fractures (Fig. 4.33). Malleolar fractures and ligamentous disruption may coexist, indicating some combination of axial compression with adduction, external rotation, or abduction.

## Ankle Tendon Injuries

Achilles tendon tears and tendonitis generally occur during athletic activity in middle-aged men. Conditions that predispose the tendon to injury include rheumatoid arthritis, systemic lupus erythematosus, diabetes mellitus, and gout. The normal Achilles tendon is a tapered structure with uniformly dark signal on all sequences. In cross section, it has a shape like the letter C that is concave toward the tibia. Complete tendon tears are evident on MRI as discontinuities with high signal on T1- and T2-weighted images (see Fig. 1.17). Partial tears are evident as thickening of the tendon with longitudinal bands of increased signal on T1- and T2-weighted MRI (Fig. 4.34). Because the Achilles tendon does not have a tendon sheath, frank fluid around the tendon is not seen. However, soft-tissue edema in the soft tissues surrounding the tendon may be seen after an acute tear.

Tibialis posterior tendon injuries are frequently chronic, classically presenting in mature women as a unilateral flatfoot deformity. The normal tibialis posterior tendon traverses the ankle posterior and inferior to the medial malleolus and then turns anteriorly along the sole of the foot to insert at the tuberosity

| TABLE 4.1 | AO-Weber Classification of Ankle Fractures | |
| --- | --- | --- |
| Type | Defining Characteristic | Associated Injuries |
| A | Lateral malleolar fracture below the level of the ankle joint space | The syndesmosis and the deltoid ligament remain intact, but there may be an associated oblique fracture of the medial malleolus. |
| B | Oblique fracture of the lateral malleolus through the syndesmosis. | Deltoid ligament tear or transverse fracture of the medial malleolus. May also have an associated posterior malleolar fracture. |
| C | Fracture of the fibula above the syndesmosis | Rupture of the syndesmosis. Deltoid ligament tear or transverse medial malleolar fracture. May also have an associated posterior malleolar fracture. |

**FIGURE 4.27.** Lateral ankle sprain as demonstrated by soft-tissue swelling (*arrow*) without fracture on the AP radiograph.

**FIGURE 4.28.** Lateral radiograph shows external rotation injury of the ankle with oblique fibular fracture (*arrow*).

of the navicular bone, with multiple fibrous slips at the plantar aspects of the navicular and medial cuneiform bones. The tibialis posterior provides dynamic support for the medial longitudinal arch of the foot, and ruptures of it are therefore associated with acquired, unilateral flatfoot deformity, often without a history of trauma. On lateral weight-bearing radiographs, loss of the longitudinal arch may be evident. On MRI, tears of the tibialis posterior are seen most frequently at or within a few centimeters of its navicular insertion, distal to the medial malleolus. The tendon

will be thickened and will have increased signal on T1- and T2-weighted MRI, with loss of continuity, surrounding edema, and fluid in the tendon sheath (Fig. 4.35). Similar MRI findings without loss of continuity may indicate tendonitis of the tibialis posterior.

Tibialis anterior tendon injuries are most commonly seen in patients whose athletic activities involve forced plantar flexion and ankle eversion; the superficial location of the tendon also leaves it vulnerable to lacerations (Fig. 4.36).

**A**    **B**

**FIGURE 4.29.** External rotation fracture dislocation of the ankle. **A, B:** Lateral and AP radiographs show displaced fractures of the medial malleolus (*long arrow*), lateral malleolus (*arrowheads*), and posterior malleolus (*short arrow*), with lateral and posterior subluxation of the talus.

A          B

**FIGURE 4.30. A:** Maisonneuve fracture (*arrow*) of the proximal fibula. **B:** Associated abduction of the lateral malleolus and tear of the syndesmosis (*arrow*).

Peroneal tendon injuries usually occur in acute injuries. An os peroneum, if present, may be fractured (Fig. 4.37) or may migrate proximally with the retracting tendon. Tears of the peroneus brevis typically occur at the level of the lateral malleolus as it makes its turn anteriorly from behind the malleolus. Longitudinal splits are more common than transverse tears (Fig. 4.38). Tears of the peroneus longus may accompany injuries of the peroneus brevis but are less common and generally do not occur in isolation.

## ■ FOOT
### Talus

Lateral osteochondral fractures of the talus may occur when forced inversion shears the lateral edge of the talar dome against the fibula (Fig. 4.39). The less common medial osteochondral fracture may follow impaction of the talus against the tibia. Clinical presentation may be nonspecific ankle pain. The terms *osteochondral defect* and

**FIGURE 4.31.** Tillaux fracture shown on axial CT (*arrow*).

**FIGURE 4.32.** Chronic anterior talofibular ligament tear (*arrow*) on axial T2-weighted fat-suppressed MRI.

**A**    **B**

**FIGURE 4.33. A:** Intra-articular axial compression fracture of the distal tibia (pilon fracture). **B:** Pilon fracture shown by CT at the level of distal tibia.

**FIGURE 4.34.** Achilles tendon tendinopathy. Axial T2-weighted MRI shows an abnormally round contour of the distal Achilles tendon with hyperintense T2 signal interspersed throughout its fibers (*arrow*).

**FIGURE 4.35.** Posterior tibial tendon tear. Axial proton density MRI shows tear within the tibialis posterior tendon with inflammation surrounding the tendon (*arrow*).

**A**    **B**

**FIGURE 4.36.** Tibialis anterior tendon tear and tendinopathy. **A:** Sagittal T1-weighted MRI of the ankle shows abnormal thickening and signal hypointensity within the partially torn tibialis anterior tendon (*arrow*). **B:** Axial T2-weighted fat saturated fast spin echo MRI of the ankle shows abnormal thickening of and signal hyperintensity within the tibialis anterior tendon, consistent with a hypertrophic partial tear (*arrow*).

*osteochondritis dissecans* are often applied to osteochondral fractures of the talar dome. Osteochondral defects may require CT or MRI for demonstration. Associated osteochondral injuries of the fibula or tibial plafond may occur. The severity of osteochondral defects ranges from a cartilage injury (stage 1), to an attached osteochondral fragment (stage 2), to a detached but nondisplaced fragment (stage 3), and, finally, to a displaced fragment (stage 4). Osteonecrosis of attached and detached fragments is common. If displaced, the fragment becomes a loose body within the joint capsule.

Subtalar dislocation, simultaneous dislocation of the talonavicular and talocalcaneal joints with the talus remaining within the

**FIGURE 4.38.** Longitudinal tear of the peroneus brevis tendon. Axial T1-weighted MRI of the ankle shows an abnormal split morphology of the peroneus brevis tendon with low signal in the surrounding tendon sheath (*arrow*).

**FIGURE 4.37.** Fractured os peroneum (*arrow*) associated with peroneus longus tear.

A                      B

**FIGURE 4.39.** Osteochondral lesions of the talar dome (different patients). **A:** Coronal proton density fat-suppressed MRI of the ankle shows a small osteochondral defect in the lateral talar dome. The central fragment is detached and partially displaced from the dome of the talus (*arrow*), and there is surrounding fluid. Subchondral bone marrow edema is also seen in the lateral aspect of the tibial plafond. **B:** Coronal T2 fat-suppressed MRI shows focal marrow edema (*arrow*) at the lateral talar dome and medial aspect of the lateral malleolus.

A                      B

**FIGURE 4.40.** Comminuted talar body fracture dislocation. The calcaneus is dislocated distally at the posterior articular facet of the subtalar joint (*arrows*). **A:** Lateral radiograph; **B:** Sagittal CT reformation.

ankle mortise, may occur with falls, motor vehicle crashes, or other severe trauma (Fig. 4.40). Most subtalar dislocations are medial, as might occur when there is an awkward landing on an inverted and plantar-flexed foot (basketball foot). Rarely, high-energy trauma such as motorcycle crashes may cause extrusion of the entire or major fragments of the talus, leaving the other bones intact and in place (Fig. 4.41).

Fractures of the body or neck occur through various poorly understood mechanisms. In more severe cases, the fracture displaces, and the subtalar joint subluxates or dislocates (Fig. 4.42). Because the vascular supply of the talus passes from distal to proximal, osteonecrosis of the proximal fragment may occur, suggested by the acute osteoporosis that accompanies fracture healing. Stress fractures of the talus are unusual, but their typical location is vertically through the neck.

A fracture of the lateral tubercle of the posterior process of the talus is called a *Shepherd fracture.*

## Calcaneus

Intra-articular calcaneal fractures are caused by axial loading, as in falls in which the heel sustains the initial impact or in head-on car crashes. Such calcaneal fractures are bilateral in 10% of cases and, because of the common mechanism of loading, may be associated with compression or burst fractures of the thoracolumbar spine and other fractures of the lower extremities. Although the loading that occurs during these injuries may be rapid and massive, resulting in gross comminution, there is a consistent pattern of injury.

**FIGURE 4.41.** Partial open talar extrusion (*arrow*) shown by coronal CT reformation.

**A**

**B**

**FIGURE 4.42.** Subtalar foot dislocation. **A:** Lateral radiograph shows abnormal alignment at the talonavicular (*short arrow*) and posterior facet (*long arrow*) joints. **B:** AP radiograph shows the talus remains within the ankle mortise, but the rest of the foot has dislocated medially as a unit. The distal articular surface (*arrow*) of the talus is bare.

**FIGURE 4.43.** Calcaneal fracture (joint depression). **A:** Lateral radiograph shows flattening of the calcaneus (*arrow*). **B:** Sagittal CT reformation shows impaction of the posterior facet (*arrow*) into the body of the calcaneus. **C:** Axial CT shows comminution of the posterior facet (*arrow*). **D:** Böhler's angle is normally 29 to 40 degrees.

The calcaneus, along with the cuboid and fifth metatarsal, forms a weight-bearing longitudinal arch on the lateral side of the foot that supports the talus and structures above. With excessive axial loading, the arch consistently breaks in the center at the tarsal sinus, where the lateral process of the talus descends like an axe. The sustentaculum tali breaks off as a separate fragment, and the arch collapses. With continued loading, the talus may depress the posterior calcaneal facet into the substance of the body of the calcaneus, which in turn may explode into a multitude of tiny fragments (joint depression type) (Fig. 4.43). Alternatively, the posterior facet and superior portion of the body may shear off horizontally as the talus is driven downward (tongue type) (Fig. 4.44). Intra-articular calcaneal fractures are usually obvious on plain films because of flattening of the normal bony longitudinal arch and the presence of many fragments. The soft tissues are often extensively injured in calcaneal fractures. Occasionally, if the fractures are impacted and not displaced, a decrease in Böhler's angle is a helpful radiographic sign. The long-term prognosis is poor: the sequelae of residual widening of the heel and posttraumatic subtalar degenerative joint disease are commonplace.

The most common of the extra-articular calcaneal fractures—those not involving the subtalar joint—is an avulsion fracture of the anterior process. This fracture occurs where the bifurcate ligament links the calcaneus to the cuboid and navicular. These injuries may occur with the inversion of the foot and are easily overlooked when the ankle is examined.

Stress fractures of the calcaneus typically occur through the tuberosity. The fracture plane is perpendicular to the stress-bearing trabeculae.

## Midfoot

The navicular is a common site for stress fractures; these are best demonstrated by MRI. Fractures of the body of the navicular occur

**FIGURE 4.45.** Intra-articular fracture (*arrow*) of the body of the navicular with central comminution and subluxation (*arrowhead*) of the navicular-first cuneiform joint.

with major trauma and may involve the various articular surfaces and joints (Fig. 4.45). Avulsion fractures may be associated with ligamentous injuries of the midfoot. Fracture dislocation of the midfoot (Chopart fracture dislocation) may occur through the talonavicular and calcaneo-cuboid articulations during incidents such as motorcycle crashes (Fig. 4.46).

## Forefoot

Dislocation of the forefoot (Lisfranc fracture dislocation) may occur after a variety of traumas, including falls, longitudinal compression with hyperflexion, and rotary loading. In most cases, multiple metatarsals are dislocated in the same direction (homolateral) laterally and dorsally (Fig. 4.47); occasionally, the second through fifth metatarsals are dislocated laterally, and the first metatarsal is dislocated medially (divergent). A transverse fracture through the base of the second metatarsal and avulsion fractures of the proximal metatarsals or distal tarsals are frequently associated.

Avulsion fractures at the base of the fifth metatarsal, proximal to the metatarsal tuberosity, are caused by tensile loading transmitted through the lateral cord of the plantar aponeurosis during sudden inversion of the foot. As a tension injury, the fracture line is oriented transversely to the direction of applied force (Fig. 4.48). These fractures are intra-articular and commonly occur with ankle trauma. The fracture fragment includes the insertion of the peroneus brevis tendon.

Fractures of the metatarsal shafts commonly occur with direct trauma. The distal shafts of the metatarsals are common locations for stress fractures, particularly those associated with running and marching. Stress fractures of the metatarsals may be radiographically occult at presentation and may require a radionuclide bone scan or MRI for demonstration. With healing, the fractures become

**FIGURE 4.44.** Comminuted intra-articular calcaneal fracture (tongue type).

**A**    **B**

**FIGURE 4.46.** Chopart fracture dislocation. **A:** AP radiograph shows medial dislocation of the talonavicular (*arrowhead*) and calcaneal-cuboid (*arrow*) joints. **B:** Sagittal CT reformation shows talonavicular dislocation (*short arrow*) with comminution and impaction fracture of the head of the talus. The cuboid articular surface (*long arrow*) does not articulate with the calcaneus on this slice.

apparent as calcified callus becomes visible. A fracture of the proximal shaft of the fifth metatarsal that is extra-articular and distal to the metatarsal tuberosity may be known by the eponym *Jones fracture* (Fig. 4.49). Jones fractures are typically stress fractures and require treatment different from that of simple avulsion fractures of the fifth metatarsal base.

Dislocations of the toes are relatively uncommon except at the MTP joint (Fig. 4.50). Stubbed toe injuries generally load

the affected digits axially, resulting in oblique fractures of the phalangeal shafts (Fig. 4.51). Alternatively, comminuted T- or Y-shaped fractures at the proximal ends of the phalanges may occur. Direct trauma to the toes from dropped objects or misadventures with wheeled or motorized conveyances are common and may result in transverse or comminuted fractures of the phalanges (Fig. 4.52).

**FIGURE 4.47.** Homolateral Lisfranc fracture dislocation (*arrow*).

**FIGURE 4.48.** Avulsion fracture of the fifth metatarsal base at the insertion of the peroneus brevis tendon (*arrow*).

**FIGURE 4.49.** Extra-articular fracture of the proximal fifth metatarsal (Jones fracture) (*arrow*).

**FIGURE 4.50.** Dorsal dislocation of the fifth MTP joint (*arrow*).

**FIGURE 4.51.** Stubbed toe injury of the fifth toe with oblique fracture (*arrow*) of the proximal phalanx.

**FIGURE 4.52.** Crush injuries of the first and second toes with transverse fractures of the distal phalanges (*arrows*).

## SOURCES AND READINGS

Armagan OE, Shereff MJ. Injuries to the toes and metatarsals. *Orthop Clin North Am.* 2001;32(1):1–10.

Berquist TH, ed. *Radiology of the Foot and Ankle.* 2nd Ed. Philadelphia, PA: Lippincott Williams & Wilkins; 2000.

Berquist TH. *MRI of the Musculoskeletal System.* 5th Ed. Philadelphia, PA: Lippincott Williams & Wilkins; 2005.

Browner B, Jupiter J, Levine A, Trafton P, Krettek C. *Skeletal Trauma: Fractures, Dislocations, Ligamentous Injuries.* 4th Ed. Philadelphia, PA: Saunders; 2008.

Bucholz RW, Heckman JD, Court-Brown C, Tornetta P. *Rockwood and Green's Fractures in Adults.* 7th Ed. Philadelphia, PA: Lippincott Williams & Wilkins; 2009.

Chew FS, Maldjian C. *Broken Bones: The X-ray Atlas of Fractures.* Seattle, WA: BareBonesBooks.com; 2009

Dunfee WR, Dalinka MK, Kneeland JB. Imaging of athletic injuries to the ankle and foot. *Radiol Clin North Am.* 2002;40(2):289–312

eMedicine. http://emedicine.medscape.com.

Fox MG. MR Imaging of the meniscus: Review, current trends, and clinical implications. *Radiol Clin North Am.* 2007;45:1033–1053.

Griffin LY. *Essentials of Musculoskeletal Care.* 3rd Ed. Rosemont, IL: American Academy of Orthopedics; 2005.

Hayes CW, Brigado MK, Jamadar DA, Propeck T. Mechanism-based pattern approach to classification of complex injuries of the knee depicted at MR Imaging. *Radiographics* 2000;20:S121–S134.

Helms CA, Major NM, Anderson MW, et al. *Musculoskeletal MRI.* 2nd Ed. Philadelphia, PA: Saunders; 2009.

Michelson JD, Myers A, Jinnah R, et al. Epidemiology of hip fractures among the elderly. Risk factors for fracture type. *Clin Orthop.* 1995;311:129–135.

Pedowitz R, Resnick D, Chung CB. *Magnetic Resonance Imaging in Orthopedic Sports Medicine.* Berlin: Springer; 2008.

Robinson CM, Court-Brown CM, McQueen MM, et al. Hip fractures in adults younger than 50 years of age. Epidemiology and results. *Clin Orthop.* 1995;312:238–246.

Rogers LF. *Radiology of Skeletal Trauma.* 3rd Ed. New York, NY: Churchill Livingstone; 2002.

Sanders TG, Medynski MA, Feller JF, Lawhorn KW. Bone contusion patterns of the knee at MR imaging: Footprint of the mechanism of injury. *Radiographics.* 2000;20:S135–S151.

Schmidt AH, Asnis SE, Haidukewych G, Koval KJ, Thorngren KG. Femoral neck fractures. *Instr Course Lect.* 2005;54:417–445.

Stoller DW. *Magnetic Resonance Imaging in Orthopaedics and Sports Medicine.* 3rd Ed. Philadelphia, PA: Lippincott Williams & Wilkins; 2006.

Wheeless CR III, ed. *Wheeless' Textbook of Orthopaedics.* http://www.wheelessonline.com.

Wojtys EM, Chan DB. Meniscus structure and function. *Instr Course Lect.* 2005;54:323–30.

# Trauma in Children

ractures in children are not the same as fractures in adults because of differences in anatomy, biomechanics, and exposure to trauma.

## EPIDEMIOLOGY

The incidence, type, and age distribution of children's fractures vary across countries and regions because of cultural and environmental differences. Fractures in children are first seen at childbirth, from birth trauma. They become more prevalent with walking (and falling) in toddlers and peak in incidence in girls at approximately 11 years of age and in boys at approximately 14 years of age. By 16 years of age, 42% of boys and 27% of girls will have sustained at least one fracture. In the United States, most fractures in children are the result of accidents while playing and sports-related injuries. Fractures are more common in boys than in girls by a ratio of nearly 2:1. The upper extremity is fractured more commonly than the lower extremity, and the left upper extremity is fractured more frequently than the right. After the first year of life, trauma is the leading cause of death in children, accounting for 50% of all deaths in children between 1 and 14 years of age. As with fractures, boys are at greater risk of dying from trauma than girls. Most trauma deaths in children are the result of head injuries.

## BIOMECHANICS

The immature, growing skeleton has cartilaginous growth plates, cartilaginous epiphyses, and a thick, strong periosteum. Immature bone is more porous than adult bone and functions less as a single mechanical unit and more as an aggregate of smaller units. Children's bone is less stiff and more malleable (ductile) than adult bone. Fracture lines do not propagate as far, and a loaded bone is more likely to bend and deform than to break and splinter. There are five general types of children's fractures: buckle fractures, plastic deformation, greenstick fractures, complete fractures, and growth plate fractures.

Cortical bone in children can fail under compressive as well as tensile loading. Failure of bone under compressive loading results in a buckle fracture. *Buckle fractures* (also called *torus fractures*) are incomplete impaction fractures in which the cortex around all or part of

the circumference of the bone is buckled (Fig. 5.1). They occur at the metaphysis, where the porosity of the bone is greatest, and are most common in preschool-aged children. On radiographs, buckle fractures can be recognized by a focal, angular protrusion of the cortex with a modest angulation of the shaft and overlying soft-tissue swelling.

With angular loading, elastic and then plastic bowing occurs (see Fig. 5.15). Traumatic plastic bowing results in a permanent bend caused by a series of microscopic shear fractures on the concave aspect without gross disruption of the cortex or trabeculae. Elastic recoil allows a bent bone to recover part of its normal shape. Plastic bowing is most often seen at the ulna, in association with fractures of the radius, and at the fibula, in association with fractures of the tibia. On radiographs, plastic bowing may be recognized by an abnormal bend in the affected bone.

When a bone is angulated beyond the limits of bowing, the convex side fails in tension and the concave side bends, resulting in an angulated, incomplete transverse fracture. Such a fracture is called a *greenstick fracture* (see Fig. 5.15). Elastic recoil usually decreases the degree of angulation; muscle pull may increase it. The periosteum is intact on the concave side of the bend but not on the convex side, leaving a periosteal hinge. Greenstick fractures are seen most often in children of elementary school age. The only anatomic sites where greenstick fractures are common are the shafts of the radius and ulna. On radiographs, greenstick fractures may be recognized by the bowing deformity of the affected bone with a transverse fracture extending through the cortex on the convex side of the bow.

Complete fractures through the bone in children resemble adult fractures. However, the displacement of complete fractures depends on whether or not the periosteum is torn. A periosteal hinge usually is present on one side, allowing angulation but not much displacement. Children's fractures are rarely comminuted. As with adult bones, the direction of loading determines the configuration of the fracture line.

## GROWTH PLATE INJURIES

The cartilage of the growth plate absorbs and dissipates some of the energy of loading, reducing the likelihood of a fracture. The growth plate is attached to the metaphysis internally by the interdigitation of the bone with the zone of calcified cartilage and externally by the

**FIGURE 5.1.** Buckle fracture (*arrows*) of the distal radial metaphysis. **A:** Lateral radiograph; **B:** PA radiograph.

periosteum. The growth plate is relatively weak compared with the capsule and ligaments of adjacent joints, and mechanisms of injury that tend to result in ligamentous joint injuries in adults typically result in growth plate fractures in children. The growth plate is particularly vulnerable to injury when loaded in torsion or shear but is relatively resistant to tension and compression. When the epiphysis is separated from the metaphysis, the plane of separation through the growth plate is in the zone of cartilage transformation between the calcified and uncalcified layers of cartilage, leaving the germinal cell layers with the epiphysis and the calcified cartilage with the metaphysis. Displacement does not occur unless the periosteum is also torn.

Injuries to the growth plate represent approximately one third of skeletal injuries in children. The most common sites of growth plate fractures are the wrist and ankle. Growth plate fractures are more common in boys than in girls. The peak incidence in boys is at 14 years of age, but the peak incidence in girls is at 11 and

12 years of age. The difference can be accounted for by the differences in the rate of skeletal maturation between boys and girls. Sometimes, a normal growth plate may be mistaken for a fracture. Keats and Smith's *Atlas of Normal Developmental Roentgen Anatomy* is a handy reference for reviewing the radiologic appearance of the skeleton at various ages; in some circumstances, it may be necessary to radiograph the contralateral body part for comparison.

Salter and Harris described five types of growth plate fractures (Fig. 5.2). Their classification should be used in describing fractures of the growth plate. The most common type of growth plate fracture is a Salter type II fracture. There are many other systems of classifying growth plate injuries of varying complexity, but the Salter-Harris system is universally understood.

A Salter type I fracture extends through the growth plate without involving the bone (Fig. 5.3). This type is usually caused by shearing, torsion, or avulsion. Because Salter type I fractures do not displace unless the periosteum is torn, they may be difficult to

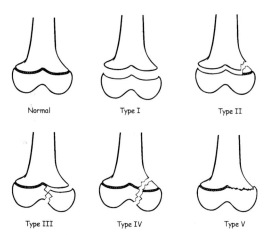

**FIGURE 5.2.** Salter-Harris classification of fractures of the growth plate.

**FIGURE 5.3.** Salter type I fracture of the distal radius. The radial growth plate appears wide (*arrow*) compared with that of the ulna.

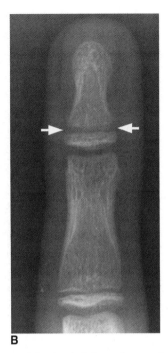

**A**          **B**

**FIGURE 5.4.** Salter type II fracture of the distal phalanx. **A:** Lateral view shows the fracture passing through the growth plate (*arrow*) and including a small piece of the metaphysis (*arrowhead*). **B:** The PA view shows widening of the growth plate (*arrows*).

demonstrate radiologically without stress views. The most common sites of Salter type I fractures are the lateral malleolus of the ankle and the distal radius.

In Salter type II fractures, the plane of the fracture passes through much of the growth plate but includes a piece of metaphyseal bone on one side (Fig. 5.4). The periosteum is intact on the side with the metaphyseal fragment but torn on the opposite side. The most common sites of Salter type II fractures are the phalanges of the fingers and the distal radius.

Salter type III fractures include a piece of the epiphysis and are intra-articular. Salter type III fractures are most common when the growth plate is partially closed, so they tend to occur in teenagers. Most Salter type III fractures are avulsion fractures that occur at sites of ligamentous or tendinous attachment. The most common sites of Salter type III fractures are the phalanges of the fingers and thumb (Fig. 5.5) and the medial malleolus of the ankle.

Salter type IV fractures involve both metaphysis and epiphysis and are intra-articular. The most common sites of Salter type IV fractures are the lateral condyle of the elbow and the medial malleolus of the ankle (Fig. 5.6). Because displacement of the fracture fragment is likely to result in premature closure of the growth plate, Salter type IV fractures have a worse prognosis than Salter type I or II fractures. Open reduction and internal fixation may be required for the treatment of these fractures.

A Salter type V injury is a crush injury of the growth plate from axial loading. These injuries are exceedingly rare and are absent from many large series of growth plate fractures. Almost by

**A**                                              **B**

**FIGURE 5.5.** Salter type III fracture of the distal femur. **A:** AP radiograph shows fracture (*arrow*) through the intercondylar portion of the epiphysis. **B:** Oblique radiograph shows widening (*arrow*) of the lateral femoral growth plate.

**FIGURE 5.6.** Salter type IV fracture of distal femoral growth plate. Intercondylar fracture lines extend through the metaphysis, physis, and epiphysis.

**FIGURE 5.8.** Coronal CT of proximal tibia shows physeal bar (*arrow*) caused by a boat propeller injury of the proximal tibial growth plate. Asymmetric growth with angular deformity has resulted.

**FIGURE 5.7.** Salter type V fracture of the distal tibial growth plate. **A:** Lateral ankle radiograph 1 year after injury shows a growth deformity (*arrow*). **B:** Coronal proton density fat suppressed MR imaging shows the prematurely closed portion of the growth plate (*arrow*).

**FIGURE 5.9.** Tibial epiphyseal fracture (*arrow*).

definition, these injuries may not be recognized until the cessation of growth is noticed (Fig. 5.7).

The growth plate is surrounded by a perichondrial ring that appears to regulate its diameter. Displacement of the perichondrial ring allows growth away from the plate laterally, resulting in a post-traumatic osteochondroma (see Chapter 9). Removal of a segment of the ring, for example, by a lawn mower blade injury, permits a bony bridge (physeal bar) to develop across the growth plate, tethering it and leading to angular deformity as growth proceeds (Fig. 5.8).

Fractures of the epiphysis in children without involvement of the growth plate may occur as osteochondral fractures or avulsion fractures (Fig. 5.9). When the fractures involve only the cartilage, they may be unrecognized. These injuries were not included in the original Salter-Harris classification.

*Apophyses* are bony prominences that typically accept traction from an attached tendon or muscle, and fractures involving apophyses are almost always avulsion fractures. Fractures of the apophyses are Salter type I or III injuries.

Common sites for apophyseal avulsion injuries include, in the upper extremity, the medial epicondyle, the olecronon process, the coronoid process, and the coracoid process, and in the lower extremity, the anterior tibial tubercle, the femoral trochanters, and the calcaneus. There are multiple sites around the pelvis that may be avulsed.

# OPEN FRACTURES

Open fractures in children are typically the result of accidents, many of which are preventable (Fig. 5.10). Open fractures account for approximately 3% of fractures in children. On radiographs, open fractures may be recognized by the presence of gas within the fracture site, a soft-tissue wound extending to the fracture site, protrusion of bone through the soft tissues, missing fragments of bone, or penetration of foreign bodies to the bone.

# FRACTURE HEALING AND TREATMENT

Fracture healing in children is rapid (Table 5.1). The younger the child and the greater the remaining growth potential of the fractured bone, the faster and more complete are the healing and remodeling. Fracture remodeling is a process of bone resorption and periosteal deposition. Fracture remodeling can round off protruding edges by bone resorption and fill in concavities by periosteal new bone. However, varus, valgus, and rotary misalignments do not improve by this process (Fig. 5.11). As growth proceeds and the bone enlarges, asymmetric activity at the growth plate and at the periosteum may tend to correct angular misalignment. Hyperemia from fracture healing may lead to overgrowth, so that a reduction may be left intentionally shorter than anatomic in anticipation of overgrowth. Nonunion of children's fractures is rare unless the fractures are intra-articular. Most fractures in children are treated by closed means, but open reduction and internal fixation by pins, wires, plates, screws, and rods are sometimes necessary.

In fractures of the growth plate, the production of growing cartilage may not be interrupted by the fracture if the blood supply to the separated epiphysis remains intact. After a fracture, the growth plate becomes wider until the normal zone of cartilage transformation is reestablished and then the plate returns to normal (Fig. 5.12). The healing process for Salter I and II fractures is much more rapid than that of a fracture through bone and may leave no scar.

**FIGURE 5.10.** Lawnmower accident in a child with open fractures (*arrows*) of the lateral foot.

**TABLE 5.1** **Radiographic Timetable of Fracture Healing in Children**

| Radiographic Finding | Time After Fracture to Initial Observation | |
| --- | --- | --- |
| | Typical | Range |
| Resolution of soft-tissue swelling | 4–10 days | 2–21 days |
| Periosteal new bone | 10–14 days | 4–21 days |
| Loss of fracture line definition | 14–21 days | 10–21 days |
| Soft callus | 14–21 days | 10–21 days |
| Hard callus | 21–42 days | 14–90 days |
| Remodeling | 1 year | 3 months to physeal closure |

*Source*: Kleinman PK. *Diagnostic Imaging of Child Abuse.* 2nd Ed. St. Louis, MO: Mosby–Year Book; 1998.

**A** **B**

**FIGURE 5.11.** Healing spiral femoral shaft fracture. **A:** Acute fracture. **B:** Follow-up after 8 weeks.

## SOFT-TISSUE INJURIES

Bruises and contusions are common in children and usually are inconsequential. Bruises around the head and neck or chest and abdomen may suggest more severe underlying injuries of the central nervous system or viscera, respectively. Unexplained multiple bruises of different ages may suggest child abuse. Because a child's bones and growth plates are usually weaker than the tendons and ligaments, strains and sprains in children are uncommon until adolescence, when adult patterns of injury begin to emerge as the growth plates close.

## HAND AND FOREARM

Fractures of the hand account for approximately 20% of all fractures of the extremities in children. The most common fractures in the hand are crush injuries of the distal phalanx and growth plate fractures of the proximal phalanx. The index and little fingers are the most likely to be fractured.

Distal phalanges are most commonly injured by closing doors and falling objects. These are generally extra-articular fractures that do not involve the growth plate and may have a transverse, longitudinal, or comminuted morphology. Forced flexion may result in fractures of the distal phalanx that involve the growth plate. Because the extensor tendon inserts at the epiphysis of the distal phalanx, and the flexor digitorum profundus tendon inserts along the metaphysis, these fractures may become angulated or displaced and assume a fixed position in flexion (mallet finger equivalent). These mallet finger–equivalent injuries may represent Salter type I or II fractures with displacement or angulation at the fracture site or Salter type III or IV fractures with retraction of the fragment by the extensor tendon and unopposed flexion by the flexor digitorum profundus.

In young children, proximal phalangeal fractures are typically Salter type I or II fractures. In adolescents, Salter type III fractures occur with avulsion of a portion of the articular surface by an attached tendon or ligament. Such fractures occur commonly at the thumb and are the children's equivalent of a gamekeeper's fracture

**FIGURE 5.12.** Healing distal radius growth plate fracture (Salter type I) with widening and irregularity of the zone of provisional calcification (*arrow*).

**FIGURE 5.13.** Salter 3 fracture (*arrow*) at the base of the proximal phalanx of the thumb (gamekeeper's fracture).

(Fig. 5.13). Salter type III avulsion fractures may also occur at other phalanges of the fingers.

The most common metacarpal fracture in children is the *boxer's fracture*, a volarly angulated fracture of the fifth (or sometimes fourth) metacarpal neck.

Fractures and dislocations involving the carpal bones are rare in children. A fracture of the scaphoid is the most common of these rare injuries. Similar to the fractures in adults, fractures across the scaphoid waist may lead to osteonecrosis of the proximal pole. Ligamentous injuries of the wrist in children are rarer than fractures of the carpal bones.

Fractures of the distal radius account for approximately 23% of all fractures of the extremities in children, making it the most common site of children's fractures. These injuries are most commonly sustained in falls onto an outstretched, dorsiflexed hand. The severity of the fracture depends on the energy involved in the fall, ranging from gravity falls from standing height, to falls in which the body has significant momentum (e.g., in roller skating), to falls from a great height. Simple buckle fractures are common in preschool-aged children with simple gravity falls (see Fig. 5.1). Buckle fractures are usually located 2 to 3 cm proximal to the growth plate. Complete fractures are seen in higher-energy injuries. When displaced, the fragments are most often displaced dorsally, resulting in a bayonet deformity. The distal radius is the most common location for

**FIGURE 5.14.** Displaced Salter II fracture of the distal radius.

growth plate fractures in children. These are most often Salter type I or II fractures (Fig. 5.14), and the epiphysis may be displaced.

Injuries to shafts of the radius and ulna may be plastic bowing deformities, greenstick fractures, or complete fractures (Fig. 5.15), depending on the magnitude and direction of loading and the maturity of the patient. Rotational deformity is usually present and evident as angulated fractures of both bones at different levels. Because the radius has a normal bowing curve and a pear-shaped cross section, interruption of the smooth curve of the radius or an apparent change in shaft diameter across the fracture site indicates radial malrotation. The bicipital tuberosity may serve as a guide to the rotation of the proximal radius. The position of the proximal fragments in complete fractures depends on the direction of muscle pull.

# ELBOW

Fractures of the bones around the elbow account for approximately 12% of all fractures of the extremities in children, making it the third most common location for fractures after the distal radius and the hand.

In children, 60% of elbow fractures are supracondylar fractures, 15% are lateral condylar fractures, and 10% are medial epicondylar avulsion fractures. Fractures may occur in combinations or in association with elbow dislocation. Isolated avulsion fractures of the proximal ulna, olecranon, or coronoid processes are rare.

The anterior humeral line, the radiocapitellar line, and the fat pad sign are radiographic clues to the presence of an elbow fracture. The anterior humeral line is a line drawn down the anterior humeral cortex on a true lateral radiograph; it should pass through the middle third of the capitellum. The radiocapitellar line is drawn through the proxima l radial shaft; it should intersect the capitellum on every radiographic projection. The elbow has anterior and posterior fat pads that abut the joint capsule. The posterior fat pad is usually not seen because it lies in the intercondylar depression. The anterior fat pad is typically visible, extending obliquely toward the

**FIGURE 5.15.** Forearm fractures. **A:** Complete fracture (*arrow*) of the radius with plastic bowing deformity (*arrowheads*) of the ulna. **B:** Greenstick fractures of the radius and ulna. **C:** Complete fractures of both the radius and ulna.

forearm. Elbow joint distention from any cause will displace both the anterior and posterior fat pads, making them visible. After trauma, the capsule is distended with blood. More than 90% of children and adolescents with a posterior fat pad sign have a demonstrable fracture. Absence of the fat pad sign in children virtually excludes an intra-articular fracture unless the injury is so severe that there is disruption of the elbow joint capsule.

The age of peak incidence of supracondylar fractures is 5 to 8 years of age, and they are rare after 15 years of age. Supracondylar fractures of the elbow occur with hyperextension, usually in a fall. The fracture extends transversely across the distal humerus through the coronoid and olecranon fossae, above the level of the condyles. The distal fragment is angulated posteriorly, so that the anterior humeral line passes anterior to the capitellum. A posterior fat pad sign is almost always present (Fig. 5.16). The fracture is usually complete, but greenstick fractures, torus fractures, and plastic bowing are possible. The typical treatment is closed reduction with casting.

Lateral condylar fractures are most common between 4 and 10 years of age. These are usually Salter type IV injuries sustained during a fall on an outstretched hand. In most cases, the fracture line begins in the metaphysis, extends across the growth plate, and, if complete, exits through the cartilaginous portion of the epiphysis (Fig. 5.17). Because the fracture usually extends through the cartilaginous portion of the growth plate, it may resemble a Salter type

**FIGURE 5.16.** Supracondylar elbow fracture with anterior (*long arrow*) and posterior (*short arrow*) fat pad signs and slight posterior angulation of the capitellum.

**FIGURE 5.17.** Lateral condylar fracture. The fracture through the metaphysis (*arrows*) crosses the growth plate and continues through the cartilaginous portion of the epiphysis (Salter type IV).

**FIGURE 5.18.** Medial epicondyle (*arrow*) avulsion in a 9-year-old boy (Salter type I).

II fracture. An incomplete fracture leaves a distal cartilaginous hinge. A minority of lateral condylar fractures involve the ossified portion of the epiphysis. A posterior fat pad sign is almost always present. The extensors of the forearm originate from the lateral condyle and may distract the distal fragment. Displaced fractures are treated with open reduction and internal fixation.

The medial epicondylar ossification center appears at approximately 5 years of age. It is the site of insertion of the common tendon of the flexor pronator muscle group and can be avulsed by muscular contraction. This often results in a displaced fracture (Fig. 5.18). Dislocation of the elbow also separates the medial

epicondyle from the distal humerus by stress applied through the medial ulnar collateral ligament. The medial epicondylar fragment may then become entrapped in the elbow joint as it opens with valgus stress. Medial epicondylar injuries are usually seen between 5 and 15 years of age; after the medial epicondyle fuses in late adolescence, this injury no longer occurs.

Radial neck fractures are not as common in children as in adults because of the greater vulnerability of the other structures in the growing elbow. The radial neck may be fractured by indirect forces applied across the humerus during a fall on an outstretched arm with the elbow extended. The injury is usually a Salter type II

**A**

**B**

**FIGURE 5.19.** Small child with pulled elbow. **A, B:** Lateral and AP radiographs show that the radiocapitellar line (*white line*) does not intersect the middle of the ossification center (*arrow*) of the capitellum.

separation of the radial head (proximal epiphysis) that may be accompanied by impaction of the lateral metaphysis and lateral angulation of the distal shaft.

Pulled elbow (nursemaid's elbow) is a common injury in ambulatory preschoolers. Longitudinal traction on the pronated hand or wrist, as an adult pulls a young child along, may dislocate the radial head and tear the attachment of the annular ligament to the radial head. The annular ligament binds the radial head to the ulna and is weakly attached until 5 years of age. The ligament may slip over the radial articular surface, preventing relocation of the radial head. The child may complain of pain and refuse to move the arm. Supination of the slightly flexed elbow during positioning for radiographs often reduces the ligament, resulting in normal radiographs. If the elbow has not been reduced, subluxation of the radial head relative to the capitellum is indicative of the injury (Fig. 5.19). In the normally located elbow, a line drawn through the proximal radial shaft should intersect the ossification center of the epiphysis of the capitellum on all views.

## SHOULDER AND HUMERUS

Injuries of the proximal humerus are mostly Salter type II fractures that occur in adolescents. In children younger than 5 years of age, Salter type I fractures usually occur. Hyperextension of the glenohumeral joint during a fall from a height is a common mechanism. The growth plate fracture leaves the humeral head normally located, but the humeral shaft angulates posteriorly and medially (Fig. 5.20). Treatment is usually sling or traction. The adult injury of anterior shoulder dislocation is seen only after the proximal humeral epiphysis has closed.

Scapular fractures in children are rare and are usually the result of severe direct violence such as motor vehicle collisions or child abuse.

Fractures of the clavicle account for approximately 6% of all fractures of the extremities in children. Most clavicle fractures are fractures of the middle portion of the shaft. The medial fragment is pulled cephalad by the sternocleidomastoid muscle, while the distal fragment is pulled caudad by the pectoralis minor muscle. Midshaft fractures may be complete or greenstick, but both unite quickly and remodel completely (Fig. 5.21). Because of the double curve of the normal clavicle, multiple views may be required to demonstrate the fracture. Rarely, injuries occur at the medial or lateral ends of the clavicle. At the medial end, an epiphyseal separation may occur and mimic a sternoclavicular dislocation. These injuries occur between 18 and 25 years of age, when the medial clavicular ossification center is present. At the lateral end, the distal tip may be fractured by a backward blow. If the periosteum becomes stripped from the clavicular shaft, the radiographic appearance may suggest acromioclavicular dislocation, but true acromioclavicular dislocation is rare in children.

## SPINE

### Acute Trauma

Cervical spine injuries in children are rare, accounting for less than 1% of all fractures in children. Most involve C1 or C2 and are sustained in motor vehicle collisions, as pedestrian or passenger, or in falls from a height. Weak neck musculature and relatively large head size predispose the upper cervical spine to injuries from acceleration-deceleration or axial distraction. The most common injuries are

**FIGURE 5.20.** Salter type II fracture of the humerus. The growth plate is widened (*arrow*) and the fracture lines extend into the metaphysis (*arrowhead*).

odontoid fractures and C1–2 fracture dislocations. Growth plates in children may make the interpretation of radiographs confusing. Growth plates have smooth, regular, sclerotic margins and are found in predictable locations (Fig. 5.22). The vertebral ring apophyses appear in adolescence and persist into young adulthood. Fracture lines are irregular, without sclerosis, and often in unpredictable locations. Forward glide of one vertebral body over the next by up to 3 mm is normal but may mimic subluxation, particularly at the C2–3 level (Fig. 5.23). The retropharyngeal soft tissues may appear thickened as a result of the child's crying. The neck may normally appear lordotic, neutral, or kyphotic, depending on positioning and the presence or

**FIGURE 5.21.** Acute fracture of the clavicle in a 14-year-old boy.

**FIGURE 5.22.** Coronal CT reconstruction of the cervical spine of a 2-year-old showing normal ossification centers.

absence of muscle spasm. After 8 to 10 years of age, the spine reaches mature proportions, and the adult pattern of injuries emerges.

Thoracolumbar fractures from acute trauma in children are even less common than cervical spine fractures. Because children's bones are more elastic and ductile, relatively greater amounts of loading can be sustained as the force is dissipated over more levels than in adults. When injuries do occur, however, they may be at multiple levels and

catastrophic. Spinal cord injury without radiographic abnormality may occur. Avulsion fractures of the spinous processes in infants are highly specific to child abuse (discussed later in this chapter).

## Spondylolysis and Spondylolisthesis

*Spondylolysis* refers to discontinuity of the pars interarticularis. Usually seen at the L4 or L5 level, this lesion is a stress fracture of the pars interarticularis caused by axial loads. Predisposing congenital and developmental factors are likely, and many patients with spondylolysis also have various minor deficiencies of the posterior elements such as dysraphic or malformed lamina. Spondylolysis is very rare in young children, has an increasing incidence that coincides with the adolescent growth spurt, and has a prevalence of 5% in the general population. Only a small fraction of children and adolescents with spondylolysis appear to develop symptoms before adulthood. Symptoms may be initiated or aggravated by strenuous activities involving the spine such as football, gymnastics, wrestling, rowing, tennis, baseball pitching, and hockey. The neurologic examination is usually normal. Spondylolysis can be demonstrated on radiographs (Fig. 5.24) and is seen best on lateral or oblique views as a radiolucent discontinuity in the pars interarticularis (the part of the posterior elements that connects the superior and inferior articular facets of a vertebra). On the oblique view, the posterior elements have an appearance that has been likened to a "Scottie dog." When spondylolysis is present, the "Scottie dog" appears to be wearing a radiolucent collar. Radionuclide bone scan may show a stress reaction (hot spot) in the absence of a demonstrable fracture, but a fracture is usually evident later. Nonunion is the common outcome. CT and MRI can demonstrate spondylolysis but should be reserved for problem solving or surgical planning.

Spondylolisthesis, anterior subluxation of the vertebral body, is a common sequela. The severity of spondylolisthesis can be graded from 1 to 4 by dividing the end plate of the lower vertebra into four equal parts on the lateral projection. If the posterior margin of the upper vertebral body has slipped forward up to one fourth

**FIGURE 5.23.** Normal cervical spine in a 6-year-old with forward glide (pseudosubluxation) at C2–3.

**FIGURE 5.24.** Spondylolysis (*arrow*) at L5 without spondylolisthesis.

of the AP length of the end plate of the lower vertebra, it is grade 1 spondylolisthesis; a slip of between one-fourth and one-half is grade 2, and so forth. Complete anterior dislocation is considered to be grade 5.

# PELVIS AND FEMUR

Fractures of the lower extremity in children occur much less frequently than fractures of the upper extremity.

The majority of fractures of the pelvis in children do not interrupt the continuity of the pelvic ring. Avulsion fractures of the apophyses typically occur with sports-related activities. The most common sites of pelvic apophyseal avulsion fractures are the ischial tuberosity (the origin of the hamstring muscles) (Fig. 5.25) and the anterior superior iliac spine (the origin of the sartorius muscle).

Fractures of the pelvic ring in children are caused by severe trauma, such as when a child pedestrian is struck by a car. The likelihood of concomitant injuries, especially of the thorax and head, is high. Depending on the child's age, the hip, trochanters, shaft, or condyles of the femur are at the level of the bumper. A preponderance of left-sided injuries occurs in the United States because a child running across a street is more likely to be hit by a car in the near lane whose driver has less time to react than a driver of a car in the far lane. In Great Britain and other countries where drivers stay on the left side of the road, there is a preponderance of right-sided injuries.

Hip dislocations are more common than fractures, probably because of the soft cartilaginous structure of the acetabulum in young children. When hip fractures do occur, they may be complicated by osteonecrosis of the femoral head and malunion. Fractures of the femoral shaft in children younger than 4 years of age are commonly the result of child abuse (Fig. 5.26). In older children, high-energy trauma, such as that sustained in motor vehicle crashes, is required to fracture the femur. Because of muscle pull, fractures of the femoral shaft tend to be shortened and displaced, with the distal fragment angulated posteriorly. Because

femoral shaft fractures tend to heal with overgrowth, reduction with overriding is a common orthopedic practice (see Fig. 5.11).

# KNEE

Knee injuries in children differ from knee injuries in adults because of the relative strength of the ligaments and the thick, energy-absorbing articular and growth cartilages. The most common intra-articular fracture is an avulsion of the anterior tibial spine by the anterior cruciate ligament. In an adult, the ligament would probably tear. The size of the ossified fragment may be large or

**FIGURE 5.26.** A 21-month-old boy with spiral fracture (*arrows*) of the femur suspicious for child abuse.

**FIGURE 5.25.** Avulsion of the anterior part of the right iliac crest apophysis (*arrows*) in a 16-year-old football player (Salter type I).

small, but the cartilaginous portion is always larger. The fracture may be complete and displaced, incomplete and undisplaced, or hinged posteriorly. A bloody effusion is consistently present.

Internal derangements of the knee in children are less common than in adults. Internal derangements are unusual in young children, and the incidence increases with age as the skeleton gains strength relative to the soft tissue structures of the knee, and as there is increased exposure to knee trauma.

Meniscal tears in children and adolescents may be repaired primarily if they extend through the vascularized periphery of the meniscus. The normal meniscus receives its blood supply from its peripheral attachment to the joint capsule.

Discoid meniscus is a developmental variant in which the meniscus is shaped like a biconcave disk rather than the letter C. The extension of meniscal cartilage into the joint makes it susceptible to degeneration and tears, and a significant proportion of adolescents with meniscal tears have a discoid meniscus. Chronic irritation of the discoid meniscus is thought to cause it to thicken and, in some cases, become slablike, shaped like a hockey puck with parallel superior and inferior surfaces. Patients typically present with snapping or chronic pain. Discoid meniscus is much more common in the lateral compartment. On MRI, a discoid meniscus can be recognized by the presence of a sheet of fibrocartilage connecting the anterior and posterior horns on sagittal images. An intact discoid meniscus should have a transverse dimension of at least 12 mm on coronal images, and the bow-tie configuration should be seen on three or more consecutive 4-mm-thick slices on sagittal images.

Osteochondral fractures may accompany lateral dislocation of the patella, with a fragment shearing off the lateral femoral condyle or off the medial facet of the patella (Fig. 5.27). Direct trauma to the medial femoral condyle, as might occur with a fall on stairs, may also result in an osteochondral fracture. A flexion-rotation injury of the knee may also cause an osteochondral fracture involving the medial or lateral femoral condyle. On radiographs, the fragments may be difficult to identify. MRI is the recommended method for identifying such fragments and has the added advantage of displaying the condition of the other structures of the knee.

Fractures of the patella are uncommon in children. Most are sleeve fractures in which tensile loading through the quadriceps mechanism distracts the patella (Fig. 5.28). The inferior fragment typically consists of a large sleeve of cartilage—including the inferior, medial, lateral, and articular surfaces—and sometimes a sliver of the ossification center. As healing occurs, this displaced ossification center enlarges and eventually fuses with the main ossification center. These intra-articular fractures have an associated knee effusion. Fractures of the patella must be distinguished from developmental variants, particularly a patella with multiple ossification centers (multipartite patella). Accessory ossification centers have rounded contours and sclerotic margins and typically occur in the superior lateral quadrant of the patella.

## TIBIA AND ANKLE

The tibia is the most frequently fractured bone of the lower extremity in children. Fractures of the tibial shaft are more common than fractures of the medial malleolus and are seen more frequently in younger children. Approximately one third of tibial shaft fractures have an accompanying fracture of the fibula. Pedestrian-automobile collisions are common with children, but because of their shorter

**FIGURE 5.27.** Previous patellar dislocation with osteochondral fragment (*arrow*) shown on sagittal proton density MRI.

stature, they tend to sustain fractures of the hip and femur rather than the lower leg.

Isolated spiral or oblique fractures of the tibial shaft are common injuries in ambulatory preschoolers (toddler's fracture) (Fig. 5.29). The fibula is usually intact. These injuries result from falls with torsion of the foot, and the traumatic episode is often innocuous or not witnessed. These fractures may be exceedingly subtle on radiographs because the low energy that produces the fractures is insufficient to displace it. The clinical presentation is failure to bear weight, limping, or simply the appearance of pain when bearing weight. Follow-up examinations show periosteal new bone, indicative of healing. Fractures from a similar mechanism occur less

**FIGURE 5.28.** Avulsion fracture of the inferior pole of the patella (*arrow*) in a 6-year-old boy. On physical examination, acute tenderness was localized to the site of fracture.

**FIGURE 5.30.** Salter type II fracture of the lateral malleolus (*arrow*). Note the soft-tissue swelling.

**FIGURE 5.29.** Toddler's fracture of the distal tibial shaft (*arrows*) in a 2-year-old.

frequently in the femur or metatarsals. Toddler's fractures must be distinguished from inflicted trauma in the battered child (discussed later in this chapter). Tibial shaft fractures from inflicted trauma are often caused by high-energy direct trauma. The clinical history and physical examination in inflicted trauma are often inconsistent with the radiologic findings.

The ankle ligaments in children are stronger than the growth plates and the bone. The ankle mortise usually remains intact, with the injuries occurring proximally in the growth plates of the tibia and fibula. The most common fractures are Salter type II fractures of the distal tibia and Salter type I or II fractures of the lateral malleolus (Fig. 5.30). Gross displacement and angulation may accompany the distal tibial fracture. The lateral malleolar fracture is seen as soft-tissue swelling and sometimes as widening of the fibular growth plate.

As the epiphyses begin to close, two unusual fractures may occur in the ankle through the partially fused growth plates. The juvenile

A

B

**FIGURE 5.31.** Avulsion fracture (*arrows*) of a portion of the lateral tibial epiphysis through a partially closed growth plate (juvenile Tillaux fracture, Salter type III) in a 15-year-old boy. **A:** Lateral radiograph. **B:** AP radiograph.

Tillaux fracture is an avulsion of a portion of the lateral tibial epiphysis after closure of the medial portion of the tibial growth plate. This avulsion occurs instead of rupture of the syndesmosis or fracture of the lateral malleolus (Fig. 5.31). The fragment may be anterior or posterior depending on whether the anterior or posterior portion of the syndesmosis was under tension. The tibial triplane fracture also occurs in the distal tibia when the growth plate is partially fused. This is a Salter type IV fracture that extends in the coronal plane through the tibial metaphysis, in the axial plane through the growth plate, and in the sagittal plane through the epiphysis (Fig. 5.32).

## ■ SPORTS-RELATED INJURIES

American football and wrestling have by far the highest injury rates among school sports. Swimming and tennis have the lowest, and soccer and gymnastics are in between. Fractures and acute soft-tissue injuries may occur during play or practice from discrete incidents

**FIGURE 5.32.** Triplane fracture. **A:** AP radiograph shows a fracture (*arrow*) in the sagittal plane through the distal tibial epiphysis. **B:** Sagittal reformatted CT image shows a fracture in the axial plane (*arrowhead*) through the partially opened physis connecting with a fracture through the metaphysis in the coronal plane (*arrow*). **C:** Coronal reformatted CT image shows a fracture in the sagittal plane (*arrow*) through the distal tibial epiphysis and a fracture in the axial plane (*arrowhead*) through the physis. **D:** Axial CT image through the distal tibial epiphysis shows fractures in the coronal and sagittal planes.

**FIGURE 5.33.** Stress fracture (*arrow*) of the tibia in a 7-year-old boy with healing.

of trauma. These are more likely to occur in contact sports if the participants are mismatched in size and ability. Chronic overuse injuries similar to those suffered by adults have become common in children who participate in organized single-sport athletics such as gymnastics and hockey. Children are also at risk for injuries peculiar to the growing skeleton, and repetitive loading of growing bones

may lead to mechanical adaptation and growth aberration. Stress fractures are common in the proximal tibia at the junction of the proximal and middle thirds (Fig. 5.33). Stress fractures often follow a change in the training regimen. Stress fractures may involve the growth plates or synchondroses such as those of the pelvis (Fig. 5.34). Children at a particular risk for such injuries are usually participants in activities in which repetitive shearing forces are applied to growth plates or synchondroses.

Avulsion fractures of apophyses by inserting tendons are most common about the pelvis but may also involve the knee, elbow, and shoulder. Avulsion fractures of apophyses and epiphyses at tendinous insertions are Salter type I injuries if the growth plates are open and Salter type III injuries if the growth plates are partially closed. These fractures are distracted because of excessive muscle pull. The most common sites of avulsion fractures are the fingers, around the pelvis, the lesser trochanter, the medial epicondyle, and the anterior tibial tubercle.

Osgood-Schlatter disease of the knee is thought to be a stress injury of the tibial apophyseal growth plate at the insertion of the infrapatellar tendon. The clinical presentation of Osgood-Schlatter disease is painful prominence of the tibial tubercle in an adolescent (11 to 15 years of age) who participates in jumping sports such as basketball. Symptoms may be prolonged and intermittent but always cease when the growth plate closes. Stress fractures of the anterior tibial apophysis may also occur, potentially resulting in avulsion of the apophysis by the infrapatellar tendon.

A stress injury of the inferior pole of the patella carries the eponym Sinding-Larsen-Johansson disease. In this condition, there is repetitive incomplete avulsion trauma to the inferior pole of the patella mediated through tension on the infrapatellar ligament (see Fig. 5.28).

**A**    **B**

**FIGURE 5.34.** Ischial stress fracture in a 14-year-old boy participating in kickboxing. **A:** Axial CT scan shows a stress fracture (*arrow*) in the right ischium. **B:** Radiograph shows healing fracture (*arrow*) after 3 weeks of rest.

# ■ THE BATTERED CHILD

The battered child has horrified and fascinated the medical profession since 1946 when Caffey, a pediatric radiologist, published his findings of a series of six infants with chronic subdural hematomas and unrecognized skeletal trauma. He suggested inflicted trauma as the cause for both. Described initially by physicians as a medical syndrome with predictable implications in terms of treatment, prognosis, and prevention, the concept of child abuse has expanded to include broad psychological, cultural, social, and legal implications. A contemporary concept of the physical abuse of children categorizes it as one permutation in a "world of abnormal rearing." Children who are raised in such a world do not complete the tasks of childhood; they are not taught many of the basic skills necessary for successful social interaction because their parents or caretakers themselves lack these skills. Inadequacies in behavior and parenting can be passed down through successive generations: Except for the rare psychotic individual, child abusers have had abnormal rearing, and many were battered as children. There is no broadly accepted, precise definition of child abuse. Some of these children are physically abused; others may be sexually molested, neglected, or unloved. This section is concerned with physical abuse inflicted in the home by a parent or caretaker.

Approximately 10% of children reported to governmental agencies as abused have radiologic evidence of injury. Approximately 10% of children younger than 5 years of age who are seen in hospital emergency departments for trauma have child abuse as the cause. Intentional trauma is one of the leading causes of death in infancy and childhood. Because the acts of violence are nearly always multiple, any physician with reasonable suspicion of child abuse has a duty to prompt further formal investigation. Moreover, failure to do so may expose the physician to criminal, civil, or professional liability. The standard for the radiologist is to report findings and suspicions to the referring physician. The referring physician is in a better position to correlate the radiologic findings with history and physical examination. However, if the radiologic findings are highly specific and the referring physician fails to report, the obligation for reporting then falls to the radiologist. Statutes requiring the reporting of suspected cases of child abuse are in place throughout the United States and Canada. The radiologist can suggest, support, or even establish the diagnosis of child abuse. Radiologic findings may range from suggestive to virtually pathognomonic (Table 5.2); normal radiographs do not exclude the possibility, however. Abused children often present with misleading histories and complaints, and an absent, inconsistent, or implausible history of injury raises the suspicion of abuse. In this circumstance, the radiologic report may become a key medicolegal document.

The skeletal survey is the usual screening examination for evidence of abuse. In children 2 years of age or younger, a full skeletal survey with the best technique available for bone detail is required. A single view of the entire baby, including skull, trunk, and extremities (babygram), is almost never adequate or satisfactory. The skull, trunk, and extremities should all be examined and are best radiographed separately. In children older than 2 years of age, radiologic findings are limited to those in whom there is a history or physical evidence of inflicted trauma; in these, radiologic screening can be limited to the specific areas of suspicion. In a few imaging departments, the radionuclide bone scan is used for screening. Compared to the skeletal survey, the bone scan has higher sensitivity but greater cost and lower specificity. A high level of technical and interpretive expertise is required to perform high-quality bone scans in young children. Many use the bone scan only when there is a high level of suspicion but a normal skeletal survey.

The most common fractures seen in child abuse are spiral fractures of the femur and tibia, fractures of the clavicle, and simple linear fractures of the skull outside the occiput. These fractures are not specific to child abuse and may also occur with accidental trauma. Child abuse is likely when injuries are discovered that are more extensive or more severe than the history given for the trauma; when the injuries are of different ages, indicating prior episodes of trauma; or when there is fracture without adequate explanation. Some skeletal injuries are highly specific to child abuse regardless of the clinical circumstance. Patterns of fractures that are specific to child abuse are caused by indirect torsional, acceleration, and deceleration forces generated when an infant is gripped around the thorax or by the extremities and shaken violently. Massive forces develop as the head and extremities flail about. Torsional and tractional forces are applied as an infant is twisted or pulled by an extremity. The radiologic alterations from such forces are found in infants and young children.

In the long bones of the extremities, radiologic-pathologic studies have shown the fundamental lesion to be a series of microfractures occurring in a plane through the immature metaphyseal primary spongiosa, which is the zone of growing bone where delicate trabeculae are first apposed to central calcified cores. The fracture fragment consists of a thin plate of bone, calcified cartilage, the growth plate, and the attached epiphysis. This fracture is recognized as a transverse subepiphyseal lucency with an adjacent linear density abutting the growth plate. If the fragment is tipped or viewed obliquely, it has a bucket-handle appearance. If the periphery is thicker than the central portion, it has a corner fracture appearance (Figs. 5.35 and 5.36). These metaphyseal lesions are injuries highly specific for intentional injury and differ from the usual Salter types of growth plate fractures, in which the fracture plane is between the calcified and uncalcified zones of cartilage. Shaking may also separate a long bone from its periosteal envelope,

## TABLE 5.2 Skeletal Injuries in Child Abuse

High specificity
  Classic metaphyseal lesions
  Rib fractures, especially posterior
  Scapular fractures
  Spinous process fractures
  Sternal fractures

Moderate specificity
  Multiple fractures, especially bilateral
  Fractures of different ages
  Epiphyseal separations
  Vertebral body fractures and subluxations
  Digital fractures
  Complex skull fractures

Low specificity
  Subperiosteal new bone formation
  Clavicular fractures
  Long-bone shaft fractures
  Linear skull fractures

*Source*: Kleinman PK. *Diagnostic Imaging of Child Abuse*. 2nd Ed. St. Louis, MO: Mosby–Year Book; 1998.

**A**

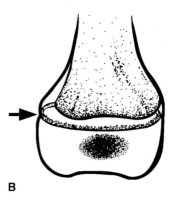

**B**

**FIGURE 5.35.** Corner fracture of child abuse. **A:** Distal femur radiograph of a 6-month-old girl shows a corner fracture (*arrow*). **B:** Diagram of the metaphyseal lesion that is pathognomonic of child abuse. The fracture plane extends through the metaphysis just beneath the growth plate. Because the bone plate is often very thin, it may only be visible in areas of overlap (*arrow*) or after the start of healing.

leading to subperiosteal hemorrhage and periosteal elevation. Once the periosteum begins to make new reactive bone, its displaced position becomes evident (Fig. 5.37).

In the head, violent shaking produces rapid rotational accelerations and decelerations of the brain within the skull. Disruption of the bridging veins between the cortical surface and the dural sinuses results in subdural hematoma, often interhemispheric. Subarachnoid hemorrhage may also occur, but not epidural hemorrhage.

If the child's head strikes a wall or other solid object while he or she is being shaken, skull fractures may occur in the occipital or posterior parietal regions. Accidental intracranial trauma is so rare in early childhood that virtually all serious intracranial injuries in infants have been intentionally inflicted. In the absence of an adequate history of massive trauma, skull fractures that are depressed, complex, or associated with dural tear are probably caused by abuse. The incidence of skull fractures in infants after accidental falls is

**FIGURE 5.36.** Healing metaphyseal fracture in a 1-month-old boy. The original extent of ossification is indicated by the *arrowhead*; the extent of the new bone made by the fractured and displaced metaphysis and growth plate is indicated by the *arrow*.

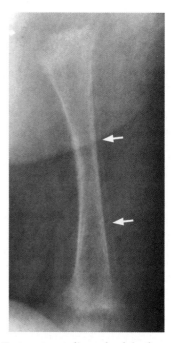

**FIGURE 5.37.** Postmortem radiograph of the femur of a 5-month-old girl shows periosteal elevation from subperiosteal hemorrhage with early reactive bone (*arrows*).

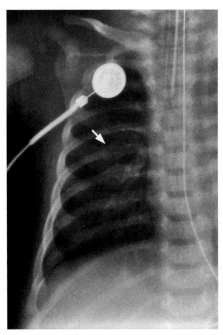

**FIGURE 5.38.** Posterior rib fractures (*arrow*) in a 5-week-old boy with advanced callus formation indicating that the fractures are at least 14 days old.

**FIGURE 5.39.** Bone scan of a 1-month-old girl shows three separate sets of rib fractures (*arrows*). The two sets of posterior rib fractures are virtually pathognomonic for child abuse.

not higher than 2%; these fractures are generally narrow, linear, and uncomplicated. Head injuries may be acutely life threatening; in survivors, posttraumatic long-term developmental effects such as mental retardation and learning disabilities are common. Fractures are best detected by plain films, and intracranial injuries are best demonstrated by MRI. Facial fractures are unusual in child abuse.

Rib fractures may result from AP compression of the rib cage when a child is grabbed around the trunk and shaken. This compression causes fractures of the inside cortex of the posterior portions of the ribs and the outside cortex of the lateral portions at multiple contiguous levels (Figs. 5.38 and 5.39). Rib fractures at these sites also may occur in motor vehicle collisions, but not as a result of falls or attempted cardiopulmonary resuscitation.

It may become critical to establish the age of a fracture by radiologic appearance in relation to the historical timing of the trauma. Dating fractures by roentgenography is imprecise. In general, a fracture with definite but slight periosteal new bone may be as recent as 4 to 7 days old. Unless immobilized or internally fixed, a fracture that is 20 days old will almost always have well-defined periosteal new bone and soft callus. A fracture with a large amount of periosteal new bone or callus is more than 14 days old. Long-bone fractures in infants heal with widespread periosteal new bone formation.

The radiologic differential diagnosis of extremity fractures in child abuse is limited.

## SOURCES AND READINGS

Beaty JH, Kasser JR. *Rockwood and Wilkins' Fractures in Children*. 6th Ed. Philadelphia, PA: Lippincott Williams & Wilkins; 2005.

Caffey J. Multiple fractures in the long bones of children suffering from chronic subdural hematoma. *AJR*. 1946;56:163–173.

Chew FS, Maldjian C. *Broken Bones: The X-ray Atlas of Fractures*. Seattle, WA: BareBonesBooks.com; 2009.

eMedicine. http://emedicine.medscape.com.

Futami T, Foster BK, Morris LL, et al. Magnetic resonance imaging of growth plate injuries: The efficacy and indications for surgical procedures. *Arch Orthop Trauma Surg*. 2000;120:390–396.

Griffin LY. *Essentials of Musculoskeletal Care*. 3rd Ed. Rosemont, IL: American Academy of Orthopedics; 2005.

Helfer RE, Kempe RS, Krugman RD, eds. *The Battered Child*. 5th Ed. Chicago, IL: University of Chicago Press; 1997.

John SD. Trends in pediatric emergency imaging. *Radiol Clin North Am*. 1999;37:995–1034.

Kao SC, Smith WL. Skeletal injuries in the pediatric patient. *Radiol Clin North Am*. 1997;35:727–746.

Keats TE, Smith TH. *An Atlas of Normal Developmental Roentgen Anatomy*. 7th Ed. Chicago, IL: Year Book; 2002.

Kleinman PK. *Diagnostic Imaging of Child Abuse*. 2nd Ed. St. Louis, MO: Mosby–Year Book; 1998.

Morrissy RT, Weinstein SL. *Lovell and Winter's Pediatric Orthopaedics*. 6th Ed. Philadelphia, PA: Lippincott Williams & Wilkins; 2005.

Ogden JA. Injury to the growth mechanisms of the immature skeleton. *Skeletal Radiol*. 1981;6:237–253.

Perron AD, Miller MD, Brady WJ. Orthopedic pitfalls in the ED: Pediatric growth plate injuries. *Am J Emerg Med*. 2002;20:50–54.

Reynolds R. Pediatric spinal injury. *Curr Opin Pediatr*. 2000;12:67–71.

Rhemrev SJ, Ekkelkamp S, Sleeboom C. Epiphyseal fractures of the proximal tibia. *Injury*. 2000;31:131–134.

Rogers LF. *Radiology of Skeletal Trauma*. 3rd Ed. New York, NY: Churchill Livingstone; 2002.

Salter RB, Harris WR. Injuries involving the epiphyseal plate. *J Bone Joint Surg Am*. 1963;45A:587–622.

Staheli LT. *Fundamentals of Pediatric Orthopedics*. 4th Ed. Philadelphia, PA: Lippincott Williams & Wilkins; 2007.

Wenger DR, Pring ME. *Rang's Children's Fractures*. 3rd Ed. Philadelphia, PA: Lippincott Williams & Wilkins; 2005.

Wheeless CR III, ed. *Wheeless' Textbook of Orthopaedics*. http://www.wheelessonline.com.

# 6 Imaging of Fracture Treatment and Healing

The seriousness of an injury is not always related to the radiographic severity of the fracture. The patient's general state of health, associated injuries and conditions, degree of soft-tissue injury, and consistency of underlying bone can have a vast influence on outcome. For example, a minimally displaced, closed femur fracture in a frail, osteoporotic woman is often life threatening, whereas a comminuted, displaced femoral fracture in an otherwise healthy child probably is not. In choosing the mode of fracture treatment, considerations other than the location and morphology of the fracture are crucial.

## FRACTURE HEALING

The natural history of an uncomplicated long-bone fracture is union through the formation of callus. This *secondary fracture healing* occurs in three stages: an inflammatory stage, a reparative stage, and a remodeling stage (Table 6.1 and Fig. 6.1). Immediately after the fracture, hematoma and devitalization of soft tissues and bone at the fracture site provoke an acute, intense inflammatory reaction. On radiographs, soft-tissue swelling and sharp fracture lines are present. By 10 to 14 days after injury, the fracture lines may have become more readily visible because of bone resorption. Acute regional osteoporosis of the involved extremity, caused by the hyperemia that accompanies inflammation, is usual (Fig. 6.2). As the hematoma organizes into granulation tissue capable of osteogenesis, the reparative phase begins. External periosteal callus is formed in the subperiosteal regions adjacent to the fracture. Fibrous tissue, cartilage, and immature bone form within the mass of granulation tissue around the fracture. This mass, called *primary* or *soft callus*, is fusiform in shape and bridges the fracture gap. In the proper environment of ample blood supply and limited motion and stress, the primary callus forms bone.

Ossification in primary callus may be seen on radiographs as early as 10 days after injury in children and 2 weeks in adults. Because external callus expands the diameter of the bone at the site of fracture healing, often by a factor of 2 or 3, mechanical stability (clinical union) is generally achieved within 6 to 12 weeks. Radiographs should show abundant, well-defined callus bridging the fracture site, with fracture lines becoming fuzzy. Bone repair continues with the formation of intramedullary (IM) callus and the eventual remodeling of woven bone to lamellar bone along the lines of stress. Remodeling of callus may take place over a period of months to years. In time, there may be scant radiographic indication of the previous fracture. By contrast, fractures of cancellous bone, particularly if impacted, tend to form internal callus rather than external callus as they heal. Healing in a fracture that is wholly confined to cancellous trabeculae may be evident radiographically only as increasing and then decreasing sclerosis at the fracture site (Fig. 6.3).

Injuries of the soft tissues heal through the process of localized necrosis, inflammation, and repair. Ligament and tendon injuries heal with a bridging scar if the ends are not too far distracted. The scar may eventually remodel along the lines of stress. Cartilage heals through a different process because of the lack of vascularization. Localized necrosis occurs, but there is no inflammatory phase. Superficial injuries that do not extend to the bone marrow heal by migration of cells from the synovial fluid or from elsewhere in the cartilage. In injuries that extend to the bone marrow, an initial blood clot is replaced by granulation tissue. The resulting fibrous scar undergoes progressive hyalinization and chondrification to become fibrocartilage.

## CLOSED FRACTURE TREATMENT

The vast majority of fractures are treated closed, that is, without open surgery. The fractures in soft tissues are reduced, and the fracture is stabilized but not completely immobilized. Muscle activity, joint motion, and load transmission promote external callus formation. The two common methods of closed fracture treatment are casts and traction.

Casts can be used to reduce and control fractures with angular deformity through three-point fixation. The cast is shaped so that it pushes at the apex of the fracture and at the opposite ends

| TABLE 6.1 | Stages of Fracture Healing | |
|---|---|---|
| **Stage** | **Time Frame** | **Tissue at Fracture Site** |
| Inflammatory | Days to weeks | Hematoma and granulation tissue |
| Reparative | Weeks to months | Callus |
| Remodeling | Months to years | Remodeling bone |

A    B    C

**FIGURE 6.1.** Fracture healing of cortical bone without fixation in an adult. **A:** Acute fracture of the humeral shaft. **B:** At 6 weeks, calcified callus is visible and the fracture lines are becoming obscured. **C:** At 12 weeks, the fracture has almost completely healed.

of the bone, tending to keep it straight. Slow-setting plaster of Paris (Fig. 6.4) is applied while reduction maneuvers are performed. Casts are typically applied over a stockinette and a layer of padding so that a radiolucent zone is present between the limb and the cast on radiographs. A second layer of cast material can be applied to provide strength and durability. Plaster casts are often covered with a layer of fiberglass for durability and may be replaced completely by fiberglass as the fracture begins to heal and the patient regains the use of the limb (Fig. 6.5). Fiberglass casts can be made into more functional braces through the addition of hinges where the cast crosses a joint. Some fractures of the thoracic and lumbar spine are treated with casts or braces that envelop the torso and stabilize the spine by compressing the soft tissues of the abdomen. The position and alignment of reduced fractures of the limbs can be maintained

**FIGURE 6.2.** Acute osteoporosis accompanying fracture healing. Radiograph 6 weeks after injury shows subchondral bone resorption (*arrow*).

**FIGURE 6.3.** Sclerosis (*arrow*) indicates healing fracture in the cancellous bone of the calcaneus.

**FIGURE 6.4.** Plaster cast applied to distal radius fracture.

in a similar manner. The shape and relative rigidity of the cast use the patient's own soft tissues to turn the cast into a fluid-filled cylinder that resists swelling and deformation. Stable fractures, when subjected to normal stresses, maintain their reduction. External supports such as casts, splints, or braces are load-sharing devices that restrict motion after a stable fracture has been reduced. Traction can be applied and maintained in a variety of ways. Skin traction, in which the limb is gripped with adhesive bandages and connected to a system of hanging weights, is seldom used except for femoral fractures in small children. Skeletal traction is applied by placing pins into the extremity distal to the fracture and connecting the pins

to weights. Dynamic traction allows the physiologic motion that is generally beneficial to the formation of periosteal callus. Traction on fractures of the clavicle and proximal humerus can be applied with a figure-of-eight harness and a long-arm cast, respectively. The upper limb itself becomes the hanging weight, and the direction of traction depends on the point of suspension along the cast. Some fractures of the cervical spine are treated with a halo brace that functions on the same principle but works against gravity by stretching the neck.

# ■ OPEN REDUCTION AND INTERNAL FIXATION

Open reduction and internal fixation (osteosynthesis) requires surgical exposure of the fracture. The fracture is reduced, the soft tissues are repaired, and the fragments are fixed with hardware. If a bone undergoes plastic deformation before fracturing, the fracture fragments may not fit back together because of the distortion in shape that preceded the fracture. Fracture fixation hardware does not substitute for the native bony structure; rather, it provides temporary mechanical stability while the natural healing process occurs.

A

B

**FIGURE 6.6.** Healing internally fixed transverse fracture of the ulna with posterior butterfly fragment. **A:** Immediate postoperative film shows a cortical plate has fixed the fragments of the transverse portion of the fracture with 1 to 2 mm distraction (*short arrow*) while the oblique fractures are compressed (*black arrow*). **B:** After 7 weeks, endosteal callus bridges the transverse fracture (*arrow*) and the oblique fractures have remodeled and disappeared.

**FIGURE 6.5.** Fiberglass cast applied to distal radius fracture.

The stability that comes with internal fixation is crucial to rapid restoration of mobility and function; many patients cannot tolerate bed rest and prolonged hospitalization. Fixation devices include screws, plates, rods, pins, nails, and wires. Many fixation devices can be inserted percutaneously under fluoroscopic guidance or through minimal incisions. A second operation is necessary to remove many types of hardware after the fractures have healed.

Internal fixation that holds bone fragments together rigidly promotes direct bony union (primary fracture healing). New intracortical haversian systems drill across the fracture site, leaving cores of new bone. Fracture callus is minimal or absent as the osteocytes remodel the fracture away (Fig. 6.6). On radiographs, primary fracture healing is seen as a gradual disappearance of the fracture line. A gap between fragments or excessive motion at the fracture site interferes with the migration of osteocytes across the fracture plane, and the fracture heals through the formation of periosteal and endosteal callus. Secondary fracture healing occurs more slowly in fractures with internal fixation because restriction of motion interferes with formation of callus.

Internal fixation devices are designed to function on the biomechanical principles of static or dynamic interfragmentary compression, bridging, or splintage. In static compression, a metal implant holds the fracture fragments together under compression. In dynamic compression, the implant transforms physiologic loading into compression at the fracture site. There is direct bony union in both types of compression. Internal fixation bridges a fracture site when it is secured to uninjured bone on either side of the fracture. Physiologic loads are transferred from the bone on one side of the fracture to the bone on the other side. If the fragments are not directly apposed and there is motion between them, periosteal and endosteal callus fills the gaps between the bones. Length and alignment are maintained while the bones heal. Internal fixation devices that function as internal splints allow motion at the fracture site and promote periosteal callus while maintaining reduction.

## ■ SCREWS

Orthopedic screws are available in a variety of sizes and shapes, often for use in specific circumstances (Fig. 6.7). The parts of a screw are the head, shaft, thread, and tip. Most types of screws have a head socketed to receive a hexagonal shaft driver and a threaded shank. The heads have a hemispheric undersurface that allows contact even when the screw is inclined. Screws used for cancellous bone have a wider thread

**A**  **B**  **C**  **D**

**FIGURE 6.7.** Common types of orthopedic screws. **A:** Compression or lag screw. **B:** Cannulated compression screw. **C:** Fully threaded screw with cancellous threads. **D:** Fully threaded screws with cortical threads.

**FIGURE 6.8.** Ankle fracture with internal fixation. Two cannulated lag screws (*long arrow*) with cancellous threads fix the medial malleolus. The cortical plate is fixed to the fibular shaft by three screws (*short arrow*) with cortical threads, and to the lateral malleolus by two cancellous screws (*arrowhead*).

diameter relative to the core shank diameter and a deeper thread pitch (larger distance between threads) than screws used for cortical bone (Fig. 6.8). Most screws are inserted into drill holes. These holes may be tapped or threaded to receive a screw, or the screw may be self-tapping and cut its own threads as it is driven into the hole.

**FIGURE 6.9.** Bioabsorbable screw. Radiograph of the foot shows lucency indicating drill hole for bioabsorbable screw fixing first and second metatarsals (*arrow*).

**FIGURE 6.10.** Headless, tapered, variable thread pitch compression screw (*arrow*) fixing scaphoid waist fracture.

Cannulated screws are hollow in the center. These allow the placement of screws over a guide wire, improving the ability of the orthopedist to place screws accurately without the need for supplementary clamp fixation of the site. Some cannulated screws are self-drilling and self-tapping and can be percutaneously inserted over a guide wire. Screws are made of metal, commonly stainless steel or titanium alloy. Bioabsorbable screws and other nonmetallic orthopedic implants for fracture fixation may be difficult to recognize on radiographs, but have markedly decreased artifacts on MRI (Fig. 6.9).

When screws are used to secure bony fragments to each other, they are called *interfragmentary screws*. Interfragmentary screws work biomechanically by converting torque applied to the screw into axial tension between the bone fragments. When screws are used to secure cortical plates or other hardware to bone, they are called *position screws* or *neutralization screws*.

Headless screws are used where the presence of a head may interfere with motion or cause soft-tissue irritation. Headless screws may be inserted below the surface of the bone, which is desirable in osteochondral fractures and intra-articular fractures. Screws with heads may also be inserted flush with the bone surface by countersinking or drilling a larger hole for the head to drop into as the screw is driven.

Compression screws, also called *lag screws*, are threaded only at the distal portion of the shank. This type of screw compresses two objects together (bone against bone or bone against another fixation device). The object into which the screw is threaded is pulled against the object through which the screw is passed. Maximal compression is obtained when the screw is oriented perpendicular to the fracture plane. A fully threaded screw fixes objects together without compressing them because the threads force them to maintain their relative positions. Screws that are fully threaded along their shanks may also be used in compression if the drill hole near the head (the glide hole) is drilled to a size that the threads pass through freely. Subsequent extraction of screws is easier if they are fully threaded. The *Acutrak screw* is a headless, fully threaded, cannulated screw with a tapered profile and a variable thread pitch (Fig. 6.10). The thread

**A**                                                    **B**

**FIGURE 6.11.** Fixation for intertrochanteric fractures. **A:** Telescoping (dynamic) hip screw fixing an intertrochanteric fracture. **B:** Percutaneous compression plate fixing an intertrochanteric fracture. Note the small size of the skin incisions, as indicated by the skin staples.

pitch is wider at one end of the screw, so that each turn of the screw compresses fragments together because of the difference in thread pitch. These screws are commonly used for internal fixation of intra-articular fractures of small bones such as the scaphoid. Were it not for the cost, they could be exceedingly useful in cabinetmaking.

Dynamic hip screws (telescoping hip screw, sliding hip screw) (Fig. 6.11) and dynamic condylar screws with side-plates are designed for dynamic compression of fractures of the proximal and distal femur, respectively. The screw fits into a sleeve in the side-plate into which it can slide or telescope. In an intertrochanteric hip fracture, for example, the screw extends through the femoral neck into the head, and the side-plate is fixed to the lateral cortex of the proximal shaft. With weight bearing, the unthreaded shank of the screw slides into the sleeve at the end of the side-plate, compressing the fracture fragments together. A smaller set screw that is threaded into the near end of the large-diameter sliding screw can be used to apply static compression to the fracture site at the time of surgery.

# WIRES AND CABLES

Kirschner wires (K-wires) are used to fix cancellous bone in situations in which a screw might also be suitable. They are introduced percutaneously, and their purchase in bone is exclusively by friction (Fig. 6.12), which makes them easier to pull out than screws. The end of the wire is typically left protruding from the skin so that the wires can be extracted when the fracture heals.

A tension band transforms tensile stress into interfragmentary compression (Fig. 6.13). Tension bands are commonly used where asymmetric muscle tension tends to distract fragments. The tension band is usually a wire loop or figure-of-eight that is placed across the fracture site along the line of tensile force. When the muscle contracts, the tension band acts like a hinge to compress the

fracture fragments together. For example, a transverse fracture of the olecranon process could be fixed by a tension band along the posterior aspect of the triceps mechanism. With contraction of the triceps muscles, the tension band functions as a hinge and converts the distractive force along the posterior aspect of the olecranon to compressive force on the opposite side (Fig. 6.14). Tension bands are also commonly used to fix transverse fractures of the patella.

**FIGURE 6.12.** K-wire fixation. Radiograph of hand shows two K-wires fixing a fracture of the proximal phalanx of the middle finger.

**FIGURE 6.13.** Biomechanical concept of tension band fixation. The band acts as a hinge, transforming tension on the olecranon into interfragmentary compression.

Cerclage wires encircle the shaft of a bone and can be used to hold fragments to the shaft. They are usually placed in combination with IM rods or cortical plates. Wires are made of stainless steel and cobalt chrome alloy and are commonly in the form of monofilament wires or high-tension braided cables with multiple filaments attached with a crimp (Fig. 6.15).

## ◼ PLATES

Cortical plates placed on the periosteal surface are secured to bone by position screws and should be considered internal splints for holding together structural defects and not load-bearing members. Compression across the fracture components is critical to protect the plate from failure. Plates function through the biomechanical principles of static compression, dynamic compression,

**FIGURE 6.15.** High tension braided cable used for cerclage at the femoral shaft. The ends of the cable are secured by a crimp (*arrow*).

buttressing, and neutralization. Static compression can be maintained by a plate when it is applied while the fracture site is being compressed during surgery (Fig. 6.16). Compression can also be applied through specially designed screw holes and eccentrically placed screws. Locking plates are cortical plates in which some of the screw holes are designed to constrain the position of the screw that is fitted to it, preventing it from toggling and fixing the relative

**FIGURE 6.14.** Tension band fixing olecranon fracture. The tension band passes through a hole drilled in the posterior ulnar cortex and hooks over the head of the K-wires.

**FIGURE 6.16.** Dynamic compression plate (*arrow*) fixing fractures of the distal radial shaft. Note the eccentric screw placement in the oval holes of the plate. Malleable plates have been used to fix fractures of the ulnar shaft.

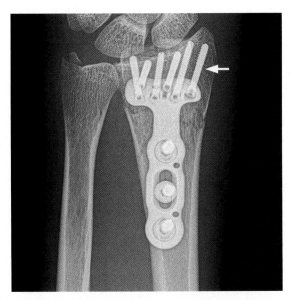

**FIGURE 6.17.** Locked T-shaped plate fixing distal radius fractures with locking screws (*arrow*) distally and nonlocking screws proximally.

**FIGURE 6.18.** Buttress plate fixating proximal metaphyseal fracture of the tibia.

positions of the plate and fracture fragment (Fig. 6.17). Small plates may be used to fix small fragments. When placed on a bone with asymmetric muscle pull such as the femur, a plate placed with initial static compression may subsequently function with dynamic compression through the tension band principle when weight bearing resumes. Plates can also be contoured to fit the particular shape of the bone to which they are applied, either at the time of manufacture or at the time of surgery. Buttress plates are broader on one end than the other and may be used to fix metaphyseal fractures of long bones such as the distal radius or the proximal tibia (Fig. 6.18). A buttress plate used dynamically transforms shearing stress directed along the longitudinal axis of the bone into compressive force across the fracture plane. Neutralization

plates counter the stresses on an internally fixed fracture but are not intended to provide interfragmentary compression. When neutralization plates are used to maintain length and position, one or more interfragmentary screws are also used to hold the fracture fragments together. The interfragmentary screws are generally oriented perpendicular to the fracture plane for maximum compression. Interfragmentary screws may also pass through one of the holes in the neutralization plate.

Recent developments in plate technology have emphasized low-profile designs for specific anatomic sites and specific types of fractures. An example is at the distal radius, a common site of fracture, where cortical plates have become much smaller and specific plates are available for various subtypes of fractures (Fig. 6.19).

**A**

**B**

**FIGURE 6.19.** Specialized cortical plates for distal radius fixation. **A:** Small cortical plates and screws fixing a comminuted intra-articular fracture. **B:** Contoured low-profile cortical plate fixing a comminuted intra-articular fracture. The unused small distal holes are designed for locking screws.

**FIGURE 6.20.** Cortical plate used as a bridge for comminuted intra-articular fractures of the distal radius and ulna.

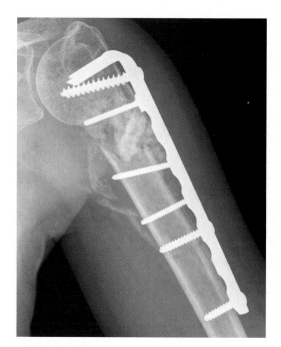

**FIGURE 6.21.** Blade plate traversing a comminuted proximal humerus fracture.

Cortical plates can be used for bridging a comminuted distal radius fracture (Fig. 6.20). In this circumstance, the bridge extends from the radial shaft, across the fracture site and the carpal bones, to the third metacarpal.

A blade plate is a cortical plate with an angled blade that is inserted sideways into the end of a bone while the plate is affixed to the cortex of the shaft with position screws. Blade plates are used at sites such as the proximal femur, the distal femur, and the proximal humerus (Fig. 6.21), where normal muscle pull would tend to destabilize

a simple plate. Blade plates have been replaced in many circumstances by telescoping screws with side-plates and by specialized IM rods.

## ■ RODS AND NAILS

IM rods or nails are used to treat long-bone fractures. In closed nailing, the rod is inserted into one end of the fractured bone and passed across the fracture site under fluoroscopic guidance.

A

B

**FIGURE 6.22.** Antegrade IM rod fixing a femoral shaft fracture. **A:** Proximal locking screws (*arrows*). **B:** Distal locking screws (*arrows*).

**FIGURE 6.23.** Femoral shaft fracture fixed by two Enders rods inserted retrograde through the condyles. Note that the distal physis has not been disturbed.

**FIGURE 6.24.** Gamma nail fixation of a subtrochanteric femur fracture.

In open nailing, the rod is passed across the fracture site under direct surgical visualization. The medullary space is usually reamed so that it can accommodate the rod, destroying the endosteal blood supply but depositing finely morselized bone and marrow elements at the fracture site; this osseous autograft enhances fracture healing. The endosteal blood supply reconstitutes in approximately 3 weeks. The periosteal blood supply is preserved. An IM rod typically functions as a load-sharing device or an internal splint. Small, flexible IM rods can be placed into small non–weight-bearing bones. Larger bones require larger, more rigid IM rods for fixation and strength. If the rod is locked on both ends by cross screws (Fig. 6.22), it ceases to function as a load-sharing device and becomes a load-bearing device. When the limb is loaded, the stresses are transferred from the bone to one end of the rod by the cross-screws, travel along the length of the rod past the fracture site, and finally are dispersed by the cross-screws at the other end, thus preventing load on the fracture site. Locking also allows control and reduction of rotary displacement. As periosteal callus is formed and the fracture begins to stabilize, one set of locking screws may be removed, allowing load sharing by the healing bone. This technique of removing the locking screws from the longer fragment is called *dynamization*.

Rods may be inserted across a fracture site in an antegrade fashion or a retrograde fashion. The direction of insertion can be identified on radiographs by the locations of the blunt and tapered ends, with the tapered end pointing in the direction of insertion and the blunt end located at the site of insertion. In children, to avoid traversing an open growth plate and risking premature closure, a pair of Enders rods may be inserted through the metaphysis and across the fracture site (Fig. 6.23).

New designs in IM rods have resulted in rods intended for fractures of specific bones, including the humerus, radius, ulna, femur, and tibia. These rods take into account the biomechanical requirements of each site as well as the unique anatomy and the technical demands of the various operative sites. For example, the gamma nail is designed specifically for subtrochanteric femur fractures (Fig. 6.24).

## ■ EXTERNAL FIXATION

External fixation allows a fractured limb to be reduced or stabilized by the manipulation of externally projecting pins or wires secured to the limb on both sides of the fracture site. Surgical trauma to the fracture site is avoided. The fixation is more rigid and allows earlier mobility than closed methods. The fractures unite by secondary bone healing. External fixation is favored for types II and III open fractures, in which distraction of the limb is appropriate and rapid surgical stabilization is necessary. The two major types of external fixators are pins attached to rods (pin fixators) and wires stretched on circular frames that are attached to rods (ring fixators). Pin fixators are secured to bone with pins that are introduced surgically or percutaneously (Fig. 6.25). Different fixator configurations can be tailored to the specific fracture site and morphology. Many fractures require external fixation in two planes for stability. Pin fixators can be applied rapidly in emergent situations and are used often for pelvic fractures in which early reduction and fixation can realign the soft tissues and avert life-threatening hemorrhage. Ring fixators (Ilizarov fixators) are secured to bone through a pair of crossed, unthreaded, transfixion

**FIGURE 6.25.** Comminuted intra-articular fractures of the distal radius and ulna. The distal radius fragments have been fixed by K-wires. The entire wrist has been stabilized by a pin-rod external fixator.

**FIGURE 6.26.** Ilizarov external fixator for treatment of nonunion (*arrow*).

wires that are stretched on a circular frame. These circular frames are attached to longitudinal connecting rods. The fragments are reduced by adjusting the position of the rings relative to each other. A nonunion may be addressed by compression to induce healing followed by distraction to restore length (Fig. 6.26). A fragment of bone can be transported axially by successive adjustments of the rings along the longitudinal rods on the order of 1 mm/day (Fig. 6.27). Modular systems of external fixation allow

the surgeon to fit hybrid frames to complex, complicated fractures using both pins and rings.

# SOFT-TISSUE HEALING AND REPAIR

Tendon and ligament healing occurs in phases. Initially, the wound fills with blood, inflammatory products, and fibrin. Proliferating granulation tissue then fills the gap, and over a period of weeks to

**A**        **B**

**FIGURE 6.27.** Hybrid pin-rod and ring external fixation for bone transport following loss of a segment of bone during an open tibial fracture. **A:** Lateral radiograph 1 month following trauma shows the large distal gap (*arrowheads*) in the tibial shaft, a proximal tibial osteotomy (*arrow*), and a bone fragment (*F*) attached to the pin-rod appliance. **B:** Lateral radiograph at 6 months shows distal transport of the fragment (*F*), narrowing the distal gap (*arrowheads*) in the tibial shaft. The osteotomy has been stretched apart as the fragment has been transported, and the gap is filled with calcifying callus (*arrow*).

**FIGURE 6.28.** Soft-tissue anchors in the distal humerus (*arrow*).

**FIGURE 6.29.** Bone graft (*arrows*) for open fracture of the ankle.

months, fibroblasts and collagen fibers begin to unite the injured ends. The healing tissue then remodels and matures as the fibroblasts and collagen fibers become oriented along the lines of stress, a process that may continue over many months. Direct repair of tendons and ligaments is generally performed by suturing the injured ends together. When a soft-tissue structure has been avulsed from a bony attachment, it may be reattached using a variety of devices, including sutures, wires, screws, pins, and soft-tissue anchors. When screws are used, washers are generally placed between the screw head and the soft tissues to increase the surface area apposed to the bone and to decrease trauma caused by the screw itself. Soft-tissue anchors are small devices that are embedded into the bone and have loops through which sutures may be passed (Fig. 6.28). Soft-tissue anchors are available in a variety of sizes, shapes, and materials, including plastic, metal, and bioabsorbable materials. With healing, the biomechanical integrity of the soft-tissue attachment is reestablished, and the fixation device is no longer needed.

# GRAFTS AND IMPLANTS

Soft-tissue grafts and bone grafts are commonly used to reconstruct severe open fractures, particularly where significant fragments of bone have been ejected from the limb at the time of trauma or debrided at the time of initial treatment (Fig. 6.29). Bone grafts used for trauma reconstruction are more commonly small pieces of corticocancellous bone rather than massive allografts. Large defects in cortical bone are generally reconstructed by bone transport rather than grafting.

Structural biomaterials as substitutes for bone is an active area of research in orthopedics. Materials gaining widespread use in the United States include genetically engineered bone growth factors, bioabsorbable hardware, and metallic implants with bone-like mechanical and physical properties.

# SPINE FIXATION

Because of the complex anatomy, the presence of the spinal cord and nerve roots, the small bones, and the large number of joints, fixation of the spinal column after trauma requires specialized hardware and techniques.

Stable injuries of the posterior column may require only fixation of the posterior elements at the levels involved. Many cervical spine injuries are treated with reduction and fusion of the posterior elements using wires and bone graft. Posterior column injuries may also be treated with pedicle screws and rods, a process in which a series of pedicle screws inserted posteriorly are attached to contoured rods. Depending on the biomechanical stresses at the level of injury, multiple levels above and below the injury may be included in the stabilization procedure (Fig. 6.30). Anterior column fractures such as compression fractures can be treated by internal fixation of the vertebral bodies above and below the level of injury with plates and screws and restoration of the height of the fractured vertebra using bone graft. The bone graft may be structural allograft or small corticocancellous chips and fragments, maintained in place by a wire fusion cage (Fig. 6.31).

Unstable injuries involving the anterior and posterior columns generally require both anterior and posterior stabilization. The rods may be placed posterior to the spine and secured to the vertebral bodies by pedicle screws above and below the level of injury. Anterior stabilization can be performed with bone graft, hardware, or a combination. At the time of surgery, the spinal canal is also decompressed.

Simple osteoporotic compression fractures may be treated by vertebroplasty. Vertebroplasty is a procedure in which methylmethacrylate cement is injected percutaneously under fluoroscopic guidance into the involved vertebral body (see Chapter 18). The injected cement is rendered radiodense so that it can be

**FIGURE 6.30.** T12 burst fracture treated with posterior fusion using pedicle screws and rods.

observed during fluoroscopy and on subsequent radiographs (Fig. 6.32).

## ■ COMPLICATIONS

Complications of fractures may be immediate or delayed (Table 6.2).

**FIGURE 6.31.** Treated T12 burst fracture. AP radiograph shows T12 corpectomy, with bone graft, and internal fixation. A fusion cage filled with bone graft has been inserted between T11 and L1.

**FIGURE 6.32.** Multiple osteoporotic compression fractures following vertebroplasty. Lateral radiograph shows osteoporosis with multiple wedging deformities, five of which have been treated by vertebroplasty.

## Failure of Fracture Healing

Fracture healing is impaired or slow when the patient is elderly or in poor nutritional condition, when the local blood supply is poor, and when the fragments are displaced rather than apposed. Intracapsular fractures (within the joint capsule) heal slowly because

| TABLE 6.2 | Fracture Complications |
| --- | --- |

Immediate complications

    Shock
    Hemorrhage
    Thromboembolism
    Disseminated intravascular coagulopathy
    Fat embolism
    Gas gangrene
    Tetanus
    Osteonecrosis
    Posttraumatic reflex sympathetic dystrophy
    Compartment syndrome
    Osteomyelitis

Delayed complications

    Failure to heal
    Posttraumatic degenerative joint disease
    Posttraumatic chondrolysis
    Remote stress injuries
    Refracture
    Chronic pain and instability
    Myositis ossificans
    Failure or migration of implant
    Synostosis

**FIGURE 6.33.** Humeral shaft fracture with atrophic nonunion and IM rod. The ends of the fragments have developed cortex (*arrow*).

**FIGURE 6.35.** Loose screws transfixing the syndesmosis for total ankle replacement. A thin zone of sclerosis (*arrows*) demarcates the region of bone resorption around the hardware.

the intracapsular part of the bone does not support periosteal callus formation, and synovial fluid lyses the blood clot. Necrotic bone fragments cannot participate in the healing process until they are revascularized. An extensive fracture heals more slowly than a limited one. A fracture through cortical bone heals more slowly than one through cancellous bone. A fracture with significant soft-tissue damage heals more slowly than one with little soft-tissue damage. An infected fracture will not heal.

Distraction of fragments or excessive motion between them may result in nonunion. Nonunion is an arrest of the healing process before there is bony union of the fragments. The bone ends become osteoporotic and atrophied or hypertrophic and sclerotic (Fig. 6.33; see Fig. 6.26). The space between the bony fragments usually contains dense fibrous tissue and sometimes may be clinically stable. Alternatively, a false joint lined with synovium and filled with synovial fluid (pseudoarthrosis) may form in the gap between ununited fracture fragments; this tends to occur when

there has been excessive motion at the fracture site. Malunion occurs when the fracture fragments heal in poor position or alignment so that functional or cosmetic problems ensue. The presence of malunion is a clinical, not a radiologic, diagnosis. Other notable variations in fracture healing include delayed union, in which there is a longer-than-average healing process, and slow union, in which the healing process is protracted but progressive.

Failure of an internally fixed fracture to heal is usually caused by a gap between fragments or excessive motion at the fracture site. The result is failure or loosening of the fixation device. Loosening is evident on radiographs by the presence of a lucent zone around the device. This lucent zone corresponds to resorption of bone, indicating that the device no longer has a stable purchase (Fig. 6.34). There is often a thin zone of sclerosis at the metal-bone interface (Fig. 6.35). Hardware that shifts in position from examination to examination may indicate loosening (Fig. 6.36). Catastrophic loss of fixation with breakage of hardware may occur when there is too

**FIGURE 6.34.** Loose plates and screws with fracture nonunions of the radius and ulna.

**FIGURE 6.36.** Loose screw (*arrow*) protruding into soft tissues.

A                                                                          B

**FIGURE 6.37.** Fractured plate at a comminuted distal radius fracture. **A:** Lateral radiograph 6 weeks after internal fixation shows mild dorsal angulation and bending of the volar cortical plate. **B:** Lateral radiograph 12 weeks after internal fixation shows progression of angulation with fracture of plate (*arrow*).

much biomechanical stress on the reconstructed part and there is progressive angulation or displacement (Fig. 6.37).

## Other Complications

Fat embolism is an acute complication that may occur when fatty marrow gains access to the venous system as a result of a fracture,

**FIGURE 6.38.** Talar neck fracture osteonecrosis. The talar dome is relatively denser than the surrounding bones, which have regional osteoporosis related to fracture healing.

usually of the long bones. Fat is liquid at body temperature and pours out of a fractured bone into the soft tissues, where it may enter the veins and travel to the lungs. Fat emboli appear to provoke a chemical pneumonitis rather than cause pulmonary infarction.

Avascular necrosis of bone may occur when the blood supply is compromised by the injury or by the fixation device. Normally, bones become osteoporotic in response to fracture healing. Avascular necrosis can be recognized on radiographs because necrotic, devascularized bone does not become osteoporotic (Fig. 6.38). Common sites of avascular necrosis after fracture include the femoral head, the proximal pole of the scaphoid, and the proximal pole of the talus. MRI may show osteonecrosis before radiographs.

Infection may occur as a complication of the primary injury or secondarily during treatment. Infection can be recognized radiographically as a nonhealing fracture with progressive bone loss, but the process may be far advanced before radiographic changes are noticeable (Fig. 6.39). External fixators are vulnerable to infection at the insertion sites of wires or pins through the skin into the bone (Fig. 6.40). Pin infections can be recognized by osteolysis at the site of insertion. Treatment of infected or potentially infected fractures typically includes debridement (the removal of contaminated or devitalized tissue) and antibiotic therapy. Antibiotic-impregnated beads may be placed directly into the site of infection (Fig. 6.41), and removed after the infection has resolved.

Untreated or unrecognized soft-tissue injuries may result in chronic pain and instability, often with devastating disability. This is a particular problem in the wrist, knee, and shoulder. MRI and arthrography are the two radiologic modalities most useful for delineating injuries to ligaments and cartilage in these regions.

A

B

**FIGURE 6.39.** Infected IM rod. **A:** Radiograph of the tibia shows lucencies and periosteal reaction (*arrow*) around the distal end of the rod. **B:** White cell scan shows intense accumulation of activity (*arrow*) around the distal end of the rod.

Posttraumatic reflex sympathetic dystrophy (complex regional pain syndrome, Sudeck atrophy) is a painful swelling of an extremity with rapid onset after an injury. The injury may be a fracture but is often minor. The site of swelling and pain is usually in the ipsilateral limb but remote from the site of trauma. The cause is thought to be neurovascular. Regional soft-tissue swelling and acute osteoporosis are evident at onset (Fig. 6.42). Soft-tissue atrophy may follow subsidence of the acute symptoms; the bone usually remains osteoporotic.

Failure of implanted orthopedic devices may lead to poor healing or chronic pain. Some implant failures have led to class action lawsuits and multimillion dollar payouts.

**FIGURE 6.40.** Infected pin-rod external fixator. Focal osteolysis (*arrows*) is present where the pins traverse the tibial cortex.

**FIGURE 6.41.** Antibiotic beads (*arrow*) at the site of an internally fixed open fracture.

**FIGURE 6.42.** Posttraumatic reflex sympathetic dystrophy. Acute osteoporosis and painful soft-tissue swelling of the entire hand 3 months after a fracture of the ipsilateral scapula.

Scars in bone may remain after removal of internal fixation devices. Small holes in the cortex from the removal of screws or pins do not fill in with bone but remodel by cortication of the edges (Fig. 6.43). During loading, stress tends to concentrate at irregularities in bone or at the sites of hardware. Subsequent fractures tend to begin at such "stress risers" (Fig. 6.44).

**FIGURE 6.44.** Tibial fracture line passes through screws from previous osteotomy.

Altered stresses and biomechanics related to a fracture may result in remote complications such as stress injuries to contralateral limbs. A fracture with mechanical fixation in place may not remodel because the site is shielded from mechanical stress. An insufficiency fracture may follow the removal of the fixation device.

**FIGURE 6.43.** Healed tracts in the proximal tibial shaft where a locked IM was used for fixation. The margins have become corticated.

**FIGURE 6.45.** Posttraumatic myositis ossificans.

**FIGURE 6.46.** Misplaced pedicle screw. Axial CT image following myelography shows a pedicle screw (*arrow*) extending into the spinal canal and neural foramen.

Posttraumatic degenerative joint disease may occur because of direct damage to the articular surfaces or the subchondral bone (see Chapter 13). Malunion and altered patterns of stress on joints adjacent to a fracture site may also lead to degenerative changes, particularly in weight-bearing joints. Posttraumatic chondrolysis is an articular complication in which there is rapid, generalized dissolution of the articular cartilage of the traumatized bones; the process is poorly understood.

Myositis ossificans is heterotopic ossification in the soft tissues. Posttraumatic myositis ossificans may follow soft-tissue injury, resulting in mature bone formation at the site (Fig. 6.45). Although mechanical problems may ensue, the heterotopic bone usually remodels and may ultimately be resorbed. Occasionally, myositis ossificans may be mistaken for sarcoma on MRI or other imaging, but clinical correlation and follow-up clarify the issue.

## Complications of Spine Fixation

Complications of spine fixation include misplacement of pedicle screws (Fig. 6.46), nerve root injury, dural sac tear, infection, and loss of fixation (Fig. 6.47). CT with myelography is often the best method for imaging the spine after fixation, although MRI can be safely used. Artifacts on MRI from metallic implants may render a study difficult to interpret.

## ■ IMAGING AFTER TREATMENT

Radiographs are the usual method of imaging fracture healing. Early radiographs may be obtained to check the accuracy of the reduction and the appropriateness of fixation device placement.

**A**    **B**

**FIGURE 6.47.** Failure of spinal fixation. **A:** Lateral radiographs show that pedicle screws inserted at L1 for posterior stabilization for superior endplate compression fracture of L2 have shifted in position, allowing the spine to collapse into kyphosis. **B:** Sagittal T1-weighted MRI excludes nonmechanical causes of failure.

**FIGURE 6.48.** Motion at fracture nonunion (*arrow*) demonstrated by AP radiograph with valgus stress.

Subsequent exams follow the healing process or investigate possible complications. The presence of hardware often requires nonstandard oblique views so that the fracture site is not obscured by the device. Sometimes, positioning under fluoroscopy may be helpful in projecting metal away from the bone, revealing the fracture site. Stress radiographs may identify motion at a fracture site, indicating nonunion (Fig. 6.48). Additional constraints on positioning for radiographs may be imposed by casts, external fixators, external supports, or traction devices.

CT is excellent for demonstrating complex fractures or for identifying small fragments; however, artifacts from metal implants may reduce image quality. Fracture hardware and small implants such as metallic sutures or vascular clips may produce major artifacts on MRI that limit its usefulness after fractures. Even when nothing has been implanted, microscopic metal debris from drills and other instruments may still produce artifacts that reduce the image quality. However, orthopedic hardware used for fracture fixation does not deflect in the magnetic fields used for MRI, and the patients may be safely scanned. Radionuclide bone scans are occasionally helpful in demonstrating the presence of physiologic activity at a fracture site. Nuclear scans with labeled leukocytes or gallium as well as positron emission tomography may occasionally be helpful when there is a question of infection.

## SOURCES AND READINGS

Beaty JH, Kasser JR. *Rockwood and Wilkins' Fractures in Children*. 6th Ed. Philadelphia, PA: Lippincott Williams & Wilkins; 2005.

Berquist TH. *Imaging of Orthopaedic Fixation Devices and Prostheses*. Philadelphia, PA: Lippincott Williams & Wilkins; 2008.

Browner B, Jupiter J, Levine A, Trafton P, Krettek C. *Skeletal Trauma: Fractures, Dislocations, Ligamentous Injuries*. 4th Ed. Philadelphia, PA: Saunders; 2008.

Bucholz RW, Heckman JD, Court-Brown C, Tornetta P. *Rockwood and Green's Fractures in Adults*. 7th Ed. Philadelphia, PA: Lippincott Williams & Wilkins; 2009.

Buckwalter JA, Einhorn TA, Simon SR. *Orthopaedic Bioscience: Biology and Biomechanics of the Musculoskeletal System*. 2nd Ed. American Academy of Orthopaedic Surgeons; 2000.

Chew FS, Pappas CN. Fracture fixation hardware in the extremities. *Radiol Clin North Am*. 1995;33:375–390.

eMedicine. http://emedicine.medscape.com.

Eustace S, Goldberg R, Williamson D, et al. MR imaging of soft tissues adjacent to orthopaedic hardware: Techniques to minimize susceptibility artifact. *Clin Radiol*. 1997;52:589–594.

Griffin LY. *Essentials of Musculoskeletal Care*. 3rd Ed. Rosemont, IL: American Academy of Orthopedics; 2005.

Koman LA, Smith BP, Ekman EF, Smith TL. Complex regional pain syndrome. *Instr Course Lect*. 2005;54:11–20.

Shellock FG. *The Reference Manual for Magnetic Resonance Safety, Implants and Devices: 2008 Edition*. Los Angeles, CA: Biomedical Research Publishing Group; 2008.

Siegel J, Tornetta P III, Borrelli J Jr, Kregor P, Ricci WM. Locked and minimally invasive plating. *Instr Course Lect*. 2007;56:353–368.

Taljanovic MS, Hunter TB, Miller MD, et al. Gallery of medical devices: Part 1: Orthopedic devices for the extremities and pelvis. *Radiographics*. 2005;25:859–870.

Taljanovic MS, Hunter TB, O'Brien MJ, et al. Gallery of medical devices: Part 2: Devices of the head, neck, spine, chest, and abdomen. *Radiographics*. 2005;25:1119–1132.

Taljanovic MS, Jones MD, Ruth JT, et al. Fracture fixation. *Radiographics*. 2003;23:1569–1590.

Tejwani NC, Wolinsky P. The changing face of orthopaedic trauma: Locked plating and minimally invasive techniques. *Instr Course Lect*. 2008;57:3–9.

Tsiridis E, Upadhyay N, Giannoudis P. Molecular aspects of fracture healing: Which are the important molecules? *Injury*. 2007;38(Suppl. 1): S11–S25.

Watson MA, Mathias KJ, Maffulli N. External ring fixators: An overview. *Proc Inst Mech Eng*. 2000;214:459–470.

Wheeless CR III, ed. *Wheeless' Textbook of Orthopaedics*. http://www.wheelessonline.com.

Zalavras CG, Marcus RE, Levin LS, Patzakis MJ. Management of open fractures and subsequent complications. *Instr Course Lect*. 2008;57:51–63.

# PART II

# Tumors

# Approach to Bone Lesions

Incidence
Cardinal Principle
Patient Factors

Location of Lesion
Rate of Growth
Tissue Characterization

Staging
Treatment
Metastases

## INCIDENCE

Malignant primary musculoskeletal tumors represent less than 1% of all cancers. Approximately 2,500 new cases of primary bone malignancies and 6,400 new cases of primary connective tissue malignancies are reported annually in the United States. A malignant tumor located in a bone is much more likely to be a metastasis or multiple myeloma than a primary sarcoma. The average practicing radiologist may see a new primary bone malignancy every few years; many clinicians never see one. Thus, it is often the radiologist who is the physician with the first and best opportunity to suggest the diagnosis and who may guide the initial evaluation and management. Because the prognosis of primary bone and soft-tissue malignancies is often related to the initial management, it is crucial for the radiologist to know both the clinical and the radiologic features of these lesions. As a general rule, patients in whom a primary malignant musculoskeletal tumor is suspected should be referred to a medical center with special expertise. Obtaining the biopsy should be the very last (not first) step in the diagnostic process and is best performed by a member of the multidisciplinary team that will provide the definitive care. A hasty attempt at biopsy that violates and contaminates the otherwise unaffected tissue planes may compromise the definitive procedure and necessitate a more extensive operation with a worse prognosis.

A situation that arises more frequently than the tumors themselves is the discovery of an incidental bone lesion for which a primary malignant bone tumor is a differential diagnostic possibility. It is more important for the radiologist to know with confidence which lesions are not aggressive tumors than to know which specific entity an aggressive bone tumor might be.

## CARDINAL PRINCIPLE

The cardinal principle in the diagnosis of solitary bone lesions is that the radiologic appearance reflects the underlying pathology of the abnormal lesional tissue and its interplay with the host bone. The radiologic images are best understood when the underlying pathologic processes are also understood; this principle applies regardless of the particular imaging modality. Knowledge regarding the histogenesis and clinicopathologic classification of many lesions is controversial and in constant flux. However,

a few pathologic entities account for the majority of these lesions (Table 7.1).

The standard radiologic approach addresses four issues: (a) patient factors, especially age; (b) location within the skeleton and within the involved bone; (c) rate of growth or aggressiveness; and (d) tissue characterization from specific features such as mineralization. Careful consideration of these factors may lead to a diagnostic conclusion that is almost certain. Often, however, the diagnosis can only be narrowed to several entities or may even be completely uncertain.

In many musculoskeletal lesions, the pathologic examination is not sufficient to provide a definitive diagnosis. In many cases, the radiologic appearance and clinical course of the lesion are equally important. Thus, if a lesion has specific radiologic features that narrow the differential diagnosis, the radiologist should be prepared to defend his or her diagnosis—even in the face of a contrary opinion from the pathologist.

## PATIENT FACTORS

Most bone lesions tend to affect particular age groups. Therefore, knowing the patient's age is often valuable in distinguishing among lesions with similar radiologic features or lesions with nonspecific

| TABLE 7.1 | Frequency of 8,591 Primary Malignant Bone Tumors in the Mayo Clinic Series |
|---|---|
| Type of Tumor | Frequency (%) |
| Myeloma | 44 |
| Osteosarcoma (including variants) | 20 |
| Chondrosarcoma (including variants) | 12 |
| Lymphoma | 8 |
| Ewing sarcoma | 6 |
| Chordoma | 4 |
| Fibrosarcoma/MFH | 4 |
| Hemangioendothelioma | 1 |
| Others | 1 |

MFH, malignant fibrous histiocytoma.
*Source:* Unni KK. *Dahlin's Bone Tumors. General Aspects and Data on 11,087 Cases.* 5th Ed. Philadelphia, PA: Lippincott-Raven; 1996.

| TABLE 7.2 | Most Frequently Encountered Types of Primary Malignant Bone Tumors at Various Ages | | |
|---|---|---|---|
| **0–9 Years** | **10–19 Years** | **20–29 Years** | **30+ Years** |
| Ewing sarcoma | Osteosarcoma | Osteosarcoma | Myeloma |
| Osteosarcoma | Ewing sarcoma | Chondrosarcoma | Chondrosarcoma |
| Primary lymphoma | Primary lymphoma | Ewing sarcoma | Osteosarcoma |
| | | Primary lymphoma | Primary lymphoma |
| | | MFH/fibrosarcoma | Chordoma |
| | | | MFH/fibrosarcoma |

For each age range, the tumor types are listed in order of frequency and account for over 90% of the primary tumors.
MFH, malignant fibrous histiocytoma.
*Source*: Unni KK. *Dahlin's Bone Tumors. General Aspects and Data on 11,087 Cases*. 5th Ed. Philadelphia, PA: Lippincott-Raven; 1996.

| TABLE 7.3 | Sex Predominance of Bone Lesions | | | | | |
|---|---|---|---|---|---|---|
| | **Male Predominance** | **Ratio[a]** | **No Predominance** | **Female Predominance** | **Ratio** |
| Malignant | PNET | >2:1 | Adamantinoma | Parosteal osteosarcoma | Slight |
| | Osteosarcoma, telangiectatic | Slight | | | |
| | Chondrosarcoma | 2:1 | | | |
| | Chordoma | 2:1 | | | |
| | Osteosarcoma, conventional | Slight | | | |
| | Ewing sarcoma | Slight | | | |
| | Myeloma | Slight | | | |
| | Lymphoma of bone | Slight | | | |
| | MFH of bone | Slight | | | |
| Benign | Simple cyst | 3:1 | Enchondroma | Giant cell tumor | Slight |
| | Osteoid osteoma | 3:1 | Fibrous dysplasia | Aneurysmal bone cyst | Slight |
| | Osteoblastoma | 2:1 | | Hemangioma | Slight |
| | Osteochondroma | 2:1 | | | |
| | Periosteal chondroma | 2:1 | | | |
| | Chondroblastoma | 2:1 | | | |
| | Chondromyxoid fibroma | 2:1 | | | |
| | Fibrous cortical defect | 2:1 | | | |
| | Nonossifying fibroma | 2:1 | | | |
| | Eosinophilic granuloma | 2:1 | | | |
| | Desmoplastic fibroma | Slight | | | |
| | Intraosseous lipoma | Slight | | | |
| | Intraosseous ganglion | Slight | | | |

[a]Ratios are approximate and rounded.
PNET, primitive neuroectodermal tumor; MFH, malignant fibrous histiocytoma.
*Source*: Unni KK. *Dahlin's Bone Tumors. General Aspects and Data on 11,087 Cases*. 5th Ed. Philadelphia, PA: Lippincott-Raven; 1996; Fechner RE, Mills SE. *Tumors of the Bones and Joints*. Washington, DC: Armed Forces Institute of Pathology; 1993.

appearances (Table 7.2). Many lesions affect a broad age range. Most bone lesions are more common in men (Table 7.3). A few precursor conditions increase the risk of developing a bone malignancy (Table 7.4).

may be difficult to localize. Although there may be considerable variability in location, tumors of a given cell type seem to arise preferentially at sites where the homologous normal cells are most active.

# ■ LOCATION OF LESION

The location of a lesion within the skeleton and within the involved bone may have considerable differential diagnostic significance (Tables 7.5 and 7.6). The site of origin of a large, extensive lesion

# ■ RATE OF GROWTH

The rate of growth of a lesion is classified according to the type of bone destruction and the type of bone proliferation in response to the presence of the lesion.

**TABLE 7.4    Precursors of Malignancy in Bone**

| Precursor Condition | Comment |
|---|---|
| Enchondroma | Very low risk with solitary lesions; higher risk with multiple lesions |
| Osteochondroma | Very low risk with solitary lesions; higher risk with multiple lesions |
| Paget disease | Higher risk with more extensive; polyostotic disease |
| Radiation injury | Low risk with 7000 rads or less |
| Osteomyelitis with chronic sinus tract | Long latency period (20+ years) |
| Bone infarct | Rare, 90% or more have multiple infarcts |
| Fibrous dysplasia | Case reports |
| Metallic implants | Case reports |
| Bone cysts | Case reports |
| Osteogenesis imperfecta | Case reports |
| Genetic predisposition | Association with mutant Rb gene and retinoblastoma |
| Synovial chondromatosis | Case reports |
| Giant cell tumor | Rare malignant recurrence after treatment |
| Osteoblastoma | Rare locally aggressive form that does not metastasize |
| Osteofibrous dysplasia | Coexistent with adamantinoma; possibly subsets of the same disease |

*Source*: Unni KK, Inwards CY. *Bones and Joints*. In: Henson DE, Albores-Saavedra J. *Pathology of Incipient Neoplasia*. 3rd Ed. New York, NY: Oxford University Press; 2001.

**TABLE 7.5    Typical Longitudinal Locations of Solitary Bone Lesions**

| Epiphysis | Metaphysis | Diametaphysis | Diaphysis |
|---|---|---|---|
| Chondroblastoma | Osteochondroma | Benign fibrous lesions | Ewing sarcoma |
| Eosinophilic granuloma | Osteosarcoma | Malignant fibrous lesions | Myeloma |
| Giant cell tumor | Enchondroma | Chondromyxoid fibroma | Lymphoma |
| Subchondral cyst | Chondrosarcoma | Simple bone cyst | |
| Brodie abscess | | Osteoid osteoma | |
| Clear cell chondrosarcoma | | Osteoblastoma | |

**TABLE 7.6    Typical Transverse Locations of Solitary Bone Lesions**

| Medullary Cavity | Cortex | Juxtacortical |
|---|---|---|
| Conventional osteosarcoma | Cortical osteoid osteoma | Osteochondroma |
| Medullary chondrosarcoma | Fibrous cortical defect | Periosteal chondroma |
| Ewing sarcoma | Adamantinoma | Parosteal osteosarcoma |
| Myeloma | | Exostotic chondrosarcoma |
| Lymphoma | | |
| Giant cell tumor | | |
| Enchondroma | | |
| Simple bone cyst | | |
| Nonossifying fibroma | | |

Bone destruction occurs when a normal bone tissue is replaced by a lesional tissue. Bone destruction is described as *geographic* when it is confined to a focal area, forming a single hole in the bone (Fig. 7.1). The demarcation between the lesion and the normal unaffected bone can be sharp or gradual. Bone destruction is described as *moth eaten* when there are multiple medium-sized holes with irregular edges randomly distributed in the area of involvement (Fig. 7.2). It is described as *permeated* when the multiple holes are so small that the overall outline of the bone may remain intact in the presence of extensive destruction

**FIGURE 7.1.** Geographic bone destruction (*arrow*) in the proximal femur (giant cell tumor).

(Fig. 7.3). In moth-eaten and permeated destruction, the transition between normal and abnormal bones is usually gradual.

Proliferative bone is a reaction to the lesion by the host bone. This reaction can be endosteal, within the bone, or periosteal, on the cortical surface. A sclerotic rim is a layer of dense endosteal reactive bone surrounding the lesion and separating it from the normal adjacent bone (Fig. 7.4). A sclerotic rim implies that the growth rate of the lesion is slow enough for new bone to form around it and confine it. An expanded cortical shell is a layer of periosteal new bone that confines a lesion that has already destroyed the cortex and expanded beyond the original contour of the bone (Fig. 7.5). The periosteal new bone is formed as the endosteal surface of the cortex is destroyed; the faster the cortical destruction and expansion of the lesion, the thinner is the cortical shell. An expanded shell may have ridges or trabeculations on the endosteal surface, reflecting an uneven growth rate. Nodules of tumor have grown more rapidly beneath the thinner areas of bone and less rapidly where the trabeculations are located. True bony septations that divide a lesion into compartments are rare. If a lesion expands so rapidly that the periosteal bone response cannot keep up, a shell will not be visible. Mottled sclerosis, scattered throughout the cancellous bone adjacent to a lesion, suggests disorganized reactive bone formation in the presence of an aggressive, fast-growing lesion.

**FIGURE 7.2.** Moth-eaten bone destruction (multiple myeloma). **A:** Humerus. **B:** Skull.

**FIGURE 7.3.** Permeated bone destruction (*arrow*) in the anterior femoral cortex with soft-tissue extension (metastasis). **A:** Lateral radiograph. **B:** Sagittal T1 fat-suppressed MRI following gadolinium contrast injection.

Cortical penetration by an intramedullary lesion is indicative of an aggressive process (Fig. 7.6) typically apparent by the presence of a soft-tissue mass. Periosteal reaction may also indicate cortical penetration. Layers of periosteal reaction may be caused by the cortical penetration of the lesion into the subperiosteal region (Fig. 7.7).

A sunburst periosteal reaction or streaks of periosteal new bone indicate penetration with reactive bone-forming periosteum being carried along by an expanding lesion (Fig. 7.8). An interrupted layer of bone at the edge of a lesion that has expanded beyond the periosteum may be present, the so-called Codman triangle.

**FIGURE 7.4.** Sclerotic rim (*arrow*) around the lesion in proximal tibia (nonossifying fibroma).

**FIGURE 7.5.** Expanded cortical shell in the fifth metacarpal (osteoblastoma).

**FIGURE 7.6.** Geographic destruction and cortical penetration with Codman triangle (*arrow*) in the distal femur (osteosarcoma). There is a medial soft-tissue mass (*arrowheads*) with a faint sunburst periosteal reaction.

**FIGURE 7.7.** Layers of periosteal reaction with Codman triangle (osteosarcoma).

**A**

**B**

**C**

**FIGURE 7.8.** Sunburst periosteal reaction (osteosarcoma). **A:** AP radiograph. **B:** Axial CT scan. **C:** T1-weighted axial MRI.

| TABLE 7.7 | Radiologic Grading of Destructive Bone Lesions | |
|---|---|---|
| AFIP System | Defining Characteristics | Simplified System |
| I-A | Geographic destruction; well-defined lucent destruction with sclerotic margin; cortex expanded up to 1 cm | Low grade; nonaggressive |
| I-B | Geographic destruction; well-defined lucent destruction without sclerotic margin or cortex expanded >1 cm | Medium grade; moderately aggressive |
| I-C | Geographic destruction; complete cortical penetration with ill-defined margin | |
| II | Geographic destruction combined with moth-eaten or permeated destruction, middle-sized holes in bone with irregular poorly defined contours | High grade; very aggressive |
| III | Moth-eaten or permeated destruction only, numerous elongated slotted holes parallel to long axis | |

*Source*: Hudson TM. *Radiologic-pathologic Correlation of Musculoskeletal Lesions*. Baltimore, MD: Williams & Wilkins; 1987.

The rate of growth reflects the biologic aggressiveness of the lesion and can be assigned a radiologic grade. The grading system devised by Lodwick at the Armed Forces Institute of Pathology (AFIP) is commonly used (Table 7.7). Growth rate I-A is geographic destruction with a complete sclerotic margin and partial or no cortical destruction; the cortex may be expanded by up to 1 cm (see Fig. 7.4). Growth rate I-B is geographic destruction with either no sclerotic rim or cortical expansion greater than 1 cm (Fig. 7.9). Growth rate I-C is geographic destruction with complete cortical penetration. Growth rate II is geographic destruction combined with moth-eaten or permeated destruction or both (see Fig. 7.6). Growth rate III is moth-eaten destruction with or without permeated destruction only (see Fig. 7.2). Higher-grade growth rates may have features of lower-grade growth rates, but not vice versa. Lesions with growth rate I-A are low grade and nonaggressive, lesions with growth rate I-B or I-C are medium grade and moderately aggressive, and lesions with growth rate II or III are high grade and very aggressive. It may be difficult to distinguish growth rate I-B from I-C and growth rate II from III, but the distinction is not important clinically.

# ◼ TISSUE CHARACTERIZATION

Many primary musculoskeletal tumors form an intercellular matrix. The internal radiologic characteristics of tumors that form a matrix are determined by the relative proportions of cells and matrix and the composition and mineralization of the matrix. Types of tumor matrices include osteoid (osseous), chondroid (cartilaginous), myxoid (proteinaceous), fat (lipomatous), and fibrous (collagenous). Identifying the type of the matrix often suggests a specific diagnosis (Table 7.8). The pattern of mineralization on radiographs, the attenuation on CT, and the signal on MRI may be helpful in identifying the tumor matrix.

A                                    B

**FIGURE 7.9.** Geographic destruction with no sclerotic margin in the distal femur (giant cell tumor). A pathologic fracture is present. **A:** Radiograph. **B:** Coronal reformatted CT.

| **TABLE 7.8** | **Matrix Mineralization in Bone Tumors** | | |
|---|---|---|---|
| | Osteoid Matrix | Chondroid Matrix | Intermediate Matrix |
| Benign | Osteoid osteoma<br>Osteoblastoma<br>Bone island<br>Osteoma | Enchondroma<br>Osteochondroma<br>Periosteal chondroma<br>Chondroblastoma<br>Chondromyxoid fibroma | Fibrous dysplasia<br>Osteoblastoma |
| Malignant | Osteosarcoma | Chondrosarcoma | Osteosarcoma |

Dense, homogeneous mineralization is typical of osteoid matrix, formed by benign and malignant bone-forming lesions (Fig. 7.10). Alternatively, osteoid matrix may have a ground-glass or intermediate pattern of matrix mineralization. Osteoid matrix is not always mineralized; therefore, the lack of densely mineralized matrix does not rule out the possibility of an osteoid-forming lesion. Nonmineralized osteoid matrix may have attenuation on CT similar to muscle and often has low signal on both T1-and T2-weighted MRI.

Calcified rings and arcs, dense punctate calcifications, and flocculent calcifications (small, loosely aggregated masses) are patterns of mineralization of chondroid matrix (Figs. 7.11–7.13), formed by benign and malignant cartilage-forming lesions. The rings-and-arcs configuration of mineralization corresponds to the calcification and ossification around the periphery of cartilaginous lobules. Chondroid matrix that is not mineralized typically has attenuation on CT that is lower than muscle but greater than water.

On MRI, chondroid matrix has low signal on T1-weighted images and high signal on T2-weighted images, similar to hyaline cartilage. Myxoid matrix may be formed by benign and malignant cartilage-forming tumors and by other benign and malignant mesenchymal tumors, including chordomas. Myxoid matrix generally does not mineralize and typically has attenuation on CT that is lower than muscle and greater than water. On MRI, myxoid matrix has high signal on T2-weighted images, presumably due to its high water content, and variable signal on T1-weighted images, presumably due to its variable protein content.

Lesions that form a fibrous matrix range from densely cellular fibrous tissue to myxoid tissue, often within the same lesion. Fibrous matrix typically does not mineralize. On CT, fibrous matrix has variable, nonspecific attenuation, depending on its composition. On MRI, fibrous matrix has variable, nonspecific signal, also depending on its composition. Fibrous dysplasia characteristically has the intermediate pattern of mineralization

**FIGURE 7.10.** Mineralized osteoid matrix (osteosarcoma). **A:** AP radiograph. **B:** Coronal T1-weighted fat-suppressed MRI with gadolinium enhancement.

**A**     **B**

**FIGURE 7.11.** Rings-and-arcs cartilage matrix mineralization (chondrosarcoma). **A:** Lateral radiograph. **B:** Axial CT scan shows the lobular morphology of the tumor and the calcifications.

(ground-glass appearance). However, this appearance results from the presence of dysplastic, microscopic bone spicules rather than the mineralization of the fibrous matrix itself. On radiographs, the ground-glass appearance may be difficult to recognize. The lesion is more dense than the marrow space but less dense than the cortical bone; CT is often helpful in identifying the matrix (Fig. 7.14). A lesion with no mineralization will have either matrix that is not mineralized or no matrix at all. Lesions without matrix may be densely cellular (e.g., Ewing sarcoma, lymphoma, and myeloma), or they may be acellular (e.g., bone cyst) (see Fig. 7.1). MRI may be diagnostic when a nonaggressive lesion can be demonstrated to be fluid filled and therefore cystic. A localized change in the character of a tumor matrix from mineralized to nonmineralized may indicate a focus of higher-grade tumor cells.

**FIGURE 7.12.** Flocculent cartilage matrix mineralization (enchondroma).

**FIGURE 7.13.** Punctate cartilage matrix mineralization (enchondroma).

**FIGURE 7.14.** Intermediate (ground glass) mineralization (*arrow*) of matrix (fibrous dysplasia) in the proximal tibia. **A:** AP radiograph. **B:** Coronal reformatted CT.

# ◼ STAGING

Staging requires full and exact anatomic delineation of the tumor tissue and its surrounding reactive tissue. This reactive tissue may contain micrometastases. The anatomic relationship of the lesion to all surrounding structures, anatomic compartments, and neurovascular bundles must be established. In addition to plain films, cross-sectional imaging is necessary. Although CT is much better than MRI for establishing a diagnosis, the two modalities are equal for evaluating the extent and anatomic setting of the tumor. Chest CT can exclude lung metastases; a radionuclide bone scan or whole-body MRI can exclude skeletal metastases.

PET and PET-CT are becoming progressively valuable tumor staging tools. Most centers in the United States are performing PET-CT, as opposed to PET alone. The PET literature showed it to be a sensitive and effective test for staging tumors of many types. The literature supporting PET-CT is lagging the rapid rate at which it is being utilized. Preliminary studies are promising and the National Oncologic PET Registry is expected to provide outcome data for a large number of tumor types and locations. Since PET alone was found to be a powerful technique in tumor staging, the addition of unenhanced thin section CT through the entire body will almost undoubtedly enrich this staging modality.

The Musculoskeletal Tumor Society and the American Joint Committee for Cancer Staging and End Results Reporting have adopted the surgical staging system described in Table 7.9 for primary malignant musculoskeletal tumors. The staging system is based on a combination of the histologic grade (designated

| **TABLE 7.9** | **American Joint Committee on Cancer Staging for Musculoskeletal Cancers** | |
|---|---|---|
| Bone | Stage I | Low grade (well or moderately differentiated); no distant metastases |
| | A | 8 cm or smaller |
| | B | >8 cm |
| | Stage II | High grade (poorly differentiated or undifferentiated); no distant metastases |
| | A | 8 cm or smaller |
| | B | >8 cm |
| | Stage III | Discontinuous tumors in the primary bone site; no distant metastases |
| | Stage IV | Distant metastases |
| | A | Lung only |
| | B | Regional lymph node metastasis or distant sites other than the lung |
| Soft tissue | Stage I | Low grade (well and moderately differentiated); no distant metastasis; any location or size |
| | Stage II | High grade (poorly differentiated and undifferentiated); no distant metastasis; superficial location or 5 cm or smaller |
| | Stage III | High grade (poorly differentiated or undifferentiated); no distant metastasis; deep location or >5 cm |
| | Stage IV | Distant metastasis, including regional lymph node metastasis |

*Source*: Greene FL, Page DL, Fleming ID, et al., eds. *AJCC Cancer Staging Manual*. 6th Ed. New York, NY: Springer-Verlag; 2002:187–200.

$G_0$ through $G_2$), the anatomic setting of the tumor itself (designated $T_0$ through $T_2$), and the presence or absence of metastases (designated $M_0$ or $M_1$). Benign lesions have three stages that are designated by Arabic numbers; malignant lesions have three stages designated by Roman numerals. Stage I lesions are low-grade malignancies, stage II lesions are high-grade malignancies, and stage III lesions are those with metastases, whether low or high grade. The additional letter designation of A or B reflects the anatomic setting. Stages I-A, II-A, and III-A are intracompartmental lesions in which the tumor is confined within a natural anatomic barrier to tumor growth, such as the cortical bone, articular cartilage, major fascial septa, or joint capsules. Stages I-B, II-B, and III-B are extracompartmental lesions in which the lesion has expanded beyond the confines of a single anatomic compartment. At presentation, 30% of musculoskeletal sarcoma patients have stage I lesions (66% of these are stage I-A, and 33% are stage I-B), 60% have stage II lesions (10% of these are stage II-A, and 90% are stage II-B), and 10% have stage III lesions. As a general observation, benign lesions in stages 1 and 2 are radiologically low grade or nonaggressive, stage 3 benign lesions and stage I malignant lesions are medium grade or moderately aggressive, and stage II or III malignant lesions are high grade or very aggressive.

# ◼ TREATMENT

Treatment of musculoskeletal tumors is individualized. Benign lesions whose radiologic appearance and clinical presentation are typical often do not require a histologic diagnosis and may be ignored, followed up, or treated according to the symptoms and natural history. Most other benign lesions can be treated with curettage or simple excision. Aggressive or malignant lesions usually require both local and systemic therapies. Although lesions such as lymphoma and Ewing sarcoma are treated with radiation (Fig. 7.15), local therapy for most malignant or aggressive lesions is surgical (Fig. 7.16). The size of the surrounding cuff of tissue that is ideally excised with the lesion is usually related to the histologic grade of the tumor. Depending on the operation chosen and the site and extent of the tumor, amputations and local limb-sparing operations may leave behind a gross tumor, a macroscopic or microscopic residual tumor, or no residual tumor at all. A contaminated biopsy site can enlarge the scope of the operation required to achieve a particular biologic goal; the biopsy site is generally resected with the tumor. Newer regimens of neoadjuvant and adjuvant therapies—including radiation therapy, chemotherapy, and immunotherapy—are aimed at reducing tumor bulk before surgery and at eliminating the residual (often microscopic) tumor and subclinical metastases after surgery. Major advances in the staging and treatment of primary bone and joint cancers have improved the 5-year survival rates for children younger than 15 years of age from 20% in 1960–1963 to 64% in 1986–1991. Primary bone sarcomas that have been resected segmentally are usually reconstructed with large allografts. If a joint is included in the resection, the reconstruction may include a prosthesis or an arthrodesis. Involvement of major vessels is not necessarily a contraindication to limb-sparing resection if a vascular graft can be successfully placed. However, in some cases, an amputation is necessary. For a benign disease in which intralesional excision is appropriate—for example, enchondroma or osteoblastoma—the resulting defect at the surgical site may be filled with material such as bone graft or methylmethacrylate cement.

After the initiation of therapy, imaging may be used to monitor the response and to screen for complications or recurrences (Fig. 7.17). For bone lesions that have undergone curettage with bone or cement grafting, MRI is commonly used to screen for

**A**    **B**

**FIGURE 7.15.** Ewing sarcoma in the proximal femur. **A:** At presentation, there is permeated destruction, layered periosteal reaction, and a large soft-tissue mass. **B:** One year later, after radiation therapy, the mass has regressed and the tumor bed has ossified.

**FIGURE 7.16.** Soft-tissue sarcoma with normal posttreatment changes. **A:** Axial T2-weighted MRI with fat suppression before surgery shows a large mass (*arrow*) in the anterior compartment with high-signal regions of necrosis. **B:** Axial T2-weighted MRI with fat suppression three months after surgery shows resection of the mass with a small seroma (*arrow*) at the surgical site. The remaining quadriceps musculature (*Q*) shows increased signal from denervation atrophy. **C:** Axial T1-weighted MRI with fat suppression following gadolinium injection shows modest enhancement around the periphery of the seroma (*arrow*).

**FIGURE 7.17.** Recurrent soft-tissue sarcoma. **A:** Axial T1-weighted MRI shows a lesion (*arrow*) with intermediate signal in the anterior subcutaneous tissues of the proximal thigh. The marker has been placed on the incision scar from previous surgery. **B:** Axial T2-weighted MRI with fat suppression shows heterogeneous high signal within the lesion. **C:** Axial T1-weighted MRI with fat suppression following gadolinium injection shows heterogeneous enhancement in the lesion.

**A**                                                    **B**

**FIGURE 7.18.** Recurrent giant cell tumor. **A:** PA radiograph shows cement in the curettage bed of the distal radius with an enlarging adjacent area of lucency (*arrow*). **B:** Coronal T1-weighted fat-suppressed MRI with gadolinium enhancement confirms an enhancing soft-tissue mass (*arrow*) consistent with the recurrent tumor.

recurrences (Fig. 7.18). CT using a metal algorithm or radiographs can be useful for monitoring the treated area of bone for periprosthetic fracture, infection, and graft incorporation. In cases where metal artifact is overwhelming, Doppler ultrasound can evaluate the surrounding soft tissues for tumor recurrence. PET is becoming progressively more utilized for tumor surveillance in cases where large amounts of metal degrade CT and MRI.

## ◼ METASTASES

Metastases to the lungs are common in patients with musculoskeletal sarcomas. The lung lesions typically have a cannonball morphology. The pulmonary metastases of matrix-forming bone tumors also form a similar matrix. In many clinical circumstances, pulmonary metastases are aggressively pursued, even when multiple. Musculoskeletal malignancies also metastasize to other bones. The metastatic lesions generally resemble the primary lesions (Fig. 7.19).

## SOURCES AND READINGS

Campanacci M. *Bone and Soft Tissue Tumors: Clinical Features, Imaging, Pathology and Treatment.* 2nd Ed. Vienna, Austria: Springer; 1999.

Daldrup-Link HE, Franzius C, Link TM, et al. Whole-body MR imaging for detection of bone metastases in children and young adults: Comparison with skeletal scintigraphy and FDG PET. *AJR.* 2001;177:229–236.

Enneking WF. *Clinical Musculoskeletal Pathology.* 3rd Ed. Gainesville, FL: University of Florida Press; 1991.

Fechner RE, Mills SE. *Tumors of the Bones and Joints.* Washington, DC: Armed Forces Institute of Pathology; 1993.

Greene FL, Page DL, Fleming ID, et al., eds. *AJCC Cancer Staging Manual.* 6th Ed. New York, NY: Springer-Verlag; 2002:187–192.

Hudson TM. *Radiologic-pathologic Correlation of Musculoskeletal Lesions.* Baltimore, MD: Williams & Wilkins; 1987.

Iagaru A, Chawla S, Menendez L, Conti PS. 18F-FDG PET and PET/CT for detection of pulmonary metastases from musculoskeletal sarcomas. *Nucl Med Commun.* 2006;27(10):795–802.

Jemal A, Siegel R, Ward E, et al. Cancer statistics, 2008. *CA Cancer J Clin.* 2008;58(2):71–96.

Kransdorf MJ, Murphey MD. *Imaging of Soft Tissue Tumors.* 2nd Ed. Philadelphia, PA: Lippincott Williams & Wilkins; 2006.

Liu PT, Valadez SD, Chivers FS, Roberts CC, Beauchamp CP. Anatomically based guidelines for core needle biopsy of bone tumors: Implications for limb-sparing surgery. *Radiographics.* 2007;27(1):189–205.

Lodwick GS. *Atlas of Tumor Radiology. The Bones and Joints.* Chicago, IL: Year Book; 1971.

Lodwick GS, Wilson AJ, Farrell C, et al. Determining growth rates of focal lesions of bone from radiographs. *Radiology.* 1980a;134:577–583.

Lodwick GS, Wilson AJ, Farrell C, et al. Estimating rate of growth in bone lesions: Observer performance and error. *Radiology.* 1980b;134: 585–590.

**FIGURE 7.19.** Metastatic osteosarcoma. CT scan shows a dense lesion with sunburst morphology in the prespinal soft tissues.

Moser RP, Madewell JE. An approach to primary bone tumors. *Radiol Clin North Am*. 1987;25:1049–1093.

Olson PN, Everson LI, Griffiths HJ. Staging of musculoskeletal tumors. *Radiol Clin North Am*. 1994;32:151–162.

Taira AV, Herfkens RJ, Gambhir SS, Quon A. Detection of bone metastases: Assessment of integrated FDG PET/CT imaging. *Radiology*. 2007; 243(1):204–211.

Temple HT, Bashore CJ. Staging of bone neoplasms: An orthopedic oncologist's perspective. *Semin Musculoskelet Radiol*. 2000;4(1):17–23.

Unni KK. *Dahlin's Bone Tumors. General Aspects and Data on 11,087 Cases*. 5th Ed. Philadelphia, PA: Lippincott–Raven; 1996.

Unni KK, Inwards CY. Bones and Joints. In: Henson DE, Albores-Saavedra J. *Pathology of Incipient Neoplasia*. 3rd Ed. New York, NY: Oxford University Press; 2001:745–767.

# CHAPTER 8

# Malignant and Aggressive Tumors

## ■ OSTEOSARCOMA

Osteosarcomas are malignant osteoid-producing sarcomas (Table 8.1). Although they are the most common of the primary bone sarcomas, there are fewer than 1,000 new cases per year in the United States. Eighty-five percent of cases occur at 30 years of age or younger, but osteosarcomas may occur at any age. Most arise de novo, but in patients older than 40 years of age, as many as 15% to 20% of osteosarcomas are associated with Paget disease, therapeutic irradiation, or bone infarct.

### Conventional Osteosarcoma

Conventional (intramedullary) osteosarcoma is found within the cancellous portion of a long or flat bone. Aggressive growth within the medullary cavity leads to early cortical penetration and invasion of the soft tissues. The typical longitudinal location is the metaphysis; the typical transverse location is eccentric within the medullary cavity. An open growth plate can act as a barrier to tumor spread, sparing the epiphysis in the immature skeleton. The common locations are the distal femur (32% of cases), proximal tibia (15%), proximal femur and femoral shaft (9%), proximal humerus (8%), and ilium (7%). Note that nearly 50% of osteosarcomas occur around the knee.

The typical clinical presentation is nonspecific: pain, swelling, and limited joint motion for a few weeks or months. Some patients present with pathologic fractures, especially those with rapidly growing, sparsely ossified tumors. An osteosarcoma may be overlooked in the presence of a healing pathologic fracture, but appreciation of the presence of bone destruction leads to the correct diagnosis. Fracture callus and osteosarcoma can be virtually indistinguishable histologically.

Most osteosarcomas are heavily or moderately ossified, with the dense blastic areas corresponding to mineralized osseous matrix made by the tumor and reactive medullary bone (Figs. 8.1 and 8.2). Lytic areas, when present, correspond to the destruction and replacement of the bone by tumor tissue containing scant or no ossification. Cortical penetration with a large soft-tissue mass is common (see Fig. 7.6). Confluent bone densities within a soft-tissue mass correspond to mineralized matrix. Reactive periosteal new

**TABLE 8.1**    **Classification of Osteosarcomas**

Central (Intramedullary)
  High-grade
    Conventional
    Telangiectatic
    Small cell
    Epithelioid
    Osteoblastoma-like
    Chondroblastoma-like
    Fibrohistiocytic
    Giant cell–rich
  Low-grade
    Low-grade central
    Fibrous dysplasia–like
    Desmoplastic fibroma–like
Surface
  Low-grade
    Parosteal
  Intermediate-grade
    Periosteal
  High-grade
    Dedifferentiated parosteal
    High-grade surface
Intracortical
Gnathic
Extraskeletal
  High-grade
  Low-grade

*Source:* Klein MJ, Siegal GP. Osteosarcoma: Anatomic and histologic variants. *Am J Clin Pathol.* 2006;125(4):555–581.

bone may have a linear, laminated, or perpendicular sunburst bone configuration, all of which are indicative of cortical penetration. Approximately 50% of osteosarcomas have features typical enough to allow a confident radiologic diagnosis. Approximately 25% of osteosarcomas are chondroblastic, with large amounts of chondroid matrix mixed with the osteoid, so that the appearance on imaging

**FIGURE 8.1.** High-grade intramedullary osteosarcoma. **A:** AP radiograph shows sclerotic lesion (*arrow*) in the distal femoral metaphysis. **B:** Coronal T2-weighted fat-suppressed MRI shows low signal (*long arrow*) in the mineralized portion of the tumor with high signal in nonmineralized portions, including a significant soft-tissue component (*arrowheads*). There is extension into the epiphysis (*short arrow*). **C:** Coronal T1-weighted fat-suppressed MRI following gadolinium injection shows enhancement in the tumor.

**FIGURE 8.2.** Osteosarcoma of the proximal tibia. **A:** AP radiograph shows a mixed lytic-blastic lesion. **B:** Coronal T1-weighted fat-suppressed MRI following gadolinium injection shows the full extent of the lesion.

**A**    **B**

**FIGURE 8.3.** High-grade intramedullary osteosarcoma with skip metastasis. **A:** Sclerotic metatastasis (*arrow*) is present in the proximal femur. **B:** Primary lesion (*arrow*) is present at the distal femur.

may resemble a chondroid or myxoid lesion. Approximately 25% of osteosarcomas are fibroblastic, with large amounts of fibrous matrix. Recurrent tumors resemble the primary. Any cloudlike, solid, dense bone formation within the medullary cavity, even in the absence of overt bone destruction and soft-tissue extension, should suggest the possibility of an osteosarcoma.

Osteosarcoma metastasizes to the lung, where the deposits may form dense, mineralized osteoid, accumulate bone-scanning agents, cavitate, and cause pneumothorax. At presentation, 10% to 20% of patients have metastases, usually to the lungs. Occasionally, skip metastases occur in the medullary cavity of the host bone, sparing an interval of normal marrow between the primary tumor and the metastasis (Fig. 8.3). A metastasis may even skip across a joint.

Osteosarcomas are rapidly growing tumors with a median doubling time of 34 days. Local recurrences are usually apparent within the first year. The current treatment consists of neoadjuvant chemotherapy to reduce the tumor mass, aggressive resection of the tumor, adjuvant chemotherapy, and resection of pulmonary metastases. Segmental limb-sparing resections may improve function without necessarily compromising local control. The disease-free, overall 5-year survival rate of those without metastatic disease at presentation (up to stage II-B) approaches 80%.

## Osteosarcoma Variants

Radiation-induced osteosarcomas have the radiologic appearance and biologic behavior of conventional high-grade intramedullary

osteosarcomas (Fig. 8.4). Approximately 5% of osteosarcomas are postirradiation in etiology. Osteosarcoma is the most common type of postirradiation musculoskeletal sarcoma.

Telangiectatic osteosarcomas represent approximately 4% of all osteosarcomas and display distinctive pathologic features. The lesions are destructive and lytic, with large extraosseous masses incompletely surrounded by thin shells of bone (Fig. 8.5). They grow rapidly and elicit relatively little bone reaction. Pathologically, telangiectatic osteosarcomas are mostly cystic and vascular, containing little or no tumor matrix or other solid tumor tissue. Fluid-fluid levels may be demonstrated on CT or MRI. Telangiectatic osteosarcomas were previously thought to be more lethal but were subsequently shown to have the same prognosis as conventional osteosarcomas with neoadjuvant chemotherapy and wide resection.

Parosteal osteosarcomas represent 6% to 9% of osteosarcomas. This variety arises on the cortical surface and affects a slightly older age group, with most patients older than 20 years of age. Virtually all are found in the metaphysis of a long bone, especially the posterior surface of the distal femoral metaphysis (66% of cases). The presentation is nonspecific, often dull, aching pain or mechanical difficulties caused by the mass itself. The lesions are commonly diagnosed and treated incorrectly for years as atypical osteochondromas that somehow recur locally. Even with late diagnosis, the prognosis is often better than for conventional osteosarcoma. The radiographic appearance is a lobulated juxtacortical mass with densely ossified tumor tissue attached to the cortex, often by a stalk; variable amounts of lucent, nonossified

A                                                 B

**FIGURE 8.4.** Radiation induced osteosarcoma of the scapula. **A:** AP radiograph shows radiation change in the clavicle and scapula, with a coarsened trabecular bone pattern. The humerus overlies a destructive lesion of the scapular spine. **B:** Axial T2-weighted fat-suppressed MRI shows heterogeneous high signal in a large scapular mass with soft-tissue extension (*arrow*).

tissue are usually present, making the lesion larger than apparent on plain radiographs (Fig. 8.6). CT or MRI can document tumor invasion of the medullary cavity by direct extension through the stalk.

Periosteal osteosarcomas are found in a periosteal location, most commonly along the shaft of the femur or tibia. These osteosarcomas are generally chondroblastic and therefore not densely ossified

(Fig. 8.7). They are predominantly radiolucent on radiographs and CT, with a lobulated morphology. A sunburst appearance is often present. On MRI, the bulk of the lesion typically has heterogeneous low signal on T1-weighted images and high signal on T2-weighted images. The age of onset is similar to conventional osteosarcomas, and periosteal osteosarcomas are of moderate histologic grade and biologic aggressiveness.

A                                                 B

**FIGURE 8.5.** Telangiectatic osteosarcoma in the proximal humerus. **A:** Radiograph shows an expansile, destructive lesion in the proximal humerus with cortical penetration (blow out). **B:** CT scan shows destruction, mineralized tumor, and soft tissue mass.

**FIGURE 8.6** Parosteal osteosarcoma. **A:** Lateral radiograph shows large, dense, lobulated mass arising from the posterior cortex of the distal femur. **B:** Axial T1-weighted fat-suppressed MRI following gadolinium injection shows regions of enhancement. **C:** Axial CT scan shows variation in mineralization of the lesion.

Other osteosarcoma variants with distinctive histologic or clinical features account for approximately 1% of all osteosarcomas. These include multifocal osteosarcoma (synchronous and asynchronous types), small cell osteosarcoma (see the section "Small Cell Osteosarcoma"), intraosseous well-differentiated osteosarcoma, intracortical osteosarcoma, and high-grade surface osteosarcoma.

# ■ CHONDROSARCOMA

Chondrosarcomas are malignant cartilage-producing tumors that arise de novo or in preexisting cartilage lesions or rests. They present a wide variation in form and aggressiveness, and low-grade malignant lesions may be almost indistinguishable morphologically from benign cartilage-containing lesions. A limited focus of malignancy may be

**FIGURE 8.7.** Periosteal osteosarcoma. **A:** Lateral radiograph shows a partially mineralized lesion arising from the tibial cortex (*arrow*). **B:** Axial CT scan shows lesion arising from the tibial cortex with soft-tissue mass (*arrow*). **C:** Axial T2-weighted MRI shows heterogeneous signal within the lesion (*arrow*).

**FIGURE 8.8.** Central chondrosarcoma in the pelvis arising from an enchondroma. **A:** Radiograph shows calcified lesion in the acetabulum (*arrow*). **B:** Coronal reformatted CT shows mildly expansile, calcified, intraosseous lesion (*arrow*). **C:** Coronal T2-weighted MRI with fat suppression shows high signal in the nonmineralized portions of the lesion (*arrow*).

embedded in a much larger mass of clearly benign tissue. At the other end of this spectrum are high-grade, frankly malignant tumors that recur and spread by local extension or metastasis. Chondrosarcomas follow a slow clinical evolution; they tend to metastasize late in the clinical course, and patients rarely present with metastatic disease.

## Medullary Chondrosarcoma

Medullary (central) chondrosarcomas are primary lesions that arise within the cancellous bone or the medullary cavity. The most common locations are the pelvis (23% of cases), femur (22%), ribs (11%), and humerus (11%). The presenting symptom is deep pain lasting for months or years. If the tumor has breached the cortex,

local swelling may be present. Presentation is over a wide age range, but most patients are between 35 and 70 years of age, and men are affected more frequently than women. The treatment is surgical. The incidence of metastasis and the prognosis are related to the histologic grade, with 10-year survival ranging from 28% for high-grade lesions to 85% for low-grade lesions. The radiographic appearance is osseous destruction with matrix mineralization characteristic of cartilage. A typical lesion would be a lucent area in the center of a long bone with endosteal scalloping, cortical thickening, and geographic margins. Often, the tumor contains punctate or flocculent calcification and ring-shaped ossification characteristic of cartilage tissue (Figs. 8.8–8.10). The lucent appearance is a result of the replacement of normal bone by noncalcified cartilage.

**FIGURE 8.9.** Low-grade chondrosarcoma of the scapula. **A:** AP radiograph shows a well-circumscribed, mildly expansile lesion in the acromion process (*arrow*) with cartilage-type calcifications. **B:** Axial CT scan demonstrates endosteal scalloping and chondroid matrix (*arrow*).

A          B          C

**FIGURE 8.10.** Low-grade chondrosarcoma of the femur. **A:** AP radiograph of the femur shows an intramedullary lesion with flocculent calcification. **B:** Coronal inversion recovery MRI shows high signal in a lobular morphology. **C:** Axial CT scan shows endosteal scalloping (*arrow*) and mineralized matrix. There is no cortical penetration.

On CT, the nonmineralized regions have a myxoid appearance with attenuation in the range of 10 to 30 Hounsfield units (HU). On MRI, these regions have high signal on T2-weighted images and variable signal on TI-weighted images. A lobular growth pattern is often evident on CT or MRI. Bone scan shows increased tracer accumulation.

## Exostotic Chondrosarcoma

Exostotic (peripheral) chondrosarcomas arise in the cartilage cap of a previously benign exostosis (osteochondroma) or from the surface of a bone involved by multiple heritable exostoses. They represent approximately 15% of chondrosarcomas. Men are affected twice as often as women. A wide age range is affected, but most patients are young adults. The tumors tend to be of low histologic grade and may be difficult to distinguish from the cartilaginous cap, but a nonmineralized soft-tissue component larger than 1 cm should raise suspicion. If a lesion recurs, it tends to be of a higher histologic grade. The radiographic appearance is that of an exostosis with an attached mass of soft-tissue density containing variable amounts of cartilaginous calcification (Fig. 8.11). CT and MRI reliably demonstrate nonmineralized cartilaginous matrix. Serial films

A          B          C

**FIGURE 8.11.** Exostotic chondrosarcoma in a patient with multiple hereditary exostoses. **A:** CT scout of pelvis shows deformity of right hemipelvis from multiple exostoses. **B:** Axial CT shows low attenuation soft-tissue mass (*arrow*) with dense calcifications. **C:** Axial T2-weighted fat-suppressed MRI shows the noncalcified areas of the mass to be of predominately high signal (*arrow*).

may document destruction of ossified portions of the underlying exostosis. These lesions appear as areas of increased tracer uptake on bone scan, with the intensity of radionuclide accumulation roughly proportional to the combined amount of enchondral ossification, osteoblastic activity, and hyperemia in the tumor. The intensity of uptake does not reliably predict whether the lesion is benign or malignant.

## Chondrosarcoma Variants

Dedifferentiated chondrosarcomas contain a limited focus of anaplastic sarcoma within a larger mass of typical low-grade chondrosarcoma. The clinical course is that of the higher-grade tumor, and the prognosis is grim. These account for approximately 11% of chondrosarcomas. Other chondrosarcoma variants with distinctive histologic or gross pathologic features comprise approximately 5% of all chondrosarcomas. These include clear cell chondrosarcoma, mesenchymal chondrosarcoma, and juxtacortical (parosteal or periosteal) chondrosarcoma.

## ■ PRIMARY MARROW CELL TUMORS
## Multiple Myeloma

Multiple myeloma is a malignant neoplasm of plasmacytes, the cells of the bone marrow that make immunoglobulins. The most common primary tumor arising in the bone, multiple myeloma, has an incidence of 14,600 per year in the United States. The age of onset is usually between 45 and 80 years. Although palliative treatments exist, the condition is uniformly fatal and without cure. Myeloma arises in the bone marrow and involves it diffusely. Bony abnormalities usually occur at multiple sites, including the vertebrae in 66% of patients, the ribs in 45%, the skull in 40%, the shoulder girdle in 40%, the pelvis in 30%, and the long bones in 25%. Myeloma lesions are sharply defined, purely lytic areas of bone destruction with no reactive bone formation. The pattern of destruction may be geographic, moth-eaten, or permeated; involvement may be so diffuse that the bones are simply osteopenic or even normal in

**FIGURE 8.12.** Multiple myeloma. Axial CT shows expansile, lytic destruction of L1 vertebral body (*arrows*) with pathologic transverse process fracture (*arrowhead*).

radiographic appearance (Fig. 8.12; see Fig. 7.2). Pathologically, the marrow and bone have been replaced by the myeloma tissue. Focal holes in the involved bones are filled with closely packed sheets of plasmacytes of varying maturity. The lesions may be expansile, penetrate the cortex, and form large extraosseous soft-tissue masses. Pathologic fractures are common. The radionuclide bone scan is typically normal or may show areas of decreased uptake ("cold" spots). These cold spots represent destruction and replacement of the bone by the myeloma tissue without the evocation of osteoblastic bone reaction. For this reason, radiographs are better than bone scans for disclosing sites of bone destruction. MRI shows the replacement of the normal marrow by the myeloma tissue (Fig. 8.13).

A

B

**FIGURE 8.13.** Multiple myeloma. **A:** Coronal T1-weighted MRI showing multiple lesions (*arrows*) in the marrow with signal intensity similar to the muscle. **B:** Coronal T2-weighted fat-suppressed MRI shows corresponding high signal intensity of the lesions (*arrow*).

**FIGURE 8.14.** Plasmacytoma. Radiograph shows expansile, lytic lesion involving the entire L3 vertebra.

Several differential points may help distinguish between multiple myeloma and osseous metastases in patients with multiple destructive bone lesions. Myeloma tissue produces osteoclast-stimulating factors that result in bone destruction that is cleanly marginated and purely lytic. Although metastases also produce osteoclast-stimulating factors, they tend to provoke the reactive bone, frequently resulting in a more ragged and irregular appearance. Myeloma may involve the intervertebral disks and the mandible, but metastases rarely do so. Metastases often involve the vertebral pedicles, but myeloma rarely does so. A large soft-tissue mass is more likely to be present with myeloma than with metastases. The bone scan is usually positive in the presence of bone metastases and often negative in myeloma.

## Solitary Myeloma

Solitary myeloma (plasmacytoma) is myeloma that has a single focus of involvement. The findings from marrow aspiration may therefore be negative, and laboratory manifestations may be absent. Virtually all patients with solitary myeloma develop multiple myeloma, but 10 years or more may pass before the progression of the disease becomes apparent. Solitary myeloma commonly presents as an expansile lesion in the spine, a rib, the pelvis, or the sacrum (Figs. 8.14 and 8.15).

## Primary Lymphoma

Lymphoma presenting as a primary tumor of the bone without concurrent regional lymph node or visceral involvement represents 5% of all extranodal (non-Hodgkin) lymphomas. Most are large-cell lymphomas of B-cell origin and are histologically similar or identical to extranodal lymphomas arising at other sites. Lymphoma may develop at any age, but most patients are adults, and men are affected more frequently than women. The common presentation is localized pain, often with a mass, and minimal or absent systemic symptoms. Approximately 50% have symptoms for a year or longer before diagnosis. Most lesions have a diaphyseal location in a long bone, especially the femur or humerus, but other frequent sites of involvement include the clavicle, ribs, and pelvis. Ill-defined, permeated, or moth-eaten destruction of the bone with little or no periosteal reaction is the usual radiographic appearance. This appearance reflects the insidious spread of tumor cells along the marrow spaces and through the cortex by way of the haversian systems, growing through and enlarging them. The lesions may be extensive

**A**    **B**

**FIGURE 8.15.** Plasmacytoma. **A:** Axial CT with soft-tissue window shows expansile, lytic lesion in the acetabulum and superior pubic ramus. **B:** Axial CT with bone window shows areas of cortical destruction.

**FIGURE 8.16.** Lymphoma of the distal femur. **A:** Lateral radiograph shows permeated destruction and mottled sclerosis. **B:** Sagittal T2-weighted fat-suppressed MRI shows a soft-tissue mass (*arrowheads*).

at presentation, often involving more than 50% of the affected bone. A large, nonmineralized soft-tissue mass may be present when there is extensive cortical destruction. Mild to moderate bone reaction is seen in approximately 45% of lesions, consisting of a mottled sclerotic reaction within the cancellous bone, new reactive periosteal bone, or both (Fig. 8.16). Sequestra are seen in 11% of the cases of primary lymphoma of the bone. Lymphoma always shows increased isotope uptake on bone scan. CT and MRI are useful for demonstrating tumor extent, especially cortical penetration and extraosseous tumor. Primary lymphomas may also occur in the muscle (Fig. 8.17). The treatment of

lymphoma involves radiation therapy, adjuvant chemotherapy, and sometimes surgery. The prognosis is related to the cell type and pattern of disease and to the extent of dissemination at presentation. With optimal treatment, the 5-year survival rate is greater than 75%.

## ■ SMALL CELL SARCOMAS

The group of small cell sarcomas includes Ewing sarcoma, primitive neuroectodermal tumor (PNET) of the bone, and small cell osteosarcoma.

**FIGURE 8.17.** Intramuscular lymphoma. **A:** Axial T1-weighted MRI shows a focal mass in the medial head of the gastrocnemius muscle (*arrow*). The remainder of the gastrocnemius muscle is atrophied (*arrowhead*). **B:** Axial T2-weighted fat-suppressed MRI shows high signal in the mass (*arrow*).

## Ewing Sarcoma

Ewing sarcoma is a tumor that consists of small, round, undifferentiated cells, probably of neuroectodermal histogenesis. Although 75% of Ewing sarcomas occur in patients younger than 20 years of age, these lesions may develop at any age. They are the most common primary bone tumor in the first decade of life, and the second most common (behind osteosarcoma) in the second decade. Patients present with local pain and swelling, fever, anemia, and elevated erythrocyte sedimentation rate; the clinical impression is often that of osteomyelitis. Up to 30% of patients have metastases at presentation. Ewing sarcoma may develop in practically any bone, although the majority of cases involve the sacrum, innominate bone, and long bones of the lower extremities. Only 3% of tumors affect the hands and feet. Most Ewing sarcomas are found in the metadiaphysis of long bones, mostly the femur, but they also occur in the diaphysis and metaphysis. Approximately one fourth occur in flat bones (pelvis and scapula). The tumor begins in the medullary space and spreads through the bone, often causing only minimal osseous destruction. The tumor penetrates the cortex by extending through the haversian systems into the subperiosteal space where the tumor may enlarge, lift the periosteum off the bone, and eventually penetrate it to form an extraosseous mass. As further destruction of the cortex occurs, a permeated pattern of bone destruction may become evident. In the long bones, the typical radiographic appearance is that of permeated intramedullary bone destruction with periosteal reactive bone (Figs. 8.18–8.20). Sclerotic bone reaction within the bone is usually not seen, but on bone scan, intense radionuclide activity is present. Pathologic fractures occur in a small number of cases. CT and MRI scanning define the extraosseous and intramedullary components of the tumor and are useful in planning radiation portals and in following response to radiation and chemotherapy. A surrounding zone of edema is commonly present. Ewing sarcoma is highly radiosensitive. Radiation and chemotherapy may be used alone or

**A**

**B**

**C**

**FIGURE 8.18.** Ewing sarcoma of the distal humerus. **A:** AP radiograph shows a lytic lesion in the distal humerus at the olecranon fossa (*arrow*). The margins of the lesion are irregular, and there is no reactive bone formation. **B:** Axial CT scan shows the destructive bone lesion (*arrow*) with anterior and posterior soft-tissue extension. **C:** Sagittal T2-weighted fat-suppressed MRI shows a mass centered at the distal humerus with large anterior and posterior soft-tissue components (*arrows*). The lesion has heterogeneous high signal. An elbow effusion is present.

**FIGURE 8.19.** Ewing sarcoma of the rib. Enhanced CT scan shows rib destruction and massive soft-tissue mass (*arrow*).

in combination with surgical excision. However, the rate of local tumor recurrence ranges from 12% to 25%. Soft-tissue extension is associated with increased risk of distant metastases and local recurrence. Five-year survival for nonmetastatic tumor confined to the bone of origin is 87%, but survival drops to 20% with extraosseous extension. Patients who survive for several years may eventually develop secondary, radiation-induced sarcomas.

Hematogenous osteomyelitis spreads through the bone in a fashion similar to Ewing sarcoma, leading to a similar radiologic appearance (see Chapter 16). Both may occur in the same age group and have similar clinical presentations.

## Primitive Neuroectodermal Tumor

PNET is a type of small cell sarcoma closely related to but pathologically distinct from Ewing sarcoma and neuroblastoma. It shares a number of cytogenetic and molecular biologic features and is identical to the malignant small cell tumor of the thoraco-pulmonary region (Askin tumor). In the extremities, PNET shares many clinical characteristics with Ewing sarcoma, with similar presentation, peak age (mean, 15 years), and male predominance of 2:1. Metastases to bone, lung, liver, bone marrow, spleen, and lymph nodes are noted at presentation in 50%. It is virtually indistinguishable from Ewing sarcoma on imaging (Fig. 8.21). There is a permeated pattern of destruction with early soft-tissue extension in a diaphyseal or metadiaphyseal location. There can be extensive periosteal reaction, often with an onion-skin or hair-on-end appearance. CT and MRI can be helpful in clarifying the extent of the disease, and the radionuclide bone scan is useful in looking for osseous metastases. PNET has a much poorer prognosis than Ewing sarcoma.

## Small Cell Osteosarcoma

Small cell osteosarcoma is a variant of osteosarcoma that has a histologic appearance similar to Ewing sarcoma and lymphoma of the bone. However, small amounts of mineralized tumor osteoid are present. The radiologic appearance is that of osteosarcoma in the majority of cases, but a significant proportion has an appearance that resembles Ewing sarcoma or lymphoma (Fig. 8.22). Similar to Ewing sarcoma, most patients are young. Small cell osteosarcomas are high-grade lesions that are treated similarly to conventional high-grade intramedullary osteosarcomas.

**A**

**B**

**FIGURE 8.20.** Ewing sarcoma of the femoral shaft. **A:** Axial CT scan shows onion-skin periosteal reaction in the femoral cortex with soft-tissue density replacing normal fatty marrow. **B:** Axial T2-weighted fat-suppressed MRI shows onion-skin periosteal reaction and surrounding edema.

**FIGURE 8.21.** PNET of the ankle. Sagittal T1-weighted MRI shows a lobulated soft-tissue mass in the posterior compartment of the ankle.

# ■ MALIGNANT FIBROUS HISTIOCYTOMA OF THE BONE

Malignant fibrous histiocytoma (MFH) is a malignant tumor of mesenchymal origin. Although MFH is the most common soft-tissue sarcoma of adults, MFH of the bone is rare. MFH of the bone is most commonly found in the fifth to seventh decades but may occur at any age. Symptoms are nonspecific, often a palpable mass with pain and tenderness. More acute pain can occur secondary to pathologic fractures, which are common. MFH of the bone can occur de novo, but 10% to 20% occur in association with other osseous abnormalities such as Paget disease and bone infarct (Fig. 8.23) or after radiation therapy. The most common sites are similar to those in osteosarcoma: the ends of long bones (75%), with a preponderance in the lower extremity. The femur (45%), tibia (20%), and humerus (9%) are the bones most often involved. The metaphyseal region is the most common location within the bone, and extension into

the epiphysis or diaphysis is frequent. The lesions have an aggressive appearance with permeated or moth-eaten destruction involving a poorly defined unifocal lesion. Cortical destruction and soft-tissue mass are almost invariably present, and cortical expansion is unusual except in the flat and irregularly shaped bones (ribs, scapula, and sternum). Periostitis is unusual unless a healing pathologic fracture is present. Mottled internal calcifications or sclerotic margins are rarely present. On CT, the lesions are predominantly muscle density (30 to 60 HU), with hypodense regions representing necrosis. MRI may be helpful to assess intraosseous versus extraosseous extension. Increased uptake is seen on bone scan. The treatment is surgical, with no clearly defined role for chemotherapy or radiotherapy. However, the prognosis is poor because of high rates of local recurrence and early metastases to regional lymph nodes and other distant sites. The reported 5-year survival ranges from 0% to 70%, depending on the stage of the lesion.

# ■ CHORDOMA

Chordomas are slow-growing malignant neoplasms that arise from notochordal remnants. They are typically seen in middle-aged men, most frequently at the ends of the spine (50% in the sacrum or coccyx, 35% in the clivus, and 15% elsewhere in the spine). Patients present with pain of insidious onset and symptoms caused by mass effect, often of long duration. Grossly, these tumors are multilobular, soft, myxoid, gelatinous masses that infiltrate locally and may eventually metastasize. In the sacrococcygeal region, the radiologic appearance is geographic bone destruction and replacement of bone by nonmineralized tumor. The margins range from sclerotic to ill-defined. The cortex is often penetrated with the formation of a large, lobular, extraosseous mass anterior to the spine (Fig. 8.24). The tumors are typically large at presentation. Because of the myxoid matrix, the attenuation on CT is typically lower than the cellular soft tissue, and MRI may show high signal on both T1- and T2-weighted images. The treatment is surgical, but complete excision is rarely possible because of their central location. A high rate of local recurrence and progressive difficulties in treating the recurrences result in a poor long-term prognosis. A secondary component of

**A**

**B**

**C**

**FIGURE 8.22.** Small cell osteosarcoma. **A:** AP hip radiograph shows a lytic lesion in the intertrochanteric region of the femur (*arrow*). **B:** Axial CT scan shows intramedullary lesion with anterior cortical breakthrough and soft-tissue mass with hyperdense mineralized region (*arrow*). **C:** Axial T2-weighted fat-suppressed MRI shows the extent of the lesion. The mineralized portion of the soft-tissue mass (*arrow*) has low signal.

**FIGURE 8.23.** MFH of the bone arising in a marrow infarct. **A:** AP radiograph of the distal femur shows permeated bone destruction (*arrow*). **B:** Axial CT scan shows bone destruction surrounding an irregularly shaped sequestrum (*arrow*) of the bone. **C:** Coronal T1-weighted MRI shows the lesion (*long arrow*) in the distal femur and a marrow infarct (*short arrow*) in the proximal tibia.

high-grade sarcoma resembling MFH (dedifferentiated chordoma) may appear after multiple recurrences.

# ADAMANTINOMA

Adamantinoma is a primary low-grade malignant tumor of the bone. It is of epithelial origin, with marked predilection for the tibia. Adamantinoma is often associated with osteofibrous dysplasia, and some authorities believe that they are subsets of the same disease. Adamantinoma of the bone is distinct from gnathic adamantinoma (ameloblastoma), although both share an epithelial origin and a microscopic resemblance. Although 50% present at ages 10 to 30 years, adamantinoma may be found at any age. Symptoms of pain are often present for more than a year, and 90% involve the tibia. A few patients have an ipsilateral fibular tumor. The radiographic appearance is that of an eccentrically located lucent lesion with lobulated expansion of the cortex and sharply defined margins (Fig. 8.25). The most common location is the tibial diaphysis

with involvement of the anterior cortex. An anterior tibial bowing deformity is common. Approximately 90% involve the cortex and medullary space, 10% are confined to the cortex, and 15% penetrate the cortex and involve the soft tissues. The treatment is surgical, with a high rate of recurrence after curettage and a lower rate after wide excision. Metastases to the lung, nodes, or bone may present many years later.

# SOFT-TISSUE SARCOMAS

The reported annual incidence of soft-tissue sarcomas in the United States is 6,400. Approximately two thirds of these are found in the extremities and limb girdles (Table 8.2), making them more common than primary bone sarcomas in the same locations. Most are of mesenchymal origin; a minority is of neuroectodermal origin. In adults, the most common lesions are MFH, liposarcoma, synovial sarcoma, leiomyosarcoma, and malignant schwannoma (Table 8.3). Fibrosarcoma is the most

**A**    **B**

**FIGURE 8.24.** Chordoma. **A:** CT shows irregular bone destruction of the lower sacrum (*arrow*). **B:** Sagittal T1-weighted MRI with fat suppression following gadolinium injection shows heterogeneous enhancement of the marrow space and extension into the surrounding soft tissues (*arrowheads*).

**FIGURE 8.25.** Adamantinoma of the tibia. Lateral radiograph shows lobulated, expansile lucent lesion with anterior tibial bowing deformity.

common lesion in patients younger than 6 years of age, and MFH (including variants) and synovial sarcoma are most common from ages 6 to 15 years. The majority of soft-tissue sarcomas present in adults. Patients complain of a palpable mass of long duration and pain or tenderness of insidious onset. Patients may delay seeking medical attention, and this long chronicity may falsely suggest an indolent process. The majority of lesions present in stage II-B or III (see Chapter 7). Soft-tissue sarcomas metastasize to the lung, liver, or bone. Soft-tissue sarcomas have nonspecific appearances on imaging, and there are no reliable criteria for distinguishing among them. Once benign soft-tissue masses with specific features such as lipoma, elasto-fibroma, ganglion, myositis ossificans, aneurysm, bursitis, and hematoma have been eliminated as possibilities, factors that suggest sarcoma include older age, location in the thigh, large size, round or ovoid shape, and involvement of the adjacent bone. Malignant soft-tissue masses usually have areas of inhomogeneity and lower density on CT that correspond to regions of necrosis and hemorrhage. Sarcomas that calcify or ossify include synovial sarcoma (Fig. 8.26), extraskeletal osteosarcoma, extraskeletal chondrosarcoma, rhabdomyosarcoma, MFH, and liposarcoma. The presence of fat within a lesion suggests a well-differentiated liposarcoma (Fig. 8.27), but higher-grade liposarcomas generally do not contain fat. Small amounts of subcutaneous or intermuscular fat may be engulfed by an aggressive sarcoma as it enlarges so that the presence of fat is not necessarily indicative of liposarcoma. On MRI, soft-tissue sarcomas usually have intermediate signal on T1-weighted

| TABLE 8.2 | Anatomic Distribution of Soft-Tissue Sarcomas in the Extremities and Limb Girdles[a] |
|---|---|
| Location | Frequency (%) |
| Lower extremity | 45 |
| Upper extremity | 16 |
| Hip and buttocks | 14 |
| Proximal limb girdle | 9 |
| Foot and ankle | 9 |
| Hand and wrist | 7 |

[a]Based on 6,796 soft-tissue sarcomas of the extremities and limb girdles, including all ages and all histologic types.
*Source*: Kransdorf MJ. Malignant soft-tissue tumors in a large referral population: Distribution of diagnoses by age, sex, and location. *AJR*. 1995;164:129–134.

| TABLE 8.3 | Most Common Soft-Tissue Sarcomas in the Extremities and Limb Girdles at Various Ages | |
|---|---|---|
| 0–5 years | 6–15 years | 16+ years |
| Fibrosarcoma | MFH (including | MFH |
| Rhabdomyosarcoma | angiomatoid | Liposarcoma |
| | MFH) | Synovial sarcoma |
| | Synovial sarcoma | Malignant |
| | | schwannoma |
| | | Leiomyosarcoma |

For each age range, the tumors are listed in order of frequency and account for over 50% of the lesions.
*Source*: Kransdorf MJ. Malignant soft-tissue tumors in a large referral population: Distribution of diagnoses by age, sex, and location. *AJR*. 1995;164:129–134.

**A**    **B**

**FIGURE 8.26.** Synovial sarcoma. **A:** Lateral radiograph of the knee shows a heavily calcified mass (*arrow*) posterior to the knee. **B:** Axial T1-weighted MRI with fat suppression following gadolinium injection shows heterogeneous enhancement.

**A**    **B**    **C**

**FIGURE 8.27.** Liposarcoma. **A:** Lateral radiograph of the thigh shows a large, lucent lesion in the posterior soft tissues. **B:** Axial CT scan shows a heterogeneous fat-containing soft-tissue mass in the posterior compartment of the thigh. **C:** Axial T2-weighted MRI with fat suppression shows high signal in some portions of the lesion with low signal resulting from fat suppression in other portions of the lesion.
*Source*: From Ramsdell MG, Chew FS, Keel SB. Myxoid liposarcoma of the thigh. *AJR*. 1998;170:1242.

A                                                                          B

**FIGURE 8.28.** Preoperative staging for soft-tissue sarcoma in the anterior compartment of the thigh. **A:** Axial T2-weighted MRI shows a tumor (*T*) occupying the entire anterior compartment. Septation and stranding are present within the lesion. **B:** Axial T1-weighted MRI with fat suppression following gadolinium injection shows rim enhancement (*arrow*), indicative of extensive necrosis of the nonenhancing regions.

images and high signal on T2-weighted images. Enhancement with intravenous contrast can be expected on both CT and MRI. The goal of imaging, once the presence of the lesion is confirmed, should be to define the lesion's size and location and the extent and anatomic relation of the lesion to muscle compartments, fascial planes, neurovascular bundles, and the bone. Staging follows the system used for bone sarcomas. The treatment of soft-tissue sarcomas is surgical, sometimes with neoadjuvant or adjuvant radiation therapy, chemotherapy, or both. Imaging of soft-tissue sarcomas for surgical planning after chemotherapy and radiation therapy may reveal extensive areas of liquefaction, hemorrhage, and necrosis (Fig. 8.28). Five-year survival rates of 25% to 60% have been reported.

## SOURCES AND READINGS

Angtuaco EJ, Fassas AB, Walker R, Sethi R, Barlogie B. Multiple myeloma: Clinical review and diagnostic imaging. *Radiology.* 2004;231(1):11–23.

Arndt CA, Crist WM. Common musculoskeletal tumors of childhood and adolescence. *N Engl J Med.* 1999;341(5):342–352.

Askin FB, Perlman EJ. Neuroblastoma and peripheral neuroectodermal tumors. *Am J Clin Pathol.* 1998;109(Suppl.):S23–S30.

Clark MA, Fisher C, Judson I, Thomas, JM. Soft-tissue sarcomas in adults. *N Engl J Med.* 2005;353:701–711

Durr HR, Muller PE, Hiller E, et al. Malignant lymphoma of bone. *Arch Orthop Trauma Surg.* 2002;122:10–16.

eMedicine. http://emedicine.medscape.com.

Enneking WF. *Musculoskeletal Tumor Surgery.* Edinburgh: Churchill Livingstone; 1983.

Fechner RE, Mills SE. *Tumors of the Bones and Joints.* Washington, DC: Armed Forces Institute of Pathology; 1993.

Ferrari S, Palmerini E. Adjuvant and neoadjuvant combination chemotherapy for osteogenic sarcoma. *Curr Opin Oncol.* 2007;19(4):341–346.

Fuchs B, Pritchard DJ. Etiology of osteosarcoma. *Clin Orthop.* 2002;397:40–52.

Guise TA. Molecular mechanisms of osteolytic bone metastases. *Cancer.* 2000;88(Suppl.):2892–2898.

Hudson TM. Radiologic-pathologic correlation of musculoskeletal lesions. Baltimore, MD: Williams & Wilkins; 1987.

Huvos AG. *Bone Tumors: Diagnosis, Treatment, and Prognosis.* 2nd Ed. Philadelphia, PA: WB Saunders; 1991.

Jacobs JJ, Roebuck KA, Archibeck M, et al. Osteolysis: Basic science. *Clin Orthop.* 2001;393:71–77.

Jemal A, Siegel R, Ward E, et al. Cancer statistics, 2008. *CA Cancer J Clin.* 2008;58(2):71–96.

Klein MJ, Siegal GP. Osteosarcoma: Anatomic and histologic variants. *Am J Clin Pathol.* 2006;125(4):555–581.

Kransdorf MJ, Murphey MD. *Imaging of Soft Tissue Tumors.* 2nd Ed. Philadelphia, PA: Lippincott Williams & Wilkins; 2006.

Lodwick GS. *Atlas of Tumor Radiology. The Bones and Joints.* Chicago, IL: Year Book; 1971.

Ludwig H, Strasser-Weippl K, Schreder M, Zojer N. Advances in the treatment of hematological malignancies: Current treatment approaches in multiple myeloma. *Ann Oncol.* 2007;18(Suppl. 9):ix64–ix70.

Mulligan ME, McRae GA, Murphey MD. Imaging features of primary lymphoma of bone. *AJR.* 1999;173:1691–1697.

Mundy G. Preclinical models of bone metastases. *Semin Oncol.* 2001;28:2–8.

Murphey MD, Flemming DJ, Boyea SR, et al. Enchondroma versus chondrosarcoma in the appendicular skeleton: Differentiating features. *Radiographics.* 1998;18:1213–1237.

Murphey MD, Robbin MR, McRae GA, et al. The many faces of osteosarcoma. *Radiographics.* 1997;17:1205–1231.

Parsons TW III, Frink SJ, Campbell SE. Musculoskeletal neoplasia: Helping the orthopaedic surgeon establish the diagnosis. *Semin Musculoskelet Radiol.* 2007;11(1):3–15.

Resnick DL, Kransdorf MJ. *Bone and Joint Imaging.* 3rd Ed. Philadelphia, PA: WB Saunders; 2004.

Saifuddin A. The accuracy of imaging in the local staging of appendicular osteosarcoma. *Skeletal Radiol.* 2002;31(4):191–201.

Unni KK. *Dahlin's Bone Tumors. General Aspects and Data on 11,087 Cases.* 5th Ed. Philadelphia, PA: Lippincott–Raven; 1996.

Vanel D. Musculoskeletal primary tumours: Treatment evaluation and detection of recurrences. *Cancer Imaging.* 2007;7 Spec No A:S150–S151.

Weber K, Damron TA, Frassica FJ, Sim FH. Malignant bone tumors. *Instr Course Lect.* 2008;57:673–688.

Wu JS, Hochman MG. Soft-Tissue Tumors and Tumorlike Lesions: A Systematic Imaging Approach. *Radiology.* 2009;253(2):297–316.

# CHAPTER 9

# Benign Lesions

Benign Bone-Forming Lesions
    Osteoid Osteoma
    Osteoblastoma
    Bone Island
Benign Cartilage Lesions
    Enchondroma
    Osteochondroma
    Osteochondromatosis
    Periosteal Chondroma
    Chondroblastoma
    Chondromyxoid Fibroma
Benign Fibrous Lesions
    Fibrous Cortical Defects and
      Nonossifying Fibromas
    Fibrous Dysplasia
    Desmoplastic Fibroma
    Aggressive Fibromatosis

Benign Fatty Lesions
    Intraosseous Lipoma
    Liposclerosing Myxofibrous
      Tumor of Bone
    Lipoma
    Elastofibroma
Langerhans Cell Histiocytosis
Giant Cell Tumor
Cystic Lesions of Bone
    Aneurysmal Bone Cyst
    Simple Bone Cyst
    Intraosseous Ganglion
    Epidermoid Inclusion Cyst
Cystic Masses of Soft Tissues
    Ganglion
    Synovial Cysts

    Bursitis
    Myxoma
Vascular Lesions
    Osseous Vascular Lesions
    Soft-Tissue Vascular Lesions
Neurogenic Lesions
    Peripheral Nerve Sheath Tumors
    Morton Neuroma
Posttraumatic Lesions
    Myositis Ossificans
    Bizarre Parosteal Osteochondromatous
      Proliferation
    Foreign Body Granuloma

This chapter describes benign neoplasms and benign tumorlike lesions that are not neoplastic in origin. A key decision that becomes easier with experience is whether a radiologic finding represents an actual lesion or merely a normal structure, an anatomic or developmental variant, or the result of previous trauma, surgery, or other disease. Atlases of normal variants are often helpful. The principal lesions one should consider in formulating a differential diagnosis for a benign lesion are listed in Table 9.1.

## ■ BENIGN BONE-FORMING LESIONS

### Osteoid Osteoma

Osteoid osteoma is a fairly common benign bone-forming neoplasm. The lesion, called a *nidus,* is small, generally ranging in size from 3 to 15 mm. When larger, the lesion is often classified as an osteoblastoma (discussed in "Osteoblastoma"). Approximately 80% of patients are between the ages of 5 and 20 years; few are older than 30 years of age. The location may be cortical, central, or, less frequently, subperiosteal. The femur is the most common site (39% of cases), followed by the tibia (23%) and upper extremity (21%). Patients present with dull, aching pain that has lasted for months to years. When located in the spine, osteoid osteomas may cause painful scoliosis of rapid onset; near a joint, they may cause reactive synovitis. The nidus consists of osteoid and fibrovascular connective tissue. The osteoid may be mineralized to a variable extent, usually in the center (Fig. 9.1). The nidus is radiolucent but may be obscured by cortical thickening and dense sclerosis from the reactive bone. Sclerosis is usually minimal around lesions located in the

cancellous bone, near a joint, or in a subperiosteal position (Fig. 9.2). Osteoid osteomas have intensely increased activity on bone scan; the activity may be more intense in the nidus ("double-density" sign). The nidus may enhance on CT and MRI, reflecting the fibrovascular tissue within it. Because of the small size of the nidus and its possible obscuration by reactive sclerosis, CT is

| TABLE 9.1 | Benign Bone Lesions | |
|---|---|---|
| | Solitary[a] | Solitary or Multifocal |
| Common | Osteoid osteoma | Bone island |
| | Simple bone cyst | Fibrous cortical defect |
| | Bone (Brodie) abscess | Osteochondroma |
| | | Enchondroma |
| | | Fibrous dysplasia |
| | | Nonossifying fibroma |
| | | Eosinophilic granuloma |
| Uncommon | Giant cell tumor | |
| | Osteoblastoma | |
| | Chondroblastoma | |
| | Periosteal chondroma | |
| | Aneurysmal bone cyst | |
| Rare | Chondromyxoid fibroma | |

[a]There may be case reports of multiple lesions.

**FIGURE 9.1.** Osteoid osteoma. **A:** Coronal T1-weighted MRI shows lesion in the subchondral bone of the lateral tibial plateau. **B:** Coronal T2-weighted fat-suppressed MRI shows the nidus (*arrow*) with surrounding edema. **C:** Axial CT scan shows central ossification within the nidus (*arrow*).

commonly used to identify and localize the nidus. Osteoid osteomas have been treated by surgical excision, but their small size makes them amenable to percutaneous radiofrequency ablation or excision under CT guidance. Failure to remove or destroy the entire nidus may lead to recurrence.

## Osteoblastoma

Osteoblastomas are uncommon lesions that are considered by some to be giant osteoid osteomas because of their histologic resemblance. They affect young persons; 80% occur in patients younger than 30 years of age. Approximately half are found in the spine and most of the remainder in the femur and tibia. Of those in the spine, most are in the posterior elements; a few also involve the vertebral body, and very few involve the vertebral body alone. Within tubular bones, osteoblastomas may be intracortical, subperiosteal, or central in location. They are larger than osteoid osteomas, generally 1 to 10 cm in diameter. There is usually much less reactive bone surrounding

an osteoblastoma than an osteoid osteoma. Patients with osteoblastomas typically present with pain of several months' duration. If the lesion is superficial, localized swelling and tenderness are present. In the spine, lesions may produce painful scoliosis; they may also interfere mechanically with the cord or with nerve roots. The radiographic appearance is a partially lucent expansile lesion with well-defined margins and a variable amount of matrix mineralization (Figs. 9.3 and 9.4; see also Fig. 7.5). The lucent area of geographic bone destruction corresponds to replacement of the bone by non-mineralized tumor tissue. The tumor osteoid may have densely solid or ground-glass mineralization. Large lesions may have an expanded cortical shell from slow endosteal cortical erosion balanced against an enlarging layer of periosteal new bone. Cortical penetration into the soft tissues is absent, but tomography may be required to demonstrate the cortical shell. The tumor tissue may have high attenuation on CT from diffuse mineralization. Osteoblastomas are hot on bone scan. Osteoblastomas usually grow slowly and respond well to excision; very few have been reported to become locally aggressive.

**FIGURE 9.2.** Osteoid osteoma (different patients). **A:** Axial CT scan shows a round nidus (*arrow*) in the lesser trochanter with moderate reactive bone formation. **B:** Axial CT scan shows a round nidus with central calcification (*arrow*) in the cortex of the femoral shaft, with exuberant reactive sclerosis. **C:** AP radiograph shows reactive scoliosis with an osteoid osteoma in the T12 vertebra (*arrow*).

**FIGURE 9.3.** Osteoblastoma. CT shows an expansile lesion in the neural arch of a lower thoracic vertebra (*arrow*).

## Bone Island

A bone island (enostosis) is a circular or oblong nodule of cortical-type bone lying within cancellous bone. Bone islands are typically 1 cm in size but range up to 4 cm. They consist of histologically normal compact bone with haversian systems. They may be found anywhere in the skeleton. Radiographically, they are homogeneous and are as dense as cortical bone. They are well defined but have peripheral spiculations that merge with the surrounding trabeculae (Fig. 9.5). Occasionally, they may change in size or remodel. On radionuclide bone scan, isotope uptake is absent or minimal. Bone islands are common and large or giant bone islands may be mistaken for other lesions such as osteoblastic tumors; they have no other clinical significance. Small bone islands are common incidental findings on CT and MRI.

## ■ BENIGN CARTILAGE LESIONS

### Enchondroma

Solitary enchondromas are benign neoplasms located within the medullary cavity that are composed of mature hyaline cartilage. They probably arise from cartilaginous rests displaced from the growth plate. Sex incidence is equal, and most patients are between 10 and 50 years of age. Typically, the lesions are asymptomatic and discovered incidentally, but many patients present with pathologic fractures. The most common locations for solitary enchondromas are the hands (approximately 50% of cases), the proximal and distal femur, and the proximal humerus. In the hands, the middle and distal portions of the metacarpals and the proximal portions of the phalanges are typically involved. Radiographically, these lesions are lucent from replacement of the bone by the nonmineralized cartilage, but the typical mineralization patterns of cartilaginous matrix may be present: dense punctate or flocculent calcifications or ring- or arc-shaped densities from enchondral ossification of lobular cartilage

**A**

**B**

**FIGURE 9.4.** Osteoblastoma. **A:** Radiograph shows a lucent lesion (*arrow*) in the femoral neck with a sclerotic margin. **B:** CT shows partial mineralization (*arrow*).

**A**    **B**

**FIGURE 9.5.** Bone island. **A:** Bone island in the cancellous bone of the coronoid process of the elbow (*arrow*) on a sagittal reformatted CT. The margins are spiculated where they blend into the normal cancellous bone. The lesion is as dense as the cortex. There is an incidental olecranon enthesophyte (*arrowhead*). **B:** Sagittal T2-weighted fat-suppressed MRI shows the bone island to have low signal intensity (*arrow*).

(Fig. 9.6; see also Figs. 7.12 and 7.13). Slow endosteal enlargement causes an expanded, thinned cortex, but cortical penetration is absent. On MRI, enchondromas have low signal on T1-weighted and proton density images but high signal on T2-weighted images

**FIGURE 9.6.** Enchondroma with lucent matrix occupying the midshaft of the fifth metacarpal. The overlying cortex is thinned. A pathologic fracture is present (*arrow*).

with foci of low signal intensity corresponding to areas of calcification. A characteristic lobular configuration is virtually diagnostic (Fig. 9.7). On radionuclide bone scan, increased isotope uptake is seen, reflecting enchondral ossification, hyperemia, and reactive bone formation.

Occasionally, it may be difficult to distinguish an enchondroma from a low-grade chondrosarcoma radiographically. Imaging findings that suggest a chondrosarcoma include deep endosteal scalloping (greater than two thirds of cortical thickness), cortical destruction and soft-tissue mass (at CT or MRI), periosteal reaction (at radiography), marked uptake of radionuclide (greater than the anterior iliac crest) at bone scintigraphy, and destruction of chondroid matrix over time. Development of chondrosarcoma from solitary enchondroma has not been proved conclusively.

Multiple enchondromatosis (Ollier disease) is a nonfamilial, nonheritable diffuse growth abnormality in which the tubular bones may be bowed and shortened to a variable extent and filled with multiple enchondromas (Fig. 9.8). The severity of involvement may range from a few lesions with mild deformities to countless lesions with severe deformities. The lesions often become stable at puberty, but their growth may continue throughout life. Individual lesions are radiologically and histologically identical to solitary enchondromas, but patients with multiple enchondromatosis have a 30% to 50% risk of developing chondrosarcoma. A lesion that becomes painful in the absence of pathologic fracture should trigger consideration of malignancy. Multiple enchondromatosis with multiple soft-tissue hemangiomas is called *Maffucci syndrome*. The hemangiomatosis may be localized or extensive and may occur anywhere in the skin or subcutaneous tissues.

**FIGURE 9.7.** Enchondroma. **A:** Coronal T1-weighted MRI shows low signal and lobular configuration (*arrow*). Deformity of the distal femoral diaphysis (*arrowhead*) is due to a sessile osteochondroma. **B:** Coronal inversion recovery MRI shows high signal in the lesion (*arrow*) and low signal in the osteochondroma (*arrowhead*).

**FIGURE 9.8.** Multiple enchondromatosis (Ollier disease) deforming the foot. Some lesions have calcified matrix.

## Osteochondroma

Osteochondromas (also called *benign exostoses)* are outgrowths of a histologically normal bone that arise in the vicinity of a growth plate. They are exceedingly common and present during late childhood and adolescence. Although any bone with enchondral ossification may be involved, the femur, the proximal tibia, and the proximal humerus account for two thirds of cases. The typical site is metaphyseal, but osteochondromas may arise anywhere near a growth plate, including accessory ossification centers. Osteochondromas are not thought to be neoplastic but result from the growth of aberrant foci of cartilage on the bony surface. As the cartilage grows, it forms a cap over a bony mass that develops by progressive enchondral ossification. The bony portion contains mature, normal cortical and medullary bone with a marrow space contiguous with the parent bone. Deep lobules of cartilage may be present, often heavily ossified. The lesion may be pedunculated on a stalk, sometimes resembling a cauliflower (Figs. 9.9 and 9.10). Osteochondromas may also be sessile and resemble an expansile lesion. The cartilage cap largely disappears by adulthood. The typical clinical presentation is a firm mass of long duration that may mechanically interfere with function. A bursa may form over the surface and produce pain; in the presence of hemorrhage in a bursa, an enlarging mass develops.

## Osteochondromatosis

Osteochondromatosis (multiple heritable exostoses, multiple osteochondromas, and diaphyseal aclasis) is one of the most common skeletal dysplasias. The condition is familial, with more severe manifestations in men. The skeleton is involved symmetrically, and the limbs are affected more than the spine. The number of exostoses varies. Deformities of the tubular bones are

FIGURE 9.9. Pedunculated osteochondroma (*arrow*) arising from the medial tibial metaphysis.

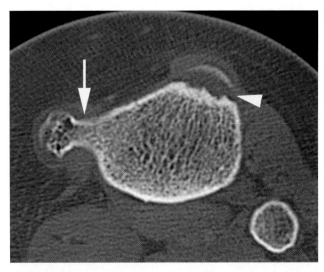

FIGURE 9.10. Axial CT scan of osteochondroma showing its marrow space to be contiguous with that of the underlying bone (*arrow*). The open tibial tubercle growth plate is visible anteriorly (*arrowhead*).

present (Fig. 9.11) and cause disproportionately short limbs, but the degree of shortness appears to be unrelated to the number of exostoses. Growth of the lesions slows as the skeleton matures, and new lesions do not appear in adulthood. Multiple exostoses are radiologically and histologically indistinguishable from solitary exostoses. Secondary development of chondrosarcoma in a

solitary exostosis or in one of the multiple exostoses is a small but definite risk, probably on the order of 1% to 2%; the onset of pain or growth in an adult suggests the possibility. The radiologic distinction between a benign exostosis and an exostotic chondrosarcoma is difficult unless growth and change in appearance can be demonstrated on serial films.

A   B

FIGURE 9.11. Multiple hereditary osteochondromatosis. **A, B:** Radiographs of the knee and shoulder show multiple bony exostoses and deformity of the tubular bones.

**FIGURE 9.12.** Periosteal chondroma of proximal humerus.

**FIGURE 9.13.** Chondroblastoma on axial CT shows a lucent lesion (*arrow*) with a sclerotic margin and cartilaginous matrix in the talus.

## Periosteal Chondroma

Periosteal chondroma is a benign neoplasm composed of a mature cartilage that is located beneath the periosteum. The cortical surface is eroded, but the medullary cavity is not involved. Most are located in the metaphysis or diaphysis of a long bone; the humerus is the most common site. The lesions are lucent and are characteristically surrounded by smoothly contoured, solid, periosteal reactive bone (Fig. 9.12). Cartilage matrix calcification may be present. Symptoms are nonspecific; local excision is curative.

## Chondroblastoma

Chondroblastoma (Codman tumor) is an uncommon benign neoplasm that consists of chondroid tissue mixed with more cellular tissues. Location in the epiphysis is characteristic (approximately 98%), often with extension into the metaphysis (Fig. 9.13). Two thirds arise in the lower extremities, and half arise around the knee. Most patients are young; 80% are between 5 and 25 years of age. When chondroblastomas occur outside the usual age group, they arise in unusual locations. The presentation is nonspecific, typically pain. The radiographic appearance is an ovoid or rounded lucent epiphyseal lesion that is eccentrically located. The margins are geographic, usually with a thin, reactive bony rim. Scattered mottled or stippled calcifications, like those of other cartilage tumors, may be present. Chondroblastomas treated by curettage usually do not recur, but some are aggressive locally.

## Chondromyxoid Fibroma

Chondromyxoid fibromas are rare, cartilage-forming neoplasms with variable amounts of myxoid and fibrous tissue. Young adults are affected most often, but there is a broad age range. The presentation is usually pain. Most chondromyxoid fibromas are found in the lower extremities. The typical radiographic appearance is an eccentric metaphyseal lucent lesion, ovoid or round and lobulated, with a sclerotic rim (Fig. 9.14). Intralesional matrix mineralization is rare. Sometimes, the rim has thickly trabeculated walls, corresponding to a grossly lobular tumor. Cortical expansion may result in a thin, perhaps imperceptible, cortical shell. The treatment is curettage.

## ■ BENIGN FIBROUS LESIONS

### Fibrous Cortical Defects and Nonossifying Fibromas

Fibrous cortical defects and nonossifying fibromas (fibroxanthomas) are histologically identical nonneoplastic lesions thought to be the result of faulty ossification at the growth plate. A causal relationship with stress or trauma has been suggested but not proved. These are self-limited, with no potential for growth or spread. Both regress spontaneously, filling in with bone from the periphery and disappearing. The lesions are present at some time in perhaps one third of all children. Fibrous cortical defects (metaphyseal fibrous defects) are seen most typically in children aged 4 to 8 years. They are located on the cortical surface of the metaphysis at the attachment of a tendon or ligament, mostly around the knee, and produce a 1- to 4-cm scalloped defect in the underlying bone. They are round or oval, lucent, and sharply marginated by a sclerotic rim (Fig. 9.15). Some have a bubbly appearance. Pathologic fractures may occur, but fibrous cortical defects are usually clinically silent and disappear within 2 years of discovery. Nonossifying fibromas can be thought of as fibrous cortical defects with somewhat different radiographic appearance; the distinction is not important for the patient. They are less common than fibrous cortical defects and are discovered in older children or adolescents. They are located eccentrically within the medullary cavity but still

**FIGURE 9.14.** Chondromyxoid fibroma. **A:** Axial CT scan shows a lucent lesion with chondroid matrix mineralization in the ischium (*arrow*). **B:** Axial T2-weighted fat-suppressed MRI showing high signal within the lesion (*arrow*).

within an expanded cortex and are lucent with a sclerotic margin. Some lesions have a trabeculated, scalloped, multilocular, or bubbly appearance (Figs. 9.16 and 9.17; see also Fig. 7.4). The size range is 1 to 7 cm, and larger lesions may fracture or cause pain. These lesions

show a variable amount of uptake on 18F-FDG PET imaging and may mimic metastatic disease, thus making review of radiographs, CT, or MRI of utmost importance to evaluate for the typical imaging appearance of these benign lesions.

**FIGURE 9.15.** Fibrous cortical defect with lobulated sclerotic border (*arrow*) and pathologic fracture (*arrowhead*). **A:** Coronal reformatted CT. **B:** Axial CT.

**FIGURE 9.16.** Nonossifying fibroma in the distal radial shaft. The lesion has a bubbly appearance with a sclerotic margin, expanded cortical shell, and no matrix calcification.

## Fibrous Dysplasia

Fibrous dysplasia is a benign fibro-osseous lesion that is neither familial nor hereditary. Fibrous dysplasia appears to be a developmental abnormality involving the proliferation and maturation of fibroblasts in which benign fibrous tissue with abnormally arranged, dysplastic trabeculae of immature woven bone replaces the normal bone. The dysplastic trabeculae are no thicker than 0.1 mm, so they are not individually visible on clinical radiographs. If present in sufficient number, however, they give the lesions a ground-glass density; if not, the lesions are radiolucent. The lesions are medullary but may replace both cancellous and cortical bones. The abnormal area may be sharply circumscribed and marginated by a thick layer of reactive bone, or it may blend gradually with the adjacent normal bone. The cortex may be either thickened or thinned, but the outer size and shape of the affected bone often are unchanged (see Fig. 7.14). Bowing deformities result from biomechanically insufficient bone and from malunion of pathologic fractures. Fibrous dysplasia has a variable radiographic appearance and often mimics the appearance of other bone lesions. Fibrous dysplasia occurs in monostotic and polyostotic forms. Approximately 80% of cases of fibrous dysplasia are monostotic. The peak age of diagnosis is 5 to 20 years. The typical sites of involvement are the proximal femur, tibia, ribs, and facial bones. Monostotic fibrous dysplasia seldom occurs in the spine or pelvis. Lesions in the long bones are often discovered because of fracture or deformity. Therapy is restricted to orthopedic management of complications. The monostotic form is not associated with other abnormalities or disease.

**A**   **B**

**FIGURE 9.17.** Nonossifying fibroma (*arrow*) expanding the distal fibula. **A:** AP radiograph. **B:** Composite T1-weighted (**left**) and gadolinium-enhanced fat-suppressed (**right**) MRI.

**A**    **B**

**FIGURE 9.18.** Polyostotic fibrous dysplasia involving the right and left distal humeri and the left proximal radius. **A:** Right side; **B:** left side.

In polyostotic fibrous dysplasia, the distribution of lesions may be monomelic, unilateral, or widespread (Fig. 9.18). The extent of bone involvement can be documented at the presentation by skeletal survey; fibrous dysplasia does not spread or proliferate, although the lesions may enlarge as the skeleton grows. Most bony lesions occur in the lower extremities, including the pelvis, legs, and feet. Rib or skull lesions are also often seen. Common deformities include leg-length discrepancy (lesions are in the longer leg); bowing deformities of long bones and ribs, including varus angulation of the proximal femur (shepherd's crook deformity); and, in the skull, frontal bossing, facial asymmetry, and inferolateral orbital displacement. Most patients have only bone lesions or bone and skin lesions; up to 30% of women with polyostotic fibrous dysplasia may have café au lait spots and precocious puberty (McCune-Albright syndrome). The clinical course ranges from asymptomatic (even in the presence of severe skeletal deformities) to multiple pathologic fractures, rapidly progressive deformities, severe pain, debilitation, and even death (Fig. 9.19). Malignant transformation has been documented but is rare. Polyostotic fibrous dysplasia with associated intramuscular myxomas (usually adjacent to the affected bone) is known as *Mazabraud syndrome*.

## Desmoplastic Fibroma

Desmoplastic fibromas are rare intraosseous fibrous lesions that are histologically identical to soft-tissue fibromatosis. They are usually seen in adolescents and young adults. Their location is typically central in the metaphysis of a long bone. They are geographic lytic lesions with a narrow zone of transition but often without a sclerotic rim. There is no matrix mineralization, but there can be a sequestrum. Endosteal erosion and modest cortical expansion are present, but cortical breakthrough usually is not. The endosteal margins characteristically

**FIGURE 9.19.** Polyostotic fibrous dysplasia involving the pelvis and lower extremities with intramedullary rod fixation of a distal femur pathologic fracture seen on coronal reformatted CT. The hip joints are chronically dislocated.

**FIGURE 9.20.** Desmoplastic fibroma of the distal radius.

have thick ridges of bone that may suggest the diagnosis in these otherwise nonspecific-appearing lesions (Fig. 9.20). They may be infiltrative and locally aggressive, but they have no metastatic potential.

## Aggressive Fibromatosis

Aggressive fibromatosis is a true neoplasm of soft tissues that arises from fascial and musculoaponeurotic coverings, sometimes at the site of a traumatic or a postsurgical scar. Nonencapsulated, poorly circumscribed, and infiltrative, aggressive fibromatosis grows insidiously and invades locally but does not metastasize. The lesion may grow large and become adherent to neighboring structures such as neurovascular bundles. Aggressive fibromatosis grossly resembles a scar tissue. It is composed of well-differentiated fibroblasts embedded in an abundant collagenous matrix with increased cellularity at the periphery. Radiographs may show soft-tissue mass, localized periosteal thickening, and frank bony destruction. Because of variable degrees of cellularity, matrix water content, and infiltration, aggressive fibromatosis may be well or poorly defined and demonstrate variable attenuation and enhancement on CT and variable signal intensity on MRI. The treatment is wide resection. Mortality is low, but local recurrences are frequent (18% to 54%).

## ◼ BENIGN FATTY LESIONS

### Intraosseous Lipoma

Intraosseous lipomas are benign bone lesions. The patients are asymptomatic, and the lesions are usually discovered incidentally. They are seen in young adults, but there is a wide age range (5 to

**A**

**B**

**FIGURE 9.21.** Intraosseous lipoma. **A:** Lateral radiograph shows a geographic lucent lesion in the calcaneus with a sclerotic margin and faint calcific densities centrally (*arrow*). **B:** Sagittal T1-weighted MRI shows an intraosseous lipoma with dark central focus corresponding to calcification (*arrow*).

85 years). They are typically found in the metaphysis or epiphysis of the long bones, skull and jaws, ribs, pelvis, and calcaneus (Fig. 9.21). They are geographic lytic lesions with a sclerotic rim. Central calcific densities are occasionally seen, representing calcification due to fat necrosis. CT and MRI demonstrate attenuation and signal intensity similar to subcutaneous fat with areas of cystic changes. If the structural stability of the bone is compromised by the lesion, treatment is curettage and bone grafting.

## Liposclerosing Myxofibrous Tumor of Bone

Liposclerosing myxofibrous tumor of bone is a benign fibro-osseous lesion of bone (Fig. 9.22). These lesions are typically seen in middle-aged adults, but there is a wide age range (15 to 85 years). Pain is the most common presenting symptom, but many lesions are discovered incidentally. The majority of the lesions (85%) are found in the femur, and 91% of the femoral lesions are located in the medullary cavity of the intertrochanteric region. Radiographs show a well-defined, geographic lytic lesion with a sclerotic margin. Most of the lesions (72%) have mineralized matrix, which include globular and linear areas of dense opacity as well as regions with small, rounded, and arc-line configurations. The potential for sarcomatous degeneration appears to be significant, perhaps as high as 10% and 16% in two relatively small pathologically proven series.

**FIGURE 9.22.** Liposclerosing myxofibrous tumor of the bone. **A:** AP radiograph of the left hip joint shows a geographic lytic lesion with a sclerotic margin (*arrow*) in the femoral neck extending into the intertrochanteric region. **B:** Axial CT scan of the pelvis shows intramedullary cavity cystic mass with a sclerotic margin (*arrow*). **C:** Coronal T1-weighted MRI shows the lesion to have both lipomatous and cystic components (*arrow*). **D:** Coronal T2-weighted MRI shows predominant cystic change (*arrow*) of the mass.

**A**

**B**

**FIGURE 9.23.** Lipoma in the flexor aspect of the arm. **A:** Radiograph shows fat lucency in biceps (*arrow*). **B:** CT shows fat within the lesion (*arrow*).

## Lipoma

Lipomas are common benign tumors consisting of mature fat. They are clinically evident as soft, painless masses that gradually enlarge. Although most are subcutaneous, they may occur in an intramuscular location. A definitive diagnosis is made by CT when the lesion has the attenuation characteristics of fat (Fig. 9.23). Fat also has distinctive signal characteristics on MRI. Unusual variants of soft-tissue lipomas include ossifying lipoma, parosteal lipoma, and atypical lipoma.

## Elastofibroma

Elastofibroma is a benign reactive fibrous lesion producing abnormal elastic fibers. This pseudotumor is believed to result from chronic mechanical friction between the tip of the scapula and the chest wall. An incidental prevalence of 2.0% was found in an elderly patient population studied by chest CT, but an autopsy series found a frequency of 11.2% in men and 24.4% in women. The characteristic location is between the chest wall and the inferior tip of the scapula, but 5% of elastofibromas are found elsewhere. Most lesions are asymptomatic, but patients may present with mass or pain. Large lesions may ulcerate or cause brachial plexus impingement. Bilateral lesions are common but are often asymmetric. On sonography, elastofibroma appears as arrays of interspersed linear or curvilinear hypoechoic strands (elastic fibers) against an echogenic background (entrapped fat). CT shows a mass of soft-tissue attenuation with striations of fat attenuation (Fig. 9.24). On MRI, elastofibroma is a poorly circumscribed, semilunar, heterogeneous soft-tissue mass with signal intensity similar to that of skeletal muscle interlaced with strands of fat. Elastofibroma may have marked enhancement after the administration of gadolinium. Surgery is curative; recurrences (7%) are probably due to incomplete excision.

## ■ LANGERHANS CELL HISTIOCYTOSIS

Langerhans cell histiocytosis is a nonmalignant, reactive process of uncertain etiology that is related to other syndromes of proliferative histiocytosis, including Hand-Schüller-Christian and Letterer-Siwe diseases. When involvement appears limited to the

**FIGURE 9.24.** Elastofibroma dorsi of the chest wall. Axial CT scan of the chest reveals the right subscapular soft-tissue mass (*arrow*) applied to the chest wall with striated appearance caused by alternating bands of soft-tissue and fat attenuation.

**FIGURE 9.25.** Langerhans cell histiocytosis. **A:** Lateral skull radiograph shows lesions with beveled edges from variable destruction of inner and outer tables. **B:** Axial CT shows the bone destruction involving inner and outer tables.

bone, the condition is often referred to as eosinophilic granuloma (of bone). An eosinophilic granuloma is a granulomatous lesion characterized by a focal proliferation of macrophages (Langerhans cells) infiltrated with eosinophils and other inflammatory cells. The lesions are more often solitary than multiple, and although the peak incidence is at ages 5 to 15 years, lesions may be found at any age. Sites of involvement include the skull and other flat bones; the spine, especially vertebral bodies; and the peripheral skeleton. Involvement of the vertebral bodies characteristically results in flattening of the vertebral body or vertebra plana. However, vertebra plana is not pathognomonic for eosinophilic granuloma. In long bones, the lesions are usually diaphyseal or metaphyseal, rarely epiphyseal, and may be up to several centimeters in size. Destruction and replacement of bone by eosinophilic granuloma produces a lytic, aggressive-appearing geographic lesion early in the clinical course (Figs. 9.25–9.27), sometimes with lamellated periosteal reaction. Late in the clinical course, lesions become well defined as they heal by becoming sclerotic and eventually remodeling. On radionuclide bone scan, the degree of isotope uptake may be high, normal, or low, depending on the bone reaction and the size of the lesion. The clinical presentation is usually localized pain or a limp, but lesions in the spine may cause neurologic symptoms, and lesions in the skull may cause chronic otic drainage. The clinical courses of both solitary and multiple eosinophilic granulomas of the bone are benign; lesions may regress spontaneously. Management may include curettage, steroid injection, low-dose radiotherapy, and, rarely, chemotherapy. There is no metastatic potential.

## ◼ GIANT CELL TUMOR

Giant cell tumor of the bone (osteoclastoma) is an uncommon lesion thought to arise from osteoclasts. The presence of giant cells is only one histologic component of the tumor, and other types of tumors may have giant cells. Giant cell tumors may occur at any age, but the typical patient is a young adult. Tumors are located almost invariably in the epiphysis, with extension to the subchondral cortex and into the metaphysis. Fewer than 2% occur adjacent to open growth plates. Giant cell tumors probably arise in the cutback zone of the metaphysis where osteoclasts are plentiful and active. Approximately 50% of tumors are found around the knee, but other long bones and the sacrum are also commonly involved. The typical radiographic appearance is a geographic, lytic tumor near the end of a long bone, extending to or very close to the

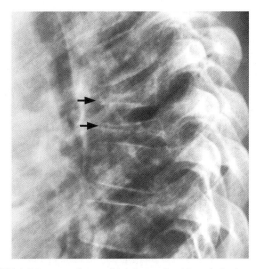

**FIGURE 9.26.** Langerhans cell histiocytosis with pathologic vertebral collapse (vertebra plana). Lateral radiograph shows collapse of T6 and T7 with kyphosis (*arrows*).

A

B

**FIGURE 9.27.** Langerhans cell histiocytosis in the femur. **A:** Radiograph shows a sharply defined lucent lesion (*arrow*) without a sclerotic margin. **B:** Sagittal T2 fat-suppressed MRI shows high signal in the lesion (*arrow*) and surrounding edema.

subarticular cortex (Fig. 9.28; see also Figs. 7.1, 7.9, and 7.18). Lytic regions correspond to nonmineralized tumor tissue, destroying and replacing cancellous bone. A lobular pattern of growth may leave ridges or trabeculations in surrounding bone. Giant cell tumors are often expansile and may have cystic blood-filled regions similar to aneurysmal bone cysts. The zone of transition from tumor to normal bone is usually sharp and abrupt but without a sclerotic margin. Some lesions erode from the epiphysis into the joint cavity and provoke synovitis. Approximately 10% of patients present with pathologic fracture. CT or MRI may be required to show the extent of tumor and the relationship to the adjacent joint. Giant cell tumors appear as areas of intense isotope uptake on bone scan and sometimes have a doughnut appearance with greater activity at the margins. The typical treatment of giant cell tumor is curettage; adjuvant treatment of the surgical bed with a high-speed burr, phenol, or cryotherapy; and packing with methyl methacrylate (bone cement). The reported overall rate of recurrence is approximately 25%. There are case reports of pulmonary metastases from giant cell tumors. Older literature suggests the existence of malignant giant cell tumors, but these likely represent primary malignant lesions such as osteosarcoma or malignant fibrous histiocytoma that have prominent giant cells at histology.

# ■ CYSTIC LESIONS OF BONE

## Aneurysmal Bone Cyst

Aneurysmal bone cysts are expansile, cystic lesions of the bone. They probably result from a vascular disturbance caused by trauma or the underlying tumor, and in one third or more of cases, an adjacent primary benign or malignant bone lesion can be recognized by the pathologist. The most common underlying lesion is giant cell tumor, and many believe that some underlying lesions may be obliterated as the aneurysmal bone cyst forms and expands rapidly. Most occur at ages 10 to 20 years, and patients typically present with pain or swelling of less than 6 months' duration. More than 50% are found in long bones, usually metaphyseal; 12% to 30% are found in the spine, often the posterior elements; and the remainder are found in the pelvis or other flat bones. Aneurysmal bone cysts are eccentric, lucent lesions that expand the host bone and give it a blown-out or ballooned appearance (hence the term *aneurysmal*) (Fig. 9.29). Sometimes, the expanded cortical shell is interrupted when periosteal bone growth is outpaced by expansion of the lesion, but the periosteum remains intact, although radiographically invisible. The walls may have trabeculations, but true septations are rare.

**FIGURE 9.28.** Giant cell tumor in the distal tibia. **A:** Mortise view radiograph shows lytic lesion extending to the end of the bone without a sclerotic border. **B:** Axial CT shows destructive lesion with regions of low density. **C:** Axial T2-weighted fat-suppressed MRI shows high signal fluid-filled spaces within the tumor.

The lesion consists of sponge-like fibrovascular tissue with cystic spaces or cavities filled with blood or serosanguineous fluid. The growth plate may be invaded. Vertebral lesions commonly involve contiguous levels or adjacent ribs. Fluid-fluid levels may be demonstrated by CT or MRI; CT attenuation values of 20 to 78 Hounsfield units (HU) reflect the fluid, blood, and solid-tissue components of the lesion (Fig. 9.30). Bone scans show increased uptake around the periphery of the lesion but none within the lesion itself. Aneurysmal bone cysts are treated in a manner similar to giant cell tumors,

unless an underlying lesion is found that requires a more aggressive treatment. The clinical course may vary from indolent and self-healing to rapid, relentless growth. Aneurysmal bone cysts have no metastatic potential.

## Simple Bone Cyst

Simple (unicameral) bone cysts are fairly common nonneoplastic fluid-filled lesions in the medullary cavity that may be related

**FIGURE 9.29.** Aneurysmal bone cyst in the metacarpal. **A:** AP radiograph shows a large expansile lesion. **B:** Composite coronal T2-weighted (**left**) and T1-weighted fat-suppressed with gadolinium (**right**) MRI shows fluid-filled spaces with high T2-weighted signal.

**FIGURE 9.30.** Aneurysmal bone cyst of the distal tibia. **A:** Axial T2-weighted MRI shows fluid-fluid levels (*arrow*). **B:** Coronal enhanced T1-weighted fat-suppressed MRI shows enhancement of the septa.

**FIGURE 9.31.** Simple bone cyst in humerus. **A:** Radiograph shows the inferior extent (*arrow*) of the lesion, but the superior extent is difficult to see. **B:** Sagittal T1-weighted and inversion recovery MRIs show low and high signal in the lesion (*arrows*), respectively.

to venous outflow obstruction. Nearly all are found in patients between 2 and 20 years of age, and they disappear with maturity. Men are affected more often than women by a 3:1 ratio. The most common sites are the proximal humerus and the proximal femur. The location transversely is intramedullary, usually occupying the entire cross section of the bone; the location longitudinally is meta-physeal, sometimes extending to the diaphysis. In young adults, cysts

may be found in the flat bones. Simple cysts have a thin lining with serous or serosanguineous fluid inside and sparse solid tissue. The internal pressure is greater than that in normal marrow. Most are unicameral (having a single compartment), but some have fibrous septa that make them multilocular. Bony ridges in the cyst wall may give the false impression of multiple cysts. The cortex is thinned and expanded, but cortical penetration or soft-tissue involvement never occurs (Fig. 9.31). The lesion is considered active if it abuts the growth plate. After the lesion has become inactive, it becomes separated from the physis as normal bone formation resumes. The lesions are radiolucent and may reach large size. A CT scan shows a homogeneous avascular lesion with attenuation values typical of cysts (15 to 20 HU). MRI shows fluid. Pathologic fracture may lead to the discovery of an unsuspected cyst (Fig. 9.32). These fractures heal with a solid layer of periosteal bone that eventually thickens the cortex. Occasionally, a bone fragment may actually fall into the cyst; such a fallen fragment is indicative of a fluid-filled lesion. Treatment of simple bone cysts may be necessary to avoid pathologic fracture and deformity. The therapy is intralesional steroid injection, curet-ting, and packing with bone chips. Approximately 20% recur after curetting; recurrent lesions may have been unrecognized multiloc-ular lesions.

## Intraosseous Ganglion

An intraosseous ganglion (juxta-articular bone cyst) is a nonneo-plastic, mucin-filled cyst lined by the fibrous tissue. Of uncertain pathogenesis, it is usually found in patients between 30 and 60 years of age. It is always located in the epiphysis and tends to be eccentric, lucent, and sharply defined, with a thin sclerotic margin. Unlike a subchondral cyst, an intraosseous ganglion does not communicate with the adjacent joint space. Curettage, with bone graft packing, if necessary, is curative.

**FIGURE 9.32.** Simple bone cyst presenting with a pathologic fracture (*arrow*).

## Epidermoid Inclusion Cyst

An epidermoid inclusion cyst may develop after a penetrating trauma displaces epidermoid elements into the substance of the bone. These cysts are usually seen at the terminal phalanx of the hand after remote trauma to the finger. They are radiolucent, sclerotically marginated, and nearly perfectly round.

## ■ CYSTIC MASSES OF SOFT TISSUES

### Ganglion

Ganglia are cystic tumorlike lesions that are usually attached to a tendon sheath, commonly found in the hands, wrists, and feet. They may be found near a joint, such as a meniscal cyst or cruciate ligament ganglion of the knee and paralabral cyst of the shoulder or hip. Ganglia can be either unilocular or multilocular cystic masses. MRI reveals a cystic mass with peripheral enhancement after the administration of gadolinium. There is a high association of meniscal and paralabral cysts with meniscal and labral tears (see Figs. 2.46 and 4.17). Once they become large, they may erode the adjacent bone, stimulate periosteal new bone formation, or cause compressive neuropathy.

### Synovial Cysts

Synovial cysts are fluid-filled juxta-articular masses. Unlike ganglia, synovial cysts are lined by a synovial membrane that may or may not communicate with the adjacent joint. The most common symptomatic synovial cyst is the Baker cyst, found in the popliteal fossa (see Chapter 13).

### Bursitis

Bursae are enclosed, flattened sacs consisting of synovial lining and a thin film of synovial fluid. They facilitate motion between apposing tissues. Bursitis is inflammation of the bursae due to trauma, repetitive stress, infection, or arthritis. In addition to normal anatomic sites, adventitial bursae may develop at sites where there is movement between apposing tissues. For example, bursae may develop over osteochondromas or other bony prominences. Similar to bursae elsewhere, adventitial bursae may become inflamed and cause symptoms.

### Myxoma

Myxomas are connective tissue tumors characterized by an abundant myxoid matrix and a paucity of stromal cells. Myxomas may appear at any age. They may be found in the subcutaneous tissue, within a muscle, or near a joint. Intramuscular myxomas predominate in women in the fifth through seventh decades of life and in the thigh. Intramuscular myxomas are well-circumscribed cystic masses of homogeneous low signal intensity on T1-weighted imaging, high signal intensity on T2-weighted imaging, and peripheral and septal enhancement after gadolinium administration. Often, myxomas have a perilesional fat rind (65% to 71%), corresponding histologically to atrophy of the surrounding muscle.

## ■ VASCULAR LESIONS

### Osseous Vascular Lesions

Benign vascular lesions of the bone are common and usually discovered incidentally in adults. Hemangioma is a benign proliferation of blood vessels, and lymphangioma is a benign proliferation of lymphatic channels; histologically, they are indistinguishable from their soft-tissue counterparts. The typical appearance of bone involvement by these lesions on radiographs is a focal, well-defined, lucent lesion surrounded by irregular, coarse, thickened trabeculae (Fig. 9.33). Abnormal vascular spaces infiltrate and replace the bone

**A**     **B**

**FIGURE 9.33.** Hemangioma involving the bony pelvis. **A:** AP radiograph shows a prominent trabecular bone pattern (*arrow*) in the right ischium. **B:** Axial CT scan shows the prominent trabeculae within a lucent, fat-filled lesion (*arrow*).

**A**                                    **B**

**FIGURE 9.34.** Intramuscular hemangioma. **A:** Coronal T1-weighted MRI of the thigh shows a heterogeneous fatty lesion (*arrow*) in the vastus medialis. **B:** Coronal inversion recovery MRI shows serpiginous structures with high signal (*arrow*).

and are surrounded by irregular, reactively thickened trabeculae. Any part of the skeleton may be affected, but most of these lesions are found in the vertebral bodies, where the thickened trabeculae are vertically oriented and give the lesion a "corduroy" appearance. On CT, they appear as a localized region of thick, vertical trabeculae interspersed with fat. This appearance is diagnostic. MRI shows the presence of fat and vascular spaces. Diffuse skeletal angiomatosis, with or without soft-tissue angiomatosis, is rare. There is no potential for malignant degeneration.

### Soft-Tissue Vascular Lesions

Hemangioma is one of the most common soft-tissue tumors, accounting for 7% of all benign tumors. Hemangioma is a benign vascular lesion that may contain nonvascular elements such as fat, fibrous and myxoid tissues, smooth muscle, thrombus, and even bone. Hemangiomas are classified histologically by the predominant type of vascular channel (capillary, cavernous, arteriovenous, or venous). Hemangiomas may be found in the subcutaneous tissue, within a muscle, or in a joint. At radiography, hemangiomas appear as a nonspecific soft-tissue mass. Phleboliths are seen in 30% of the hemangiomas, most frequently in cavernous hemangiomas. CT reveals a soft-tissue mass with associated fat overgrowth and serpentine vascular components, which may enhance after the administration of contrast. Sonography shows a complex mass with high vessel density (>5 per cm$^2$) and a peak arterial Doppler shift exceeding 2 kHz (sensitivity, 84%; specificity, 98%). MRI is considered the best modality for evaluating hemangiomas. Characteristic MRI features include lobulation, septation, central low-signal-intensity dots, and marked

enhancement after gadolinium administration (Fig. 9.34). The septated-lobulated appearance on T2-weighted images correlates with fibrous and fatty septa (low signal) between endothelial-lined vascular channels (high signal). The central low-intensity dot sign on T2-weighted imaging may represent fibrofatty septa seen in cross section, hyalinized or thrombosed vascular channels, smooth muscle components, fast flow within blood vessels, calcification, or ossification. Many forms of therapy have been used to control or cure hemangiomas: steroids, radiation therapy, sclerosing agents, interferon alpha-2a, pentoxifylline, and surgical excision. Hemangiomas may have association with several syndromes or bone lesions.

## ■ NEUROGENIC LESIONS

### Peripheral Nerve Sheath Tumors

Benign peripheral nerve sheath tumors (schwannoma and neurofibroma) can arise from any central or peripheral nerve. They are found in young adults between the third to fifth decades of life. Most are found incidentally, but others, when large, may cause pain, soft-tissue mass, and neurologic findings. They present as a fusiform soft-tissue mass related to the neurovascular bundle. The affected nerve is seen entering and exiting the mass. In neurofibroma, the nerve is central or obliterated by the mass. In schwannoma, the nerve is eccentric to the mass (Fig. 9.35). On T1-weighted images, the "split fat" sign describes a rim of fat around the tumor. On T2-weighted images, the "fascicular" or "target" sign describes a ringlike structure with central low signal intensity and peripheral high signal intensity. Treatment is surgical excision.

**A**          **B**

**FIGURE 9.35.** Schwannoma (different patients). **A:** Sciatic nerve schwannoma (*arrow*) shown by a sagittal T1-weighted MRI. **B:** Tibial nerve schwannoma with high signal (*arrow*) surrounding a lower-signal center (*arrow*), the target sign, shown by axial T2-weighted fat-suppressed MRI.

## Morton Neuroma

Morton neuroma is a benign tumorlike lesion that is perineural fibrosis of the plantar digital nerve. It has a marked predilection for middle-aged women (as high as 18:1). It has been hypothesized that the wearing of high-heeled shoes compresses the nerve against the intermetatarsal ligaments. Patients complain of pain radiating into the toes or leg that is elicited by exercise and relieved with rest. Sonography reveals a hypoechoic mass that shows increased vascularity on power Doppler mode. MRI shows a focal low-intensity mass surrounded by fat on T1-weighted images, high signal on T2-weighted images, and intense enhancement after gadolinium administration. A fluid-filled intermetatarsal bursa is often seen proximal to the neuroma. Various treatment options exist, including modification of the patient's footwear, neurolysis, steroid injection, ultrasound therapy, surgical release of the transverse metatarsal ligament for decompression, and surgical excision of the neuroma.

## ◼ POSTTRAUMATIC LESIONS

### Myositis Ossificans

*Myositis ossificans* commonly refers to posttraumatic heterotopic ossification in the muscles and other soft tissues after blunt trauma and hemorrhage. Most common in the quadriceps muscles or around the elbow, it progresses over a few weeks from hematoma to ill-defined calcification to well-organized cortical and trabecular bones. The process is similar to the formation and maturation of fracture callus and may be initially confused with sarcoma (Fig. 9.36). However, myositis ossificans evolves over a period of weeks into

an organized, peripherally calcified mass as it begins to ossify. The ectopic bone may ultimately blend with the underlying bone, sometimes causing mechanical problems. Myositis ossificans may complicate acute or chronic bony or soft-tissue trauma and may occur in association with neurologic diseases of a wide variety, including paralysis and coma. A localized form that occurs without a history of significant trauma is called *myositis ossificans circumscripta*. Treatment is rarely indicated.

**FIGURE 9.36.** Postoperative hematoma with early peripheral myositis ossificans (*arrow*) on axial spoiled gradient echo MRI.

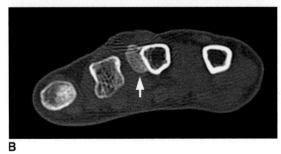

A                                                    B

**FIGURE 9.37.** BPOP. **A:** Radiograph shows mineralized parosteal mass (*arrow*) at the third metacarpal. **B:** Axial CT scans show the absence of contiguous marrow space between the lesion (*arrows*) and the underlying bone.

## Bizarre Parosteal Osteochondromatous Proliferation

Bizarre parosteal osteochondromatous proliferation (BPOP), or Nora lesion, is a form of heterotopic ossification observed most commonly in the bones of the hands and feet. It may also occur in the long tubular bones and rarely in the skull. It presents as a painless, palpable mass. A history of trauma is inconstant. Radiographically, it mimics a pedunculated or sessile osteochondroma. The main distinction is the absence of medullary continuity between the lesion and the adjacent bone (Fig. 9.37). Yuen et al. (1992) proposed a hypothesis uniting the concepts of florid reactive periostitis and BPOP. The initial stimulus is often due to trauma. Hematoma in the soft tissue develops into myositis ossificans. Subperiosteal hemorrhage or proliferation matures into a localized fusiform periostitis. If the periosteum is breached, the reactive process can extend into the soft tissue, forming a BPOP.

## Foreign Body Granuloma

Foreign body granuloma is a common cause of a soft-tissue mass in an extremity, particularly in the plantar aspect of the foot. A granulomatous reaction may be provoked by organic material such as wood or plant thorns as well as glass, plastic, or metal. The patient often does not recall the episode of penetrating trauma. CT is better than MRI for identification of a foreign body. On MRI, a metallic foreign body is suggested when there is a blooming artifact on gradient echo sequences. In the bone, foreign body granuloma causes osteolysis and is usually associated with total joint replacements (see Chapter 17).

## SOURCES AND READINGS

Bancroft LW, Kransdorf MJ, Peterson JJ, O'Connor MI. Benign fatty tumors: Classification, clinical course, imaging appearance, and treatment. *Skeletal Radiol.* 2006;35(10):719–733.

eMedicine. http://emedicine.medscape.com.

Enneking WF. *Musculoskeletal Tumor Surgery.* Edinburgh: Churchill–Livingstone; 1983.

Fechner RE, Mills SE. *Tumors of the Bones and Joints.* Washington, DC: Armed Forces Institute of Pathology; 1993.

Goodin GS, Shulkin BL, Kaufman RA, McCarville MB. PET/CT characterization of fibroosseous defects in children: 18F-FDG uptake can mimic metastatic disease. *AJR.* 2006;187(4):1124–1128.

Hoover KB, Rosenthal DI, Mankin H. Langerhans cell histiocytosis. *Skeletal Radiol.* 2007;36(2):95–104.

Hudson TM. *Radiologic-Pathologic Correlation of Musculoskeletal Lesions.* Baltimore, MD: Williams & Wilkins; 1987.

Huvos AG. *Bone Tumors: Diagnosis, Treatment, and Prognosis.* 2nd Ed. Philadelphia, PA: WB Saunders; 1991.

Keats TE, Anderson MW. *Atlas of Normal Roentgen Variants that May Simulate Disease.* 8th Ed. St. Louis, MO: Mosby–Year Book; 2006.

Kransdorf MJ, Murphey MD. *Imaging of Soft Tissue Tumors.* 2nd Ed. Philadelphia, PA: Lippincott Williams & Wilkins; 2006.

Kransdorf MJ, Sweet DE. Aneurysmal bone cyst: Concept, controversy, clinical presentation, and imaging. *AJR.* 1995;64:573–580.

Kransdorf MJ, Peterson JJ, Bancroft LW. MR imaging of the knee: Incidental osseous lesions. *Magn Reson Imaging Clin N Am.* 2007;15(1):13–24.

Kudo S. Elastofibroma dorsi: CT and MR imaging findings. *Semin Musculoskelet Radiol.* 2001;5(2):103–105.

Liu PT, Chivers FS, Roberts CC, Schultz CJ, Beauchamp CP. Imaging of osteoid osteoma with dynamic gadolinium-enhanced MR imaging. *Radiology.* 2003; 227(3):691–700.

Murphey MD, Choi JJ, Kransdorf MJ, et al. Imaging of osteochondroma: Variants and complications with radiologic-pathologic correlation. *Radiographics.* 2000;20:1407–1434.

Murphey MD, Nomikos GC, Flemming DJ, et al. Imaging of giant cell tumor and giant cell reparative granuloma of the bone: Radiologic-pathologic correlation. *Radiographics.* 2001;21:1283–1309.

Propeck T, Bullard MA, Lin J, et al. Radiologic-pathologic correlation of intraosseous lipomas. *AJR.* 2000;175:673–678.

Resnick D. *Diagnosis of Bone and Joint Disorders.* 4th Ed. Philadelphia, PA: WB Saunders; 2002.

Ryzewicz M, Manaster BJ, Naar E, Lindeque B. Low-grade cartilage tumors: Diagnosis and treatment. *Orthopedics.* 2007;30(1):35–46.

Schmidt H, Freyschmidt J. *Köhler/Zimmer Borderlands of Normal and Early Pathologic Findings in Skeletal Radiography*. 4th Ed. New York, NY: Thieme; 1993.

Stull MA, Kransdorf MJ, Devaney KO. Langerhans' cell histiocytosis of bone. *Radiographics*. 1992;12:801–823.

Sundaram M, Wang LH, Rotman M, et al. Florid reactive periostitis and bizarre parosteal osteochondromatous proliferation: Pre-biopsy imaging evaluation, treatment and outcome. *Skeletal Radiol*. 2001;30: 192–198.

Unni KK. Dahlin's bone tumors. *General Aspects and Data on 11,087 Cases*. 5th Ed. Philadelphia, PA: Lippincott–Raven; 1996.

Yuen M, Friedman L, Orr W, et al. Proliferative periosteal processes of phalanges: A unitary hypothesis. *Skeletal Radiol*. 1992;21:301.

# Metastatic Tumors

Incidence
Tumor Spread
Radiologic Appearance
Screening for Metastases

Hematologic Malignancies Involving
    the Bone Secondarily
    Leukemia
    Hodgkin Lymphoma
    Non-Hodgkin Lymphoma

Pathologic Fracture
Soft-Tissue Metastases
Percutaneous Needle Biopsy
Treatment
Radiotherapy Changes

his chapter describes the radiology of tumors that are metastatic to bone or soft tissue.

## INCIDENCE

More than 95% of adult patients with malignant disease involving bone have metastases rather than myeloma or primary bone sarcomas. The prevalence of bone involvement in autopsy series of cancer patients ranges from 3% to 85%, depending on the site of origin and the thoroughness of the postmortem search. With improving cancer treatments and longer patient survival, more and more cancer patients will have skeletal involvement by the end of their clinical course. Most skeletal metastases occur in middle-aged and elderly patients with primary cancers of the prostate, breast, lung, or kidney. In men, prostate malignancies account for 60% of patients with skeletal metastases; in women, breast malignancies account for 70% (Table 10.1). In children with osseous metastases, neuroblastoma is the most common primary lesion (Table 10.2).

The relative incidence of primary tumors that are likely to metastasize to the bone may be affected in the future by the rising incidence of lung cancer among women (due to smoking), the decrease in the proportion of advanced breast cancers (due to screening mammography), and the increasing incidence of breast and prostate cancers overall (due to an aging population). Most skeletal metastases are subclinical and asymptomatic. When symptomatic, they present as bone pain or pathologic fractures. Bone pain ranges in severity from minimal to extreme and intolerable, but skeletal metastases are themselves rarely a cause of death.

In the radiologic evaluation of metastatic bone tumors, less emphasis is placed on complete anatomic delineation of individual lesions and more on discovering sites of disease and planning and following the course of palliative therapy. Sometimes, a skeletal metastasis is the initial presentation of malignant disease in a patient whose primary site is asymptomatic or minimally symptomatic. Occult primary tumors that present with bone metastases are usually kidney, lung, and gastrointestinal tract lesions. Only in select cases does locating the primary tumor benefit the patient, because in most instances, the prognosis has already become unalterable by metastatic dissemination. In most cases, the primary tumor is never located, even at autopsy. Biopsy of the skeletal metastasis in these circumstances often shows adenocarcinoma without organ-specific features.

**TABLE 10.1  Frequency of Primary Sites Among Adults with Skeletal Metastases**

| Primary Site | Frequency (%) |
| --- | --- |
| Women | |
| Breast | 70 |
| Lung | 6 |
| Kidney | 4 |
| Uterus | 4 |
| Thyroid | 3 |
| Others/unknown | 13 |
| Total | 100 |
| Men | |
| Prostate | 60 |
| Lung | 14 |
| Kidney | 6 |
| GI tract | 3 |
| Others/unknown | 17 |
| Total | 100 |

**TABLE 10.2  Primary Tumors in Children That May Metastasize to Bone**

Neuroblastoma
Leukemia
Lymphoma
Ewing sarcoma
Osteosarcoma
Malignant soft-tissue sarcomas
Retinoblastoma
Embryonal rhabdomyosarcoma
Medulloblastoma
Wilms tumor

# TUMOR SPREAD

Tumor cells gain access to the skeleton by (a) hematogenous spread through the arterial circulation, (b) retrograde venous flow, and (c) direct extension. The portions of the skeleton that contain red marrow have a rich vascular supply, and tumor emboli frequently lodge within the sinusoidal channels found there. Tumor spread through retrograde venous flow occurs in the valveless vertebral plexus of Batson. This venous plexus interconnects the spine, the ribs, and the pelvis, providing access to the axial skeleton. Blood flow through the plexus may be transiently reversed by increased intra-abdominal pressure caused by activities such as coughing. Direct extension is much less frequent than hematogenous spread; when it occurs, it is usually an extension of an intrathoracic tumor to the chest wall, an intrapelvic tumor to the pelvic wall, or a retroperitoneal process to the lumbar spine. For practical purposes, lymphatic spread of tumor to the bone does not occur.

Metastases in the cancellous bone of the axial skeleton and in the cancellous metaphyseal bone of the proximal femur and proximal humerus account for nearly 90% of lesions, a distribution that is related to hematogenous spread. Metastases to the spinal column usually involve the vertebral body rather than the posterior elements. They are more common in the lumbar region than the thoracic region and least common in the cervical region. Metastases are distinctly uncommon distal to the knees or elbows. Approximately 90% of patients with bone metastases have multifocal involvement.

Skeletal metastases are common around joints, especially the hips, shoulders, knees, and intervertebral disks. Periarticular metastases with subchondral, intra-articular, or synovial extension may have a clinical presentation that simulates inflammatory arthritis. Lesions in the hands or feet are relatively rare and usually come from primary lung cancers. The intervertebral disk is a relative barrier to the spread of tumor, so that the usual pattern of vertebral metastatic involvement is vertebral destruction with preservation of the disk, even when multiple contiguous vertebral levels have tumor. It is very unusual for the disk to be involved by tumor. Coexistent degenerative disk disease is frequent and may be caused or exacerbated secondarily by the presence of tumor. In the subchondral region of the vertebral body, a metastasis may interfere with the nutrition of the disk or weaken the end plate so that the disk material herniates through. The former process produces degenerative disk disease, and the latter produces a Schmorl node.

# RADIOLOGIC APPEARANCE

The appearance of a bone metastasis on radiographs reflects the balance of bone destruction and bone formation (Table 10.3). Metastatic tumors secrete osteoclast-stimulating factors; the osteoclasts excavate a defect in the bone where the metastasis establishes itself. The osteoclasts are not part of the tumor mass but can be found at the periphery, sometimes separated by the fibrous tissue. Growth of the tumor is preceded by osteoclastic bone resorption. When bony trabeculae have been completely engulfed, tumor can destroy the bone directly by elaborating enzymes. Osteoclast proliferation and osteoclastic bone resorption occur in all bone metastases, regardless of whether they also form the bone. Bone formation may occur as stromal bone formation or as reactive bone formation. In those tumors associated with an acellular fibrous

| TABLE 10.3 | Typical Radiologic Appearances of Metastases from Specific Primary Tumors | |
|---|---|---|
| **Primary Tumor Site** | **Appearance on Radiographs** | **Appearance on Bone Scan** |
| Breast | Lytic, mixed, or blastic | Increased isotope uptake |
| Prostate | Blastic, occasionally mixed or lytic | Increased isotope uptake |
| Lung | Lytic, mixed, occasionally blastic | Increased isotope uptake |
| Kidney | Lytic, expansile or blow-out | Often decreased isotope uptake |
| Thyroid | Lytic, expansile or blow-out | Often decreased or normal isotope uptake |

stroma, osteoprogenitor cells form the bone under the influence of osteoinductive humoral factors secreted by the tumor. Metastases from prostatic carcinoma produce a fibrous stroma and form the bone in this way; metastases from breast and lung carcinomas do not. In reactive bone formation, immature woven bone forms at the same time that bone destruction occurs. Proposed mechanisms for reactive bone include a mechanical response to weakening of the bone by the growing metastasis, an attempt by the bone to contain the lesion, or perhaps an uncoupling of the humoral factors that normally control the bone formation and resorption.

Lytic lesions correspond to destruction and replacement of the bone by nonmineralized tumor, without appreciable bone formation. The pattern of destruction may be geographic, permeated, or moth-eaten, and although there is a rough correspondence to increasing biologic aggressiveness, all patterns may be present in the same patient when extensive disease is present (Figs. 10.1 and 10.2). Because 30% to 50% of bone mineralization must be lost before a lesion becomes visible on the plain film, widespread lytic metastases may be inapparent on radiographs. Blastic lesions correspond to

**FIGURE 10.1.** Hypervascular renal cell carcinoma metastasis (*arrow*) destroying the sternum and proximal left clavicle with large soft-tissue mass on axial CT.

**A**                                                                 **B**

**FIGURE 10.2.** Lytic metastases from breast carcinoma. **A:** Huge destructive lesion (*arrow*) in the ilium. **B:** Lytic lesion (*arrow*) in the anterior two thirds of the L3 vertebral body.

bone formation in or around tumor implants through reactive bone proliferation or ossification in fibrous stroma. Reactive apposition of the new bone on cancellous bone surfaces results in a dense, blastic appearance. Proliferation of new endosteal bone is seen as endosteal thickening or irregular densities projected over the marrow cavity. Deposition of periosteal new bone causes cortical thick-

ening or layers of periosteal new bone. Metastatic lesions usually do not stimulate periosteal new bone, and when they do, the periosteal bone tends to be scanty. The pattern of reactive bone proliferation generally reflects the tumor's growth rate, with highly anaplastic, fast-growing tumors and marrow element malignancies (myeloma and leukemia) provoking no radiographically appreciable reactive

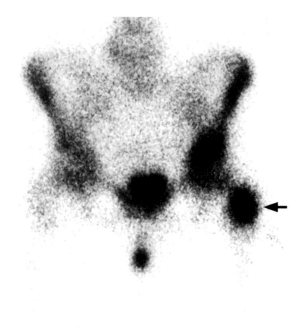

**A**                                                                 **B**

**FIGURE 10.3.** Blastic metastases from breast carcinoma in the intertrochanteric region of the femur. **A:** A homogeneously dense blastic lesion (*arrow*) with poorly defined margins. **B:** Bone scan shows increased radionuclide accumulation in the lesion (*arrow*) and in the ipsilateral acetabulum.

**FIGURE 10.4.** Diffuse blastic metastases from prostate carcinoma throughout the pelvis and proximal femurs.

bone. Blastic metastases tend to have a dense homogeneous appearance with margins that fade imperceptibly into the normal bone (Figs. 10.3 and 10.4). Mixed lesions contain both lytic and blastic areas, reflecting bone destruction and bone formation in different portions of the same lesion (Fig. 10.5). In fact, both processes occur simultaneously in virtually all metastases.

**A**

**B**

**FIGURE 10.5.** Metastasis from breast cancer detected by PET/CT. **A:** CT scan shows mixed lytic-sclerotic lesion (*arrow*) in the left iliac wing, adjacent to the sacroiliac joint. **B:** Fused FDG-PET/CT image shows high standard uptake value (*arrow*) in the lesion. CT-guided biopsy confirmed the diagnosis.

**FIGURE 10.6.** Bone scan shows multiple metastases from breast carcinoma.

Radionuclide bone scan is more sensitive than radiographs for detecting metastases but has lower specificity. Radionuclide bone scanning agents such as technetium-99m methylene diphosphonate accumulate in new reactive or stromal bone (Fig. 10.6; see Fig. 10.3). The metastasis itself may not accumulate the tracer unless the primary lesion forms the bone or cartilage. Most lytic lesions, as well as all blastic and mixed lesions, have enough new bone formation to appear as areas of intense uptake on scans. If the activity in the reactive and stromal bones is equal to that of a normal bone or if the metastasis is in the marrow space but does not affect the bone, the scan is falsely negative. If a bone is destroyed and replaced by tumor without provoking detectable reactive bone, an area of decreased uptake may result. Anaplastic, purely lytic lesions tend to have decreased uptake. A "superscan," that is, diffuse increased radionuclide accumulation throughout the entire skeleton, can indicate diffuse osseous metastatic disease.

Positron emission tomography (PET) using 18-fluorodeoxyglucose (18F-FDG), a radioactive-labeled glucose analog that permits imaging based on the metabolic rate, has considerable utility in oncologic imaging. With regard to screening for skeletal metastases, compared with the radionuclide bone scan, PET with 18F-FDG appears to have a higher sensitivity and higher specificity for detection of osteolytic metastases. Osteoblastic metastases and osteosarcoma metastases appear to have lower metabolic rates than osteolytic metastases, and the radionuclide bone scan appears better than PET in these circumstances. PET/CT has the additional advantage of combining the sensitivity and specificity of PET with the spatial resolution of CT (see Fig. 10.5).

**FIGURE 10.8.** Marrow space metastasis in the left femur (*arrow*) from lung cancer demonstrated by CT. The bone scan was negative in the region of this lesion.

**FIGURE 10.7.** Multiple blastic metastases from thyroid carcinoma on CT. Radiographs and bone scan were normal.

CT may show the extent of bone involvement more clearly than radiographs (Fig. 10.7). Delineation of the extent of cortical involvement is important when prophylactic internal fixation is contemplated. In addition, CT may show tumor in the marrow spaces in the absence of bone destruction. Increased attenuation in the medullary cavity reflects replacement of the fatty marrow by tumor, edema, or reactive mesenchymal tissue (Fig. 10.8).

On MRI, metastatic lesions are seen as focal areas of abnormal signal replacing the normal marrow signal (Fig. 10.9). Metastases are usually distinguishable from normal tissue unless the metastases are so extensive that normal marrow signal is absent. On T1-weighted images, metastatic foci have low signal intensity; on T2-weighted images, they have high signal intensity; following intravenous gadolinium, they enhance. Opposed phase MR sequences can be used to assess for obliteration of the normal marrow fat which is typically seen with tumors. When fat and water are present in the same voxel, such as with red bone marrow, then signal dropout will be seen on the out-of-phase image compared with the in-phase image. Metastases obliterate the marrow fat, thus having roughly the same signal intensity between in-phase and out-of-phase images (Fig. 10.10). MRI is more sensitive than bone scan and has superior anatomic detail. Whole-body MRI has been used for detection of bone metastases in children and young adults, using spin echo T1-weighted and inversion recovery sequences. MRI is the best examination for investigating acute spinal cord symptoms in patients with known metastatic disease and for screening the spine when the bone scan is negative and profound osteopenia is present (Fig. 10.11). MRI may also be particularly helpful in making decisions about staging and treatment when a solitary lesion is found on a screening bone scan and radiographs are normal.

Metastases may appear in any transverse or longitudinal location within an involved bone, including marrow space, cortex, or surface, and epiphysis, metaphysis, or diaphysis. Intracortical or subperiosteal locations are common for metastases (Fig. 10.12) but rare for primary bone tumors.

**A**

**B**

**FIGURE 10.9.** Metastases to the lumbar spine, pelvis, and femurs from breast carcinoma. **A, B:** Coronal T1-weighted and inversion recovery MRI shows scattered, focal lesions in the marrow.

**FIGURE 10.10.** Metastasis from lung carcinoma on axial T1-weighted fast spoiled gradient dual echo MRI. **A:** In-phase image shows a rounded lesion in the left sacrum (*arrow*) and heterogenous marrow in the right ilium (*arrowhead*). **B:** Opposed phase image demonstrates lack of signal dropout of the metastasis (*arrow*) from lack of residual marrow fat and normal signal dropout of the red marrow in the right ilium (*arrowhead*). Purely fatty replaced marrow in the left hemipelvis is due to prior radiation and does not drop out due to lack of interspersed cellular marrow elements.

**FIGURE 10.11.** Widespread spine metastases from breast carcinoma. **A:** Lateral radiograph shows osteopenia and compression fractures in the thoracic spine. **B:** Sagittal T2-weighted MRI shows widespread replacement of the normal marrow signal by high signal lesions.

**A**

**B**

**FIGURE 10.12.** Cortical metastasis. **A:** CT shows destructive lesion in the posterior cortex of the femur with irregular periosteal reaction (*arrow*). **B:** Axial T2-weighted MRI shows the lesion (*arrow*) with surrounding edema.

**FIGURE 10.13.** Child with metastases from neuroblastoma. The bones are diffusely abnormal with loss of the normal trabecular pattern and cortical edges.

In young children, skeletal metastases tend to be widespread and generally symmetric in their involvement of the skeleton (Fig. 10.13). Osteolysis and permeated destruction are prominent, and collapse of vertebral bodies is frequent.

## ◼ SCREENING FOR METASTASES

Screening for skeletal metastases in patients with known primary malignancies is usually accomplished with bone scanning; 30% of metastatic lesions detected by bone scan are missed by radiographs, and 2% of metastatic lesions detected by radiographs are missed by scans. Because most patients have multiple lesions, it is rare for a patient with osseous metastases to have an entirely normal bone scan. The bone scan can be falsely negative or nondiagnostic in debilitated patients with a poor host response or in patients who have had radiotherapy.

When bone metastases are known to be present, response to therapy can be documented by serial bone scans. With successful treatment, lesions with increased isotope uptake tend to become normal, and the number of lesions decreases. Sometimes, in the presence of clinical improvement, an increase in lesion intensity is seen after therapy. This "flare phenomenon" presumably corresponds to healing of metastatic lesions with increasing formation of the reactive bone. Follow-up scans in 2 to 3 months clarify the situation by showing the expected decrease in activity. Growth of lesions and the onset of new lesions indicate worsening of the disease. When additional lesions are suspected in specific areas of new, worsening, or recurrent pain, plain radiographs are usually obtained first. If these are negative, depending on the circumstances, further imaging evaluation may include

**FIGURE 10.14.** Metastasis from colon carcinoma not evident on radiographs. **A:** Composite sagittal T1-weighted and inversion recovery MRI shows replacement of the marrow at L3 (*arrows*) with low T1 signal and increased signal on fluid sensitive sequence. **B:** Anterior bone scan demonstrates vague increased tracer uptake in L3 (*arrow*). **C:** CT prior to biopsy demonstrates subtle sclerosis of the vertebral body.

bone scan, CT, PET/CT, or MRI, or some combination of these (Fig. 10.14).

In patients with known primary malignancies and focal symptoms, it is reasonable to obtain radiographs as an initial screening examination for metastatic disease. Some treatment protocols may be based on the burden of disease as shown by radiographic osseous survey, despite the greater sensitivity and specificity of other imaging modalities.

## ■ HEMATOLOGIC MALIGNANCIES INVOLVING THE BONE SECONDARILY

Marrow element malignancies tend to infiltrate and involve the skeleton diffusely and do not have the discrete multifocal tumor deposits more typical of metastases from primary tumors of parenchymal organs. Primary marrow element tumors (multiple myeloma, Ewing sarcoma, primitive neuroectodermal tumor, and primary lymphoma of the bone) are discussed in Chapter 8.

**FIGURE 10.15.** Child with leukemia. Transverse metaphyseal lucencies (*arrows*) are present, corresponding to marrow space packing with leukemic infiltrates.

**FIGURE 10.16.** Child with leukemia. Diffuse periosteal reaction (*arrows*) and metaphyseal lucencies are present.

## Leukemia

Leukemia is a neoplasm of leukocytes that may involve bone secondarily. Leukemia is the most common malignancy in children. Leukemic infiltration of many organs and tissues, including the marrow spaces, is present and may have a diffuse or nodular character. Packing of the marrow spaces with leukemic cells causes

pressure atrophy of cancellous trabeculae and is seen radiographically as diffuse osteopenia. In children, lucent metaphyseal bands may occur, reflecting zones of trabeculae that are thinner and sparser than normal in areas of rapid bone growth (Fig. 10.15). Although often seen in children with leukemia, these lucent metaphyseal bands are nonspecific and simply reflect the presence of systemic

A

B

**FIGURE 10.17.** Acute lymphoblastic leukemia in a young child. **A:** Coronal T1-weighted MRI (**left**) shows replacement of the marrow; coronal T2-weighted fat-suppressed MRI (**center**) shows high signal throughout the marrow spaces; and coronal T1-weighted fat-suppressed MRI following gadolinium injection (**right**) shows diffuse enhancement. **B:** Axial T2-weighted MRI through the leg shows periosteal reaction (*arrow*) and surrounding edema.

disease or even normal variation. Nodular collections of leukemic cells cause focal areas of medullary, cortical, or subperiosteal bone destruction.

Leukemic infiltration can extend through the cortex by way of the haversian systems, enlarging them by eroding the bone. This causes the cortex to appear fuzzy and osteopenic, often with lucent streaks. Infiltration of subperiosteal spaces lifts the periosteum and stimulates bone formation (Fig. 10.16). Periosteal bone formation that occurs as the periosteum is being lifted results in perpendicular sunburst bone spicules as the periosteum leaves a trail of reactive bone behind. Even if radiographs of the bone are normal, widespread marrow space involvement is the rule and can be confirmed by MRI bone marrow aspiration. On MRI, leukemia is evident as marrow replacement and periosteal reaction (Fig. 10.17).

## Hodgkin Lymphoma

Hodgkin Lymphoma is a malignant tumor of lymph nodes. Secondary bone involvement is detected clinically in 5% to 21% of patients, but a much higher incidence can be demonstrated by marrow biopsy or at autopsy. Bone involvement usually occurs by direct extension from tumor-filled nodes so that the lumbar spine is affected most commonly. Pressure erosion of the cortical surface by enlarged periaortic nodes, without actual invasion, causes scalloping of the anterior aspects of the vertebral bodies. Hematogenous spread may occur as well. Extensive osteoblastic reaction is usual, but lytic and mixed lesions may occur. Ill-defined permeating lesions reflect spread of tumor through the medullary spaces and haversian systems. Partial collapse of involved vertebral bodies is possible, representing pathologic compression fractures. A densely sclerotic vertebral body, a so-called ivory vertebra, is a classic radiographic sign with the differential diagnosis of lymphoma, blastic metastasis, Paget disease, and, rarely, myelosclerosis, fluorosis, or osteopetrosis.

## Non-Hodgkin Lymphoma

Bone involvement is seen in 5% to 15% of patients with non-Hodgkin (extranodal) lymphoma. The prevalence of bone marrow involvement in autopsy series is much higher. The radiographic appearance of secondary involvement of the bone by lymphoma is identical to that of primary involvement (see Chapter 8).

## ■ PATHOLOGIC FRACTURE

Pathologic fractures through bones involved by metastases are common. The most common sites of pathologic fracture are the vertebral bodies, ribs, pelvis, proximal femur, and proximal humerus (Figs. 10.18 and 10.19). Metastases of lytic, blastic, and mixed radiographic appearance all cause weakening of the bone.

In the spine, compression fractures with vertebral collapse occur, presumably as a result of gradual destruction of the trabeculae that bear the compressive loads. Involvement of the posterior elements may render some vertebral fractures unstable. An epidural mass may be present and may block the spinal canal. MRI or myelography with CT can demonstrate the epidural mass, indicate the status of the spinal cord, and delineate the extent of vertebral disease. In the long bones, destructive lesions with full-thickness cortical penetration lead to pathologic fractures. Gaps in the cortex weaken the bone by causing uneven and aberrant distribution of the

**FIGURE 10.18.** Pathologic fracture (*arrows*) transversely through lytic metastasis in the humeral shaft.

stresses of loading, impeding the normal biomechanical dispersion of force. Weakening is gradual as cortical bone is infiltrated, eroded, and destroyed. Blastic lesions also destroy the cortex, and the reactive bone and stromal bone that give blastic lesions their radiodensity are structurally unsound. The bone may fracture under the stresses of normal activity. Cortical weakening makes the bone most vulnerable to tensile forces; therefore, in the long bones, pathologic

**FIGURE 10.19.** Prostate carcinoma with pathologic avulsion fracture of lesser trochanter (*long arrow*). Brachytherapy seeds (*short arrow*) are present in the prostate.

fractures are usually transverse. The onset of pain at a site of metastatic involvement may indicate the presence of microfractures in a weakened cortex.

The goal of treatment of osseous metastases is to palliate pain and prevent pathologic fracture; curative resection is generally not realistic. Prophylactic internal fixation of metastatically involved bone is often considered. The clinical decision revolves around the patient's concerns and level of activity, the localization and multiplicity of bone involvement, and the extent of destruction. Fixation is generally indicated for lytic lesions if they are greater than 2.5 cm in size or involve more than half the circumference of the bone. Pathologic fractures are usually treated surgically. Prosthetic replacements allow the removal of the tumor-destroyed bone. Methyl methacrylate is often used to buttress destroyed portions of the bone and fill in bony defects. Radiotherapy can interfere with secondary healing by destroying chondrogenesis. The primary osteogenesis that occurs with internal fixation is more resistant to radiation, so that radiotherapy generally does not interfere with healing of internally fixed fractures. If the patient's life span is long enough, pathologic fractures will heal, but the healing process may be prolonged. Median survival after discovery of a pathologic fracture through an osseous metastasis, combined for all primary sites, is approximately 18 months.

# ■ SOFT-TISSUE METASTASES

Although the skeletal muscle mass of the human body accounts for a large percentage of the total body weight, nearly 50%, in clinical experience, skeletal muscle is an uncommon site for metastases. Muscle is resistant to both primary and metastatic cancers. The cited factors for this resistance include contractile activity, local changes in pH, oxygenation, accumulation of lactic acid and other metabolites, blood flow per unit weight (mL/min/g), intramuscular blood pressure, and local temperature. Weiss experimentally showed that cancer cell survival is greatest in denervated muscle that is unable to contract as opposed to electrically stimulated muscle. His experimental work supports the hypothesis that the rapid death of most cancer cells after delivery to some target organs is a consequence of their mechanical interactions within the microvasculature. Muscle metastases have been reported in sites of previously documented skeletal muscle trauma.

**FIGURE 10.20.** Soft-tissue metastasis from lung cancer. Contrast-enhanced CT scan shows a rim-enhanced soft-tissue metastasis (*arrow*).

Autopsies in two series of patients showed that the prevalence of metastases to muscle was 16.0% and 17.5%. Neoplasms with the highest incidence of metastases to muscle were carcinoma, leukemia, and lymphoma. The diaphragm, rectus muscle of the abdomen, deltoid muscle, psoas muscle, and intercostal muscles were most commonly involved. Patients with muscle metastases were 26 to 84 years old (mean age, 62 years old). Most patients present with pain in the involved muscles or a clinically palpable mass and have advanced-stage neoplasms.

On unenhanced CT scans, muscle metastasis is revealed as an enlargement of a muscle. Occasionally, the findings may be subtle because the tumor is isodense to the surrounding muscle, and contralateral asymmetry is necessary to make the diagnosis. On contrast enhanced CT, skeletal muscle metastases appear as rim-enhancing intramuscular lesions with central hypoattenuation (Fig. 10.20). On MRI, muscle metastases have high signal intensity on STIR or T2-weighted sequences, lobulated morphology, large areas of central necrosis, and extensive peritumoral edema (Fig. 10.21). MRI findings of carcinoma metastatic to muscle are

**A**        **B**

**FIGURE 10.21.** Metastases to muscle from lung cancer. **A:** Axial T2-weighted fat-suppressed MRI shows high signal (*arrow*) in the lateral compartment muscles of the leg. **B:** Axial T1-weighted fat-suppressed MRI following gadolinium injection shows moderate enhancement (*arrow*) in the lesion.

**FIGURE 10.22.** Insufficiency fractures (*arrows*) of the right ilium and right sacral wing shown by coronal CT reformation in a patient with previous pelvic irradiation for cervical cancer. Note the straight, vertical margins (*small arrows*) of the bilateral iliac sclerosis, demarcating the margins of the radiation port.

not pathognomonic, and the differential diagnosis must include soft-tissue sarcoma, hematoma, and abscess.

Metastases to skin, subcutaneous tissues, and lymph nodes may present as soft-tissue masses. On CT, such lesions tend to be isodense to muscle and may enhance. Soft-tissue metastases typically have low signal on T1-weighted MRI, high signal on T2-weighted MRI, and enhancement after gadolinium injection.

# PERCUTANEOUS NEEDLE BIOPSY

In the evaluation of a patient with one or more focal lesions in the setting of a known primary tumor or no known primary tumor, percutaneous needle biopsy is often the invasive procedure of choice. Typically performed under CT or sonographic guidance, the diagnostic yield is high, and the morbidity is low. Virtually any anatomic site may be accessible to needle biopsy, and some sites that would be problematic for the surgeon are straightforward for the interventional bone radiologist. A variety of specialized needles are available for obtaining core specimens of the bone or soft-tissue lesions. An extraosseous component of a malignant bone tumor is as representative of the tumor as is the bone tumor itself. A frozen section of a core biopsy or cytologic preparation of a fine-needle aspiration may provide an immediate pathologic diagnosis. Specific benign diagnoses that may account for clinical symptoms or radiologic abnormalities may be made from needle biopsy specimens by the experienced pathologist. Aspiration of bone marrow from the iliac crest in many patients may find tumor cells, but these correspond to circulating tumor cells that have been shed into the bloodstream. They do not necessarily become established skeletal metastases. Aspiration specimens may also be sent for bacteriology.

# TREATMENT

The basic treatment modalities for osseous metastases, with or without pathologic fractures, are radiation therapy, chemotherapy, and surgical stabilization. Palliative radiation of symptomatic lesions without pathologic fracture provides pain relief in approximately 80% of patients. If a pathologic fracture is present, pain relief may be experienced by approximately 60% of patients; without internal fixation, the pathologic fractures may progress to nonunion.

# RADIOTHERAPY CHANGES

Therapeutic irradiation is a common means of treating osseous metastases. Sites of bone pain confirmed as abnormal by roentgenography or bone scan in patients with known metastases are often treated palliatively by radiation. Irradiated osseous lesions heal by sclerosis and filling-in of lytic areas. Radiation effects are independent of the radiation source. In the immature skeleton, radiation in total doses of 2,000 cGy or greater impairs the bone growth. The epiphysis is especially sensitive; radiation causes direct cellular injury to chondrocytes and possibly vascular damage to fine physeal blood vessels. The greater the growth potential at the time of irradiation, the more profound is its effect. If an entire growing bone is irradiated, loss of bone growth in the whole bone results in a small bone. Focal doses affect the irradiated portion; for example, angular deformities could result from an asymmetrically irradiated growth plate. Radiotherapy also increases the risk for epiphyseal plate trauma, including the occurrence of slipped capital femoral epiphysis and avascular necrosis.

In the mature skeleton, the primary change is radiation necrosis, a phenomenon that is dose related. Radiographs and CT show irregular sclerosis in the irradiated bone. Insufficiency fracture is a relatively common complication of radiation necrosis (Fig. 10.22). On bone scan, the irradiated bone may initially show increased radionuclide accumulation from hyperemia and new bone formation.

**FIGURE 10.23.** Radiation changes in the marrow on sagittal T1-weighted MRI. Fatty replaced bone marrow in L2 and L4 (*arrowheads*) denotes the radiation portal surrounding a lung carcinoma metastasis (*arrow*) at L3. The remainder of the levels have normal marrow signal.

**FIGURE 10.24.** Radiation changes in muscle 6 months after treatment. **A:** Axial T1 MRI shows previous resection of soft-tissue sarcoma from the lateral portion of the anterior compartment (*arrow*). **B:** Axial inversion recovery MRI shows high signal in the lateral thigh soft tissues, including muscle and subcutaneous tissues, with a linear demarcation (*arrows*) that corresponds to the radiation portal. **C:** Axial T1 fat-suppressed MRI following gadolinium contrast injection shows enhancement (*arrows*) of the affected soft tissues.

After several weeks or months, the bone scan shows decreased radionuclide accumulation because of decreased bone formation and decreased vascularity. On MRI, the irradiated bone has the signal characteristics of fatty marrow. The anatomic location and extent of these changes conform to the size and shape of the radiation portal (Fig. 10.23).

In patients who received radiotherapy before 2 years of age, induced tumors are usually benign. The most common are exostoses (osteochondromas); these are histologically and biologically indistinguishable from those that occur naturally. Fibrosarcoma or malignant fibrous histiocytoma, chondrosarcoma, and other unusual sarcomas are much less likely to occur. Malignant tumors may occur in older patients who have received radiotherapy. The following criteria must be satisfied to make the diagnosis of a radiation-induced sarcoma: (a) the sarcoma arises within the irradiated field, (b) the latent period is at least 4 years, and (c) the sarcoma is histologically different from a previous tumor or the radiation was delivered in the absence of a malignant diagnosis. The latent period averages 11 years. The presence of pain, soft-tissue mass, and progression on serial films should raise suspicion and lead to biopsy.

Radiation myositis may occur following external beam radiation and is manifested on MRI as muscle edema and inflammation that peaks several months after treatment (Fig. 10.24). The margins of the abnormality will correspond to the radiation field and may extend straight across different muscle groups and other soft tissues. Atrophy and volume loss are late effects of radiation myositis.

## SOURCES AND READINGS

Berger FH, Verstraete KL, Gooding CA, et al. MR imaging of musculoskeletal neoplasm. *Magn Reson Imaging Clin North Am.* 2000;8:929–951.

Bui-Mansfield LT, Chew FS, Lenchik L, et al. Nontraumatic avulsions of the pelvis. *AJR.* 2001;178:423–427.

Damron TA, Heiner J. Management of metastatic disease to soft tissue. *Orthop Clin North Am.* 2000;31:661–673.

eMedicine. http://emedicine.medscape.com.

Fogelman I, Cook G, Israel O, Van der Wall H. Positron emission tomography and bone metastases. *Semin Nucl Med.* 2005;35(2):135–142.

Galasko CSB. *Skeletal Metastases.* London: Butterworths; 1986.

Glockner JF, White LM, Sundaram M, et al. Unsuspected metastases presenting as solitary soft tissue lesions: A fourteen-year review. *Skeletal Radiol.* 2000;29:270–274.

Herring CL, Harrelson JM, Scully SP. Metastatic carcinoma to skeletal muscle—a report of 15 patients. *Clin Orthop.* 1998;355:272–281.

Hudson TM. *Radiologic-Pathologic Correlation of Musculoskeletal Lesions.* Baltimore, MD: Williams & Wilkins; 1987:421–440.

Kagan AR, Bassett LW, Steckel RJ, et al. Radiologic contributions to cancer management. Bone metastases. *AJR.* 1986;147:305–312.

Lipton A. Future treatment of bone metastases. *Clin Cancer Res.* 2006 Oct 15;12(20 Pt 2):6305s–6308s.

Magee T, Rosenthal H. Skeletal muscle metastases at sites of documented trauma. *AJR.* 2002;178:985–988.

Mollabashy A, Scarborough M. The mechanism of metastasis. *Orthop Clin North Am.* 2000;31:529–535.

Orr FW, Lee J, Duivenvoorden WC, et al. Pathophysiologic interactions in skeletal metastasis. *Cancer.* 2000;88(Suppl.):2912–2918.

Panicek DM, Schwartz LH. MR imaging after surgery for musculoskeletal neoplasm. *Semin Musculoskelet Radiol.* 2002;6:57–66.

Plaza JA, Perez-Montiel D, Mayerson J, et al. Metastases to soft tissue: A review of 118 cases over a 30-year period. *Cancer.* 2008; 112:193–203.

Resnick D. *Diagnosis of Bone and Joint Disorders.* 4th Ed. Philadelphia, PA: WB Saunders; 2002.

Taira AV, Herfkens RJ, Gambhir SS, Quon A. Detection of bone metastases: Assessment of integrated FDG PET/CT imaging. *Radiology.* 2007; 243(1):204–211.

Virk MS, Lieberman JR. Tumor metastasis to bone. *Arthritis Res Ther.* 2007;9(Suppl. 1):S5.

# PART III

# Joint Disease

# Approach to Joint Disease

his chapter describes a pragmatic approach to the radiology of joint disease, based on anatomy, pathophysiology, and radiographic analysis. This approach draws heavily on the work of Forrester, Brower, and Resnick (Table 11.1). Detailed discussions of specific clinical forms of arthritis are presented in Chapters 12 and 13.

## ◼ GENERAL PRINCIPLES

Radiographs mirror the pathologic processes that affect the joints and the functional adaptations that may follow. In general, the radiologic diagnosis of arthritis can be highly specific and reliable when classic changes are present in the expected distributions but much less specific in the early stages before the disease process has fully evolved. Regardless of the approach, however, several frustrations are unavoidable: A specific radiologic diagnosis is not always possible; many types of joint disease overlap in their radiologic and clinical features; two or more diseases may coexist in the same patient; and, finally, clinical disease may precede radiologic abnormalities and vice versa, sometimes by years.

Diseases that affect joints do so by three broad pathophysiologic mechanisms, each with a distinctive radiographic appearance: degeneration, inflammation, and metabolic deposition. For practical purposes, one mechanism is usually predominant. Degeneration of a joint refers to mechanical damage and reparative adaptations; in essence, the joint is worn away. Inflammation

### TABLE 11.1    Approach to Radiographic Analysis of Arthritic Changes in the Hand

| A | Alignment |
|---|---|
| B | Bone mineralization |
|   | Bone production |
| C | Cartilage (joint space) |
|   | Calcification |
| D | Distribution |
| E | Erosions |
| S | Soft-tissue swelling |

*Source*: Data from Brower AC. *Arthritis in Black and White*. 2nd Ed. Philadelphia, PA: WB Saunders; 1997 and Forrester DM, Brown JC. *The Radiology of Joint Disease*. 3rd Ed. Philadelphia, PA: WB Saunders; 1987.

### TABLE 11.2    Characteristic Radiographic Signs of Arthritis

| Pathophysiology | Characteristic Radiographic Signs |
|---|---|
| Inflammation | Acute erosions |
|   | Osteoporosis |
|   | Soft-tissue swelling |
|   | Uniform loss of articular space |
| Degeneration | Osteophytes |
|   | Subchondral sclerosis |
|   | Uneven loss of articular space |
|   | Chondrocalcinosis |
| Metabolic deposition | Lumpy-bumpy soft-tissue swelling |
|   | Chronic bony erosions with overhanging edges |

of a joint may be acute, chronic, or both; the joint is dissolved by the inflammatory process. Metabolic deposition refers to the infiltration of a joint by aberrant metabolic products. Each of these mechanisms affects joints in radiographically distinctive ways (Table 11.2).

## ◼ SYNOVIAL JOINTS

Most articulations of the appendicular skeleton are synovial joints. In the axial skeleton, the facet joints of the spine, the atlantoaxial (C1–2) joint, the uncovertebral joints of the cervical spine, and the lower two thirds of the sacroiliac joints are synovial.

### Soft Tissues

Synovial joints have a joint cavity and are enclosed by a joint capsule consisting of an inner synovial layer (the synovium), a middle subsynovium, and an outer fibrous layer (Fig. 11.1). The synovium is a cellular secretory mucosa that produces synovial fluid. Synovial fluid is viscous because of a high concentration of hyaluronic acid. Joint capsules have an active blood supply with a large capillary surface area. The synovium has a mesenchymal rather than epithelial origin; therefore, no basement membrane or other structural barrier is present between the synovial fluid and the capillary bed. The change from synovium to fibrous capsule is gradual; there are no distinct

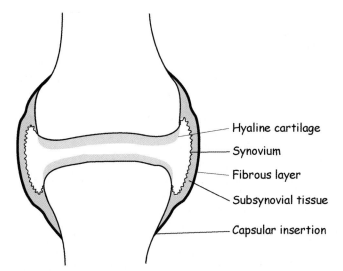

**FIGURE 11.1.** Anatomy of a synovial joint.

Hyaline cartilage
Synovium
Fibrous layer
Subsynovial tissue
Capsular insertion

**FIGURE 11.3.** "Sausage digit" soft-tissue swelling (psoriatic arthritis).

boundaries between the layers. Joint capsules are densely innervated. Tendon sheaths invest tendons and reduce friction during motion. Bursae are located where complete freedom of motion between structures is necessary, for example, where a tendon passes directly over the periosteum. Because tendon sheaths and bursae are synovial structures, diseases that affect synovial joints may also involve them.

Soft-tissue swelling at a joint may reflect capsular distention from effusion, synovial hypertrophy, soft-tissue edema, or a mass. Symmetric, fusiform swelling suggests an inflammatory process with effusion, synovial edema, synovial hypertrophy, or some combination thereof (Fig. 11.2). Inflammatory distention of a tendon sheath may also produce soft-tissue swelling, but the swelling extends beyond the joint. In a digit, this kind of swelling

produces an appearance that has been likened to a sausage (sausage digit). Generalized soft-tissue swelling may be caused by subcutaneous edema or hyperemia and suggests inflammation (Fig. 11.3). Lumpy-bumpy swelling that is not symmetric or centered near a joint suggests masses and may be caused by metabolic deposition disease with masslike deposits of metabolic products in the periarticular soft tissues (Fig. 11.4). Soft-tissue prominences at joints that

**FIGURE 11.2.** Fusiform soft-tissue swelling at the PIP joint (rheumatoid arthritis).

**FIGURE 11.4.** Lumpy-bumpy soft-tissue swelling (tophaceous gout).

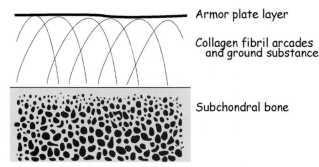

**FIGURE 11.5.** Structure of articular cartilage.

are found on physical examination may actually result from bony or cartilaginous enlargements; the overlying soft tissues may be normal. Heberden and Bouchard nodes are swellings of this kind at the distal interphalangeal (DIP) and proximal interphalangeal (PIP) joints of the hand, respectively, and are characteristic of a degenerative process. Calcification in the soft tissues may affect cartilage, skin, muscles, tendons, or other connective tissues and is associated with connective tissue diseases. Soft-tissue atrophy or loss is present in various conditions.

## Cartilage

The ends of the articulating bones, that is, the joint surfaces, are covered with hyaline articular cartilage. Hyaline cartilage is composed of a collagen fibril framework and a ground substance. One set of densely packed collagen fibrils is oriented parallel to the articular surface, forming an armor-plate layer with tiny surface pores that allow the passage of water and small electrolytes. A second, less densely packed set of collagen fibrils is oriented in arcades,

linking the armor-plate layer to the subchondral bone (Fig. 11.5). The ground substance is a gel that consists of water and large proteoglycan aggregate macromolecules that are loosely fixed to the collagen framework. The proteoglycan macromolecules are too large to pass through the pores of the armor-plate layer. The physical and chemical properties of these macromolecules allow them to attract and bind water, providing sufficient swelling pressure beneath the armor-plate layer to "inflate" the articular cartilage, even during weight bearing. During motion, a thin layer of water is expressed through the small surface pores, providing a frictionless surface for a lifetime of mobility. Articular cartilage has a load-dampening ability that spreads transmitted loads over a greater area of the subchondral bone. Under rapid, transient loading, articular cartilage has elastic properties. Under a steady load, it creeps and deforms like a sponge. The portion of cartilage that is adjacent to the subchondral bone is calcified. Interdigitations between the calcified cartilage and the subchondral bone provide a strong mechanical coupling. Chondrocytes are the cells whose metabolic activity maintains the specialized structures of articular cartilage. Less than 1% of articular cartilage volume is composed of cells. Because cartilage is avascular and alymphatic, chondrocytes derive their nutrients by diffusion from the synovial fluid. Articular cartilage has only a limited ability to repair itself. Deep injuries may repair with cartilage that is densely fibrous.

Cartilage abnormalities are inferred from the radiolucent gap between articulating bones, the articular space, or the joint space. The articular cartilage fills this space. A potential space exists where the articulating surfaces meet. Loss of articular cartilage causes the joint space to narrow. Cartilage loss within a joint can be diffuse and concentric—indicating an inflammatory process (with enzymatic dissolution of cartilage)—or focal and uneven, indicating a mechanical one (Fig. 11.6). If there is complete

**FIGURE 11.6.** Asymmetric joint space narrowing, osteophytes, and subchondral sclerosis (osteoarthritis).

**FIGURE 11.7.** Severe PIP joint subchondral bone erosions (psoriatic arthritis).

**FIGURE 11.8.** Bony ankylosis (psoriatic arthritis).

cartilage loss, the ends of the bones may become eroded, making the joint space appear wider. The ends of the bone may form a pseudoarthrosis (Fig. 11.7), or fibrous or bony ankylosis (fusion) of the joint may occur (Fig. 11.8). Widening of the articular space may indicate abnormal cartilage proliferation or intra-articular fluid. Weight-bearing views may be necessary to assess accurately

**FIGURE 11.9.** Chondrocalcinosis of the menisci (*arrowheads*).

**FIGURE 11.10.** Chondrocalcinosis of the articular cartilage (*arrow*).

the degree of cartilage loss at the knee. Asymmetric cartilage loss may result in changes in radiographic joint space narrowing with changes in position.

Calcification of cartilage is called *chondrocalcinosis*. Chondrocalcinosis may involve fibrocartilage structures such as the menisci of the knee (Fig. 11.9) or the triangular fibrocartilage complex of the wrist. Articular cartilage also may calcify (Fig. 11.10).

## Bone

Bone changes in arthritis include bone loss and bone proliferation. Osteoporosis is the loss of bone through osteoclast action and may be generalized or regional, acute or chronic. Osteoporosis reflects hyperemia from synovial inflammation or from the disuse of a body part. Acute osteoporosis is recognized by the resorption of bone from subchondral trabeculae, a location where blood flow and metabolic activity are the greatest. The process of osteoporosis affects the trabecular bone and the cortex. However, because the surface area subject to osteoclastic resorption is greater in the trabecular bone, the acute process is more evident there. If the process continues, tunneling may become evident in the cortex and can be recognized as being porotic and thin. In noninflammatory articular disease, the normal mineralization of bone is maintained. Arthritic conditions are commonly treated with corticosteroids, which may cause osteoporosis.

Bone erosions represent focal losses of bone from the cortical surface. Erosions with loss of the cortex indicate an acute, aggressive process. In rheumatoid arthritis, for example, the cortical bone is eroded by the action of enzymes produced by inflamed synovial tissues (pannus). These enzymes literally dissolve the bone and produce acute erosions without cortex (Fig. 11.11). Erosions with cortex indicate a nonaggressive, chronic process in which the bone remodels along the border of the erosion. The chronic erosions seen in metabolic deposition disease are caused by abnormal masses of metabolic products causing the adjacent bone to remodel because of mechanical pressure. The bone may attempt to encircle the deposit; such an incomplete attempt leaves an overhanging edge

**FIGURE 11.11.** Acute marginal erosions (*arrows*), diffuse joint space narrowing, and osteoporosis (rheumatoid arthritis).

(Fig. 11.12). Other masslike processes in the joint may also cause chronic erosions of the bone. The characteristic initial site of erosions in arthritis is at the margin of the articular cartilage where a gap between the cartilage and the attachment of the synovium leaves a "bare area" of bone contained within the joint capsule.

**FIGURE 11.12.** Chronic erosion and overhanging edges (tophaceous gout).

**FIGURE 11.13.** Subchondral cyst formation (rheumatoid arthritis) (*arrow*).

Once cartilage has been destroyed, erosions may extend over the entire articular surface.

Subchondral cysts, also called *geodes*, occur when cracks or fissures in the articular surface allow the intrusion of synovial fluid into the subchondral cancellous bone or when necrosis of the subchondral bone is followed by collapse (Fig. 11.13). Subchondral cysts may also result from erosions of the articular surface by inflamed synovial tissues. Subchondral cysts are seen in virtually all types of arthritis and have no particular differential diagnostic significance. Proliferative new bone may represent attempts at cyst healing.

Proliferative bone formation at arthritic synovial joints occurs in four ways. Periostitis is the periosteal apposition of a new bone to the cortical surface (Fig. 11.14). Sclerosis, also called *eburnation*, is

**FIGURE 11.14.** Periostitis (psoriatic arthritis) (*arrows*).

a new bone apposed to the trabeculae of the existing bone, usually in a subchondral location (immediately beneath the articular cartilage) but sometimes on the surface after the cartilage is gone. Osteophytes occur in the presence of cartilage loss and represent new excrescences of cartilage and bone that enlarge the articular surface at its margins. Bony proliferation may also occur at the attachment of joint capsules (discussed in the "Entheses").

## Alignment

Alignment becomes abnormal when joint capsules or ligaments are torn or lax, the normally balanced tension across joints becomes unbalanced, or articular surfaces lose their normal size or shape. The result is deformity, subluxation, dislocation, and loss of function. Continued use of a damaged, malaligned joint leads to functional adaptation and secondary anatomic changes; ultimately, it may become difficult to distinguish these functional adaptations from the primary arthritic process. Loss of function and pain are the major causes of morbidity in arthritis.

Alignment deformities in the hand may lead to a functional disability of great clinical significance. Deformities of the hand result from loss of the balanced muscular tension and ligamentous restriction that maintain its normal alignment. Common deformities of the digit include the swan neck deformity (PIP hyperextension with DIP flexion) (Fig. 11.15A), the boutonniere deformity (PIP flexion with DIP hyperextension) (Fig. 11.15B), the mallet finger (isolated DIP flexion), and the hitchhiker thumb or Z-shaped collapse of the thumb (metacarpophalangeal [MCP] joint flexion, interphalangeal [IP] joint hyperextension). Subluxations and dislocations of individual joints may be seen, or the entire hand may collapse into a zigzag deformity (radial deviation of wrist with ulnar deviation of the MCP joints). These deformities reflect loss of normal functional anatomy from any underlying cause, one of which may be arthritis.

Abnormalities of alignment resulting from articular disease are common at the wrist, knee, and foot. Alignment deformities of the wrist may follow or precede actual articular changes on radiographs; these misalignments may have great clinical significance because normal wrist function is a prerequisite for normal hand function. The ligamentous instability patterns that may follow traumatic disruption of the carpal ligaments (see Chapter 2) may also result from the arthritic involvement of the carpal ligaments. Selective involvement of the medial or lateral tibiofemoral compartment of the knee with asymmetric thinning of cartilage may lead to varus or valgus deformity. In the foot, various digital deformities similar to those occurring in the hand may be found.

## ◼ INTERVERTEBRAL DISK JOINTS

Intervertebral disk joints are present along the anterior portion of the spine. An intervertebral disk joint comprises cartilaginous end plates covering the articulating surfaces of adjacent vertebral bodies, a central nucleus pulposus, and a circumferential annulus fibrosus (Fig. 11.16). In the child, the nucleus pulposus has a gelatinous character; in the adult, the nucleus pulposus has converted to fibrocartilage. The annulus fibrosus contains an outer zone of collagenous fibers and an inner zone of fibrocartilage. The annulus fibrosus is anchored to the cartilaginous end plates, the vertebral rim, and the periosteum of the vertebral body. The anterior longitudinal ligament is applied to the anterior aspect of the vertebral column with firm attachments to the periosteum near the corners of the vertebral bodies. A posterior longitudinal ligament is applied to the posterior aspect of the vertebral bodies. The same structure and physiology are found at the symphysis pubis.

In the anterior column of the spine, one may evaluate alignment, intervertebral spaces, and bone changes. Soft-tissue changes in the axial skeleton are difficult to recognize. Abnormalities of alignment include intervertebral subluxation, exaggerated kyphosis or lordosis, kyphosis or lordosis at inappropriate levels, and scoliosis. Films of the patient in flexion, extension, or lateral bending may be required to demonstrate abnormal mobility or loss of mobility.

The intervertebral disk spaces should be proportionate to the width of the vertebral body. They are relatively small in the cervical

**FIGURE 11.15.** Rheumatoid arthritis. **A:** Swan neck deformity. **B:** Boutonniere deformity.

Sagittal Section

**FIGURE 11.16.** Anatomy of an intervertebral disk joint.

| TABLE 11.3 | Vertebral Phytes: Associations With Specific Diseases |
|---|---|
| **Type of Phyte** | **Associated Condition** |
| Syndesmophytes | Ankylosing spondylitis |
| Diffuse, flowing paravertebral ossification | DISH |
| Osteophytes | Degenerative disk disease, spondylosis deformans |
| Focal paravertebral ossification | Psoriatic arthritis (common), Reiter syndrome (uncommon) |

region but gradually become thicker in the thoracic and lumbar regions. Narrowing is characteristic of degenerative disk disease, and calcification or gas in the disk space is pathognomonic.

The morphology of bony outgrowths along the spine, called *vertebral phytes*, may be of great diagnostic value (Table 11.3). Ossification in the periphery of the annulus fibrosus may lead to a shell of bone that bridges the intervertebral space (Fig. 11.17). These are called *bridging syndesmophytes* and are characteristic of ankylosing spondylitis. Ossification of the anterior longitudinal ligament along multiple contiguous levels is characteristic of diffuse idiopathic skeletal hyperostosis (DISH). This ossification is often exuberant and adjacent to, but separate from, the vertebral body (Fig. 11.18). Osteophytes are horizontal extensions of the vertebral end plates that have a triangular configuration (Fig. 11.19). If sufficiently large osteophytes are present at adjacent end plates, they may form an extra-articular bridge across the intervertebral space. Small osteophytes are associated with degenerative conditions. Large, focal, paravertebral

**FIGURE 11.17.** Syndesmophytes (*arrow*) formed by the ossification of the outer layers of the annulus fibrosus (ankylosing spondylitis).

soft-tissue ossifications are seen in psoriatic arthritis and Reiter syndrome. These bony excrescences often become coalescent and contiguous with the vertebral bodies, resulting in extra-articular

**A**  **B**

**FIGURE 11.18.** Diffuse, flowing ossification (*arrows*) of the paravertebral soft tissues (DISH). **A:** Sagittal CT reformation shows the ossification (*arrows*) extending over multiple contiguous levels. **B:** Axial CT shows the ossification (*arrow*) is asymmetric.

**FIGURE 11.19.** Triangular osteophytes (*arrows*) of spondylosis deformans with degenerative disk changes. The disk space is narrowed and the subchondral bone is sclerotic.

bridges along the lateral aspect of the spinal column (Fig. 11.20). Typically, they occur along the lateral aspects of the vertebral bodies and do not involve multiple, contiguous levels on the same side.

# ENTHESES

An enthesis is the site of bony insertion of a tendon, ligament, or articular capsule. Tendons, ligaments, and articular capsules are strong bands or sheets of collagen fibers in a parallel arrangement. Near the attachment to bone, chondrocytes are interspersed between the collagen fibers. The collagen fibers in the bands or sheets become more compact, then cartilaginous, and finally calcified as they enter the bone (Fig. 11.21). The interdigitation of calcified cartilage and bone provides a strong attachment. Entheses have an active blood supply and a prominent innervation. Enthesopathy is a disease at an enthesis. Enthesophytes and the calcification and ossification of an enthesis are the principal radiographic signs of enthesopathy (Fig. 11.22). Ossification usually proceeds from the bony attachment into the substance of the inserting structure. MRI may directly demonstrate inflammatory and degenerative changes of tendons and ligaments much earlier than radiographs. Normal tendons and ligaments have low signal on both T1- and T2-weighted MRI. Fluid, edema, and myxoid change within tendons or ligaments are identifiable as regions of high signal.

# DISTRIBUTION OF DISEASE

There are two clinical situations: monarticular arthritis (one joint affected) and polyarticular arthritis (many joints affected). The differential diagnosis of monarticular arthritis is rather limited (Table 11.4). Each type of polyarticular arthritis has a predilection for specific sites in the skeleton and can often be recognized simply from the distribution of involvement (Table 11.5). The explanation for the highly specific distributions of disease is unknown. There are some joints in the hand and foot where involvement can be virtually diagnostic of specific types of degenerative or inflammatory polyarticular arthritis (Table 11.6).

In the hand, degenerative involvement of multiple DIP joints suggests osteoarthritis, whereas inflammatory involvement suggests psoriatic arthritis. Degenerative involvement of multiple MCP joints suggests pyrophosphate arthropathy, whereas inflammatory involvement of the MCP joints suggests rheumatoid arthritis.

**A**

**B**

**FIGURE 11.20.** Ossification in the paraspinal soft tissues leading to a bridging phyte (*arrows*) (reactive arthritis). **A:** AP radiograph. **B:** Axial CT and coronal reformation.

Bone    Cartilaginous    Non-cartilaginous

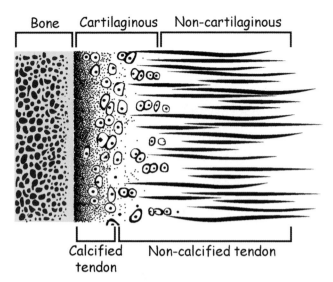

Calcified    Non-calcified tendon
tendon

**FIGURE 11.21.** Anatomy of an enthesis.

Degenerative involvement of the first carpometacarpal (CMC) joint suggests osteoarthritis. Inflammatory involvement of multiple intercarpal joints suggests rheumatoid arthritis, psoriatic arthritis, or gouty arthritis. Degenerative involvement of the radiocarpal joint suggests pyrophosphate arthropathy. In the foot, degenerative involvement of the first metatarsophalangeal (MTP) joint suggests osteoarthritis. Inflammatory involvement of the combination of multiple MTP and IP joints suggests psoriatic arthritis or Reiter syndrome, whereas inflammatory involvement of multiple MTP joints without IP joint involvement suggests ankylosing spondylitis or rheumatoid arthritis. Degenerative involvement of the first

**FIGURE 11.22.** Enthesophyte (*arrow*) at the insertion of the triceps tendon.

| TABLE 11.4 | Common Causes of Monarticular Arthritis |
| --- | --- |

Crystal related
Hemophiliac arthropathy
Rheumatoid (including juvenile chronic arthritis)
Infectious
Synovial lesions (chondromatosis, PVNS)
Traumatic

tarsometatarsal (TMT) joint suggests osteoarthritis. Inflammatory involvement of multiple intertarsal joints suggests rheumatoid arthritis. Degenerative involvement of the talonavicular joint suggests pyrophosphate arthropathy.

# ■ LABORATORY FINDINGS

Abnormal findings on laboratory examinations are integral to the diagnosis of joint diseases. They are most valuable when correlated with radiographs and other clinical information. Material for laboratory analysis is usually obtained from blood or the joint. Synovial fluid can be obtained by needle aspiration. Samples of the synovial membrane, articular cartilage, or periarticular soft tissues are usually obtained by biopsy.

Rheumatoid factor (RF) is a group of nonspecific autoantibodies found not only in the serum of patients with rheumatoid arthritis but also in that of patients with other acute and chronic inflammatory diseases. These include viral infections such as AIDS, mononucleosis, and influenza; chronic bacterial infections such as tuberculosis and subacute bacterial endocarditis; parasitic infections; neoplasms after chemotherapy or radiotherapy; and various hyperglobulinemic states. The sensitivity and specificity of detecting RF vary with the particular method of measurement. The most common method is the latex fixation test, in which the patient's serum is challenged with latex particles coated with heat-treated human immunoglobulin G. A positive result—that is, agglutination of the latex particles because of the presence of RF—makes the patient seropositive or RF positive. A negative result also has a clinical importance because it is one factor that distinguishes rheumatoid arthritis from the clinically overlapping group of seronegative spondyloarthropathies. The strength of a positive result has therapeutic and prognostic significance. Nevertheless, only 80% of patients with classic rheumatoid arthritis are RF positive, as are 30% of patients with nonrheumatic diseases, 25% of patients with other rheumatic diseases, and 5% of the normal population.

ANA are a heterogeneous population of serum antibodies that react to various human nuclear components, including DNA. They are detected by an immunofluorescence screening test. A positive ANA test is an empiric marker for connective tissue disease. The test is positive in nearly all patients with systemic lupus erythematosus, scleroderma, and mixed connective tissue disease and in approximately 80% of patients with polymyositis/dermatomyositis. The actual pathogenetic significance is unclear. Changes in serum ANA levels may parallel the clinical course and be used to follow the activity of the disease.

**TABLE 11.5**    **Distribution of Polyarticular Arthritis**

| Arthritis | Symmetry | Predominant Sites of Involvement |
|---|---|---|
| Rheumatoid arthritis | Symmetric | Hand (PIPs, MCPs), wrist (pancompartmental), elbow, shoulder, hip, knee, foot (multiple intertarsal, MTPs), and cervical spine |
| Ankylosing spondylitis | Symmetric | SI joint, ascending to lumbar, thoracic, and cervical spine, hip, and foot (MTPs) |
| Reiter syndrome | Asymmetric | SI joint, foot (MTPs, IPs, calcaneus), and lumbar spine |
| Psoriatic arthritis | Asymmetric | Hand (often entire rays), wrist, foot (MTPs, IPs, calcaneus), lumbar spine, and SI joint |
| Primary osteoarthritis | Asymmetric | Hand (DIPs, PIPs, first CMC), knee (especially medial compartment), hip (superolateral or medial), and foot (first MTP, first TMT) |
| CPPD deposition disease | Asymmetric | Wrist (radiocarpal), shoulder (glenohumeral), knee (especially patellofemoral), elbow, ankle, and foot (talonavicular) |
| Gout | Asymmetric | Hand (random joints), elbow, knee, and foot (first MTP and random joints) |

**TABLE 11.6**    **Polyarticular Arthritis: Sites that Suggest Specific Diseases When Involved by Degenerative or Inflammatory Changes**

| Involved Site(s) | Type of Joint Changes Degenerative | Inflammatory |
|---|---|---|
| Hand and Wrist | | |
| Multiple DIP joints | Osteoarthritis | Psoriatic arthritis |
| Multiple MCP joints | CPPD deposition disease | Rheumatoid arthritis |
| First CMC joint | Osteoarthritis | |
| Multiple intercarpal joints | | Rheumatoid arthritis |
| | | Psoriatic arthritis |
| | | Gouty arthritis |
| Radiocarpal joint | CPPD deposition disease | |
| Foot | | |
| First MTP joint | Osteoarthritis | |
| Multiple MTP and IP joints | | Psoriatic arthritis |
| | | Reiter syndrome |
| Multiple MTP joints | | Ankylosing spondylitis |
| | | Rheumatoid arthritis |
| First TMT joint | Osteoarthritis | |
| Multiple intertarsal joints | | Rheumatoid arthritis |
| Talonavicular joint | CPPD deposition disease | |

HLA antigens represent a polymorphic group of inherited antigens found on the surface membranes of cells; HLA antigens have an uncertain biologic role. The genes for HLA antigens are located on the sixth chromosome in the major histocompatibility complex. Although it is well established that certain specific HLA antigens are associated with certain rheumatic diseases, the precise relationship of these genetic markers to disease is unclear. HLA antigens may influence not only the likelihood of a disease but also the age of onset, severity, and individual clinical features. There are three major associations of HLA antigens with rheumatic diseases: (a) HLA-B27 with ankylosing spondylitis, Reiter syndrome, psoriatic arthritis, and enteropathic arthritis; (b) HLA-Cw6 with psoriasis and psoriatic arthritis; and (c) HLA-DR4 with rheumatoid arthritis. The strongest association is between HLA-B27 and ankylosing spondylitis. The prevalence of this antigen in patients with ankylosing spondylitis is 90%, compared with 9% in the general white population.

## SOURCES AND READINGS

Brower AC. *Arthritis in Black and White.* 2nd Ed. Philadelphia, PA: WB Saunders; 1997.

eMedicine. http://emedicine.medscape.com.

Firestein GS, Budd RC, Harris ED Jr, et al. *Kelley's Textbook of Rheumatology.* 8th Ed. Philadelphia, PA: Saunders; 2008.

Forrester DM, Brown JC. *The Radiology of Joint Disease.* 3rd Ed. Philadelphia, PA: WB Saunders; 1987.

Frediani B, Falsetti P, Storri L, et al. Quadricepital tendon enthesitis in psoriatic arthritis and rheumatoid arthritis: Ultrasound examinations and clinical correlations. *J Rheumatol.* 2001;28:2566–2568.

Griffin LY. *Essentials of Musculoskeletal Care.* 3rd Ed. Rosemont, IL: American Academy of Orthopedics; 2005.

Groshar D, Rozenbaum M, Rosner I. Enthesopathies, inflammatory spondyloarthropathies and bone scintigraphy. *J Nucl Med.* 1997;38:2003–2005.

Koopman WJ, Boulware DW, Heudebert G. *Clinical Primer of Rheumatology.* Philadelphia, PA: Lippincott Williams & Wilkins; 2003.

Koopman WJ, Moreland LW, eds. *Arthritis and Allied Conditions: A Textbook of Rheumatology.* 15th Ed. Philadelphia, PA: Lippincott Williams & Wilkins; 2004.

McGonagle D, Gibbon W, Emery P. Classification of inflammatory arthritis by enthesitis. *Lancet.* 1998;352:1137–1140.

Resnick D, ed. *Diagnosis of Bone and Joint Disorders.* 4th Ed. Philadelphia, PA: WB Saunders; 2002.

Resnick D, Niwayama G. Entheses and enthesopathy. Anatomical, pathological, and radiological correlation. *Radiology.* 1983;146:1–9.

Salvarani C, Cantini F, Olivieri I, et al. Magnetic resonance imaging and polymyalgia rheumatica. *J Rheumatol.* 2001;28:918–919.

CHAPTER

# 12

# Inflammatory Arthritis

his chapter covers those clinical forms of arthritis and connective tissue disease that present on radiographs with a preponderance of inflammatory changes.

## RHEUMATOID ARTHRITIS

Rheumatoid arthritis is a systemic autoimmune disease manifested in the musculoskeletal system by inflammatory polyarthritis of the small synovial joints. The pathogenesis is not understood, and no causative agent has been proved. Genetic factors affect susceptibility to and expression of the disease. Rheumatoid arthritis is usually distinguished from other arthritides by the presence of rheumatoid factor (RF) in the serum (see Chapter 11). Rheumatoid arthritis has a prevalence of 1% in the general population, with women affected more often than men by a 3:1 ratio. High RF titers often correlate with more severe disease. The typical age range of presentation is 25 to 55 years. In 70% of cases, the onset is insidious and occurs over weeks to months; in 20%, the onset occurs over days to weeks; and in 10%, the onset is acute and occurs over hours to days. The acute onset mimics the onset of septic arthritis. The clinical course of rheumatoid arthritis is progressive in 70% of cases, leading to disabling, destructive disease. The clinical progression may be rapid or slow. In 20%, the disease is intermittent with remissions generally lasting longer than exacerbations, and in 10%, remissions last several years. The clinical diagnosis is based on criteria that include morning stiffness, symmetric swelling of the proximal interphalangeal (PIP) joint, metacarpophalangeal (MCP) or wrist joints, rheumatoid nodules, serum RF, and specific radiographic findings.

### Pathologic-Radiologic Features

The underlying pathologic change in rheumatoid arthritis is chronic synovial inflammation with hyperemia, edema, and production of excess fluid. Chronicity leads to hypertrophy and fibrosis. Hypertrophic, chronically inflamed synovium is called *pannus*. Pannus dissolves the cartilage and bone by the actions of enzymes along its advancing margin. Commonly seen early radiographic findings include fusiform periarticular soft-tissue swelling—corresponding to synovial hypertrophy and joint effusion—and acute erosions at the margins of the joint. Articular cartilage may also be dissolved by enzymes released into the joint space, causing uniform narrowing of the joint space on radiographs. Synovial hyperemia causes juxta-articular osteoporosis. There is a characteristic lack of reactive bone formation. Common late radiologic findings include chronic generalized osteoporosis, progression of marginal erosions to severe erosions involving subchondral bone, synovial cyst formation, subluxations and abnormalities of alignment, and secondary osteoarthritis. Not all findings are present at any one time in individual patients; observation of combinations of these findings should lead to the correct diagnosis. The distinctive radiographic pattern of chronic osteoporosis, marginal erosions, and little if any reactive bone formation is the hallmark of rheumatoid arthritis. Although the appendicular skeleton tends to be extensively involved, the axial skeleton is usually spared except for the upper cervical spine. Bilaterally symmetric clinical involvement is usual, but the severity of radiologic involvement is not necessarily symmetric, especially when radiographs are obtained early in the clinical course. Secondary degenerative changes may occur if the inflammatory process remits for several years. Both rheumatoid arthritis and primary osteoarthritis are common conditions; patients with both diseases may have confusing radiographic findings.

Sonography and MRI are more sensitive than radiography in detecting synovitis, the primary abnormality in rheumatoid arthritis. Subchondral bone marrow edema may occur with synovitis, and both are precursors of bone erosions. Erosions will not occur in the absence of synovitis. MRI criteria for diagnosing rheumatoid arthritis include periarticular contrast enhancement of the wrist or the MCP or PIP joints in both hands, marrow edema, erosions, joint effusion, synovial sheath effusion, and cartilage irregularity and thinning. Gadolinium helps distinguish nonenhancing joint fluid from enhancing synovial proliferation and pannus. Successful treatment of early rheumatoid arthritis with disease-modifying antirheumatic drugs that suppress synovitis may be evident on MRI as the reversion of synovitis and marrow edema to normal. MRI is also helpful in the evaluation of the complications of rheumatoid arthritis at the craniocervical junction and elsewhere.

## Hand and Wrist

There is considerable variability in the distribution of radiographic abnormalities in rheumatoid arthritis, and the findings on radiographs may not correlate with the clinical features. The earliest radiographic changes are fusiform soft-tissue swelling and juxta-articular osteoporosis (Figs. 12.1 and 12.2). In the hand, rheumatoid arthritis classically involves the MCP and PIP joints. The earliest bone erosions are generally at the MCP joints (Fig. 12.3), often the second and third on the radial side. The PIP joint of the middle finger is another site of typical early involvement. Oblique radiographs may show subtle subchondral bone resorption. Fusiform soft-tissue swelling, juxta-articular osteoporosis, concentric loss of cartilage space, and acute marginal erosions may be seen (Fig. 12.4). Compressive erosions and remodeling of bone may result from the collapse of osteoporotic bone by muscle tension; this is especially common at the MCP joints. Loss of the normal balanced tension at the digits results in various alignment deformities, including the swan neck and boutonniere deformities of the fingers (see Fig. 11.15) and the Z-shaped deformity of the thumb (Fig. 12.5). Superficial erosions of the cortex may occur beneath the inflamed tendon sheaths, especially along the outer aspect of the distal ulna, the dorsal aspect of the first metacarpal, and the proximal phalanx of the first digit.

In the wrist, pancompartmental involvement is usual (Fig. 12.6). The earliest bone changes are erosions at the ulnar and radial styloid processes and at the waists of the capitate and scaphoid bones. On MRI, erosions are evident as focal defects in the bone that are low to intermediate signal on T1-weighted images and high signal on T2-weighted images (Fig. 12.7). On T1-weighted images after gadolinium enhancement, the pannus within the erosions enhances. Malalignment in advanced disease results from loss of balanced muscular tension and ligamentous restriction. Involvement of tendons can be demonstrated by MRI (Fig. 12.8). On T2-weighted images, synovial sheaths show fluid and high signal. On T1-weighted images after the gadolinium injection, the inflamed synovium shows enhancement. The posttraumatic ligamentous instability patterns of the wrist described in Chapter 2 are often seen in advanced rheumatoid arthritis.

## Other Peripheral Joints

In the elbow, synovial hypertrophy and effusion provide a fat pad sign. As in other joints, periarticular osteoporosis, uniform joint space narrowing, and erosions are seen. In the glenohumeral joint, erosions are especially prominent around the proximal humerus, and rotator cuff tear or atrophy causes superior subluxation of the humeral head and adaptive changes in the inferior surface of the acromion from the humeral head (Figs. 12.9 and 12.10). Resorption of the distal clavicle and widening of the acromioclavicular joint are

**FIGURE 12.1.** Rheumatoid hand. A boutonniere deformity is present at the middle finger. Erosions are present at the PIP joint of the middle finger (*short arrow*) and the MCP joints of the index, ring, and little fingers (*arrowheads*). Fusiform soft tissue swelling is present at the PIP joint of the ring finger (*long arrow*).

**FIGURE 12.2.** Rheumatoid arthritis with early erosive changes at the MCP joints.

**A**    **B**    **C**

**FIGURE 12.3.** Rheumatoid arthritis involving the MCP joint of the ring finger. **A:** Radiograph shows early subchondral bone erosion (*arrow*). **B:** Coronal T2-weighted fat-suppressed MRI shows effusion (*arrow*). **C:** Coronal T1-weighted fat-suppressed MRI following gadolinium injection shows enhancement (*arrow*).

frequently observed in rheumatoid arthritis. In the knee, meniscal invasion by pannus occurs early and may be detectable on MRI. Typical inflammatory changes may be superimposed on secondary degenerative changes, but the proliferative bone response is disproportionately modest in comparison to the loss of joint space (Fig. 12.11). On MRI, effusions, erosions, diffuse cartilage loss, bone marrow edema, and pannus may be demonstrated at the knee (Fig. 12.12). The hip is less frequently involved than the knee. Concentric uniform loss of joint space with axial migration is usual, but superior migration similar to that in osteoarthritis may also occur.

**FIGURE 12.5.** Hand deformities in rheumatoid arthritis. PA radiograph shows boutonniere deformity of the ring finger, Z-shaped deformity of the thumb, proximal dislocation of the first CMC joint, volar dislocation of the MCP joint of the little finger, and ulnar translocation of the carpus.

**FIGURE 12.4.** Rheumatoid arthritis with juxta-articular osteoporosis.

**FIGURE 12.6.** Rheumatoid wrist. **A:** Early findings include juxta-articular osteoporosis and subtle erosions, including the scaphoid waist (*arrow*). **B:** The same patient 6 years later has severe erosions and subluxations. Ulnar translocation is present. The bones are diffusely osteoporotic, with no proliferative changes. The scaphoid waist erosion has become large (*arrow*).

Acetabular protrusion (protrusio acetabuli), fibrous ankylosis, subchondral cysts, erosions, and secondary reparative and degenerative changes are common. If steroids are administered, osteonecrosis of the femoral head is a potential complication. In the foot, changes may be seen early at the metatarsophalangeal (MTP) and interphalangeal (IP) joints of the great toe (Fig. 12.13). Although the usual changes of rheumatoid arthritis that are found elsewhere in the skeleton may be present in the foot, erosions tend to be small and infrequent. Soft-tissue involvement may lead to hallux valgus and planovalgus deformity of the foot. In the heel, retrocalcaneal bursitis, Achilles tendonitis, and plantar fasciitis may cause swelling and calcaneal erosions (Fig. 12.14). Spontaneous Achilles tendon rupture may occur.

## Spine

In the spine, the upper cervical spine is the only common site of involvement. As many as 70% of patients with rheumatoid arthritis

**FIGURE 12.7.** Rheumatoid arthritis involving the carpal bones. **A:** Coronal T1-weighted MRI shows erosions. **B:** Coronal T1-weighted fat-suppressed MRI following gadolinium injection shows enhancement in the erosions, corresponding to inflammatory pannus.

**FIGURE 12.8.** Rheumatoid arthritis of left ankle with tenosynovitis. Axial T1-weighted fat-suppressed MRI following gadolinium administration shows thickened synovium with intense uptake (*arrowhead*). Effusion (*e*) is noted in the anterior ankle, and longitudinal split tears of the posterior tibialis tendon (*white arrow*) and peroneus brevis tendon (*black arrows*) are noted.

are affected symptomatically at some time, and up to 85% of those with classic rheumatoid arthritis have radiographic changes at the upper cervical spine. The atlantoaxial articulation (C1–2) has a synovial joint anteriorly where the odontoid process articulates with the anterior arch of C1 and is stabilized posteriorly by the transverse ligament. A bursa is interposed between the odontoid process and the transverse ligament. Synovitis at these sites may cause erosions of the odontoid process and rupture of the transverse ligament (Figs. 12.15 and 12.16), resulting in a widened predental interval. One consequence is atlantoaxial instability, with imminent danger of quadriplegia or death. Below the level of C2, the cervical spine may be diffusely involved by joint space narrowing. Inflammatory pannus at the synovial uncovertebral joints (joints of Luschka) may extend into the intervertebral disks. The thoracic spine and lumbar spine are usually spared. Sacroiliac (SI) joint involvement is infrequent and, when present, is mild and asymmetric.

## Extra-Articular Manifestations

Extra-articular manifestations of rheumatoid arthritis include rheumatoid nodules, development of cutaneous fistulas, infections, hematologic abnormalities, vasculitis, renal disease, pulmonary disease, and cardiac complications.

## ◼ CONNECTIVE TISSUE DISEASE

### Systemic Lupus Erythematosus

Systemic lupus erythematosus (SLE) is a chronic systemic disease, the pathogenesis of which is related to immune complex deposition. It is more common in women by an 8:1 ratio, and there is a component of genetic susceptibility. The fluorescent ANA test is virtually always positive at the onset of clinical disease. Manifestations in the musculoskeletal system are common and may precede other systemic manifestations by months or years. Nonerosive symmetric polyarthritis with a distribution similar to that of rheumatoid arthritis is present in 75% to 90% of patients with SLE. Early findings on radiographs are fusiform soft-tissue swelling and juxta-articular osteoporosis, but there should be no joint space

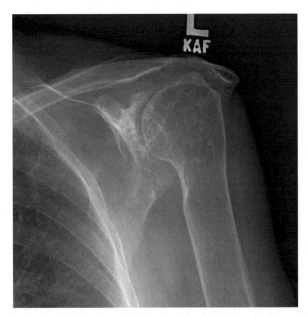

**FIGURE 12.9.** Radiograph of the shoulder in advanced rheumatoid arthritis shows osteopenia, erosion of the distal clavicle, and remodeling of the undersurface of the acromion and medial humeral shaft.

**FIGURE 12.10.** Rheumatoid shoulder with osteoporotic bones and secondary glenohumeral degenerative change. The distal clavicle is eroded and remodeled.

**FIGURE 12.11.** Rheumatoid knees. The bones are osteoporotic. Uniform joint space loss is present with minimal proliferative bone changes. Some secondary osteoarthritic changes are present in the lateral compartment of the left knee.

narrowing or erosions. A deforming nonerosive arthropathy is also common in SLE. The hands are typically involved at the MCP and IP joints (Figs. 12.17 and 12.18). Thumb, wrist, and foot involvement are more common than shoulder and knee involvement, and 10% of patients may develop atlantoaxial subluxation. These deformities are initially reducible, and radiographs may be normal. Fixed deformities and secondary degenerative changes may develop with time. Osteonecrosis may involve the femoral head, femoral condyle, humeral head, and other sites, and commonly

has a symmetric distribution. Myositis, tendon weakening and spontaneous rupture, and soft-tissue calcification are other musculoskeletal manifestations.

## Scleroderma

Scleroderma (progressive systemic sclerosis) is a multisystem fibrosing autoimmune connective tissue disease of variable clinical course. Characteristically, the skin becomes fibrotic, thickened,

**A**                                                                 **B**

**FIGURE 12.12.** Rheumatoid knee. **A:** Sagittal T2-weighted fat-suppressed MRI shows large effusion and Baker cyst with synovial thickening (*arrows*). Diffuse cartilage loss and subchondral edema are present. **B:** Coronal T1-weighted fat-suppressed MRI following gadolinium shows synovial and subchondral enhancement.

**FIGURE 12.13.** Rheumatoid foot. The great toe is deviated laterally, and the remaining MTP joints are subluxated. Erosions are present at all of the MTP joints and the IP joint of the great toe; the other joints appear spared. Some erosions appear sclerotic, suggesting clinical quiescence.

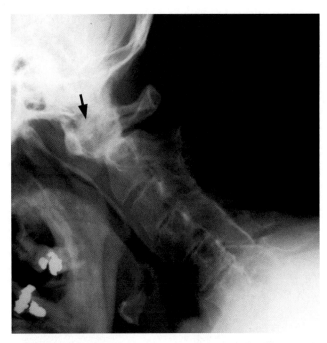

**FIGURE 12.15.** Rheumatoid arthritis. Atlantoaxial subluxation is present with a wide gap between the anterior arch of C1 and the odontoid process (*arrow*).

and taut. Gastrointestinal and renal involvement is prominent. Radiologic manifestations in the musculoskeletal system are present in most patients. These abnormalities are usually seen in the hands and consist of soft-tissue atrophy, soft-tissue calcification, resorption of the phalangeal tufts, and distal interphalangeal (DIP) joint erosions. Osseous destruction and bony erosions

are common in the phalangeal tufts (Fig. 12.19). Soft-tissue atrophy results in cone-shaped fingertips. Subcutaneous calcifications are typically present in multiple digits and elsewhere in the extremities; the calcium deposits are dystrophic and consist of calcium hydroxyapatite deposits at sites of local tissue damage. Calcification may also occur in tendons and tendon sheaths, in joint

**FIGURE 12.14.** Rheumatoid arthritis. Swelling of the retrocalcaneal soft tissues is present with a large erosion in the adjacent bone (*arrow*).

**FIGURE 12.16.** Rheumatoid arthritis. Sagittal T2-weighted MRI shows pannus (*arrow*) eroding the odontoid process and causing mass effect on the spinal cord.

A

B

**FIGURE 12.17.** Systemic lupus erythematosus with alignment deformities. **A, B:** Lateral and PA radiographs show swan neck deformities of the ring and little fingers, with PIP hyperextension of the middle finger.

**FIGURE 12.18.** Systemic lupus erythematosus with severe subluxations. Erosions are absent.

**FIGURE 12.19.** Scleroderma with calcium hydroxyapatite deposits in the thumb and atrophy of the soft tissues.

A                                                          B

**FIGURE 12.20.** Dermatomyositis. **A:** Axial STIR MRI shows muscle edema (high signal) symmetrically distributed in the gluteal and adductor muscles. **B:** Axial T1-weighted fat-suppressed MRI following intravenous gadolinium shows enhancement that corresponds to the regions of edema.

capsules, and even within the joint cavity. Synovial fibrosis without inflammation may cause flexion contractures.

## Dermatomyositis and Polymyositis

Dermatomyositis and polymyositis are diseases of unknown etiology affecting the striated muscle by diffuse, nonsuppurative inflammation and degeneration. The pathogenesis involves an autoimmune mechanism. In dermatomyositis, the skin is also involved. Multiple clinical classifications are based on various features, particularly progressive muscle weakness and rash. There is an associated risk of malignancy in patients older than 40 years of age with

dermatomyositis, especially men. The diagnosis is made by serum enzyme studies, electromyography, and muscle biopsy. Early imaging findings of dermatomyositis and polymyositis can be made on MRI. T2-weighted MRI shows high signal in the involved muscles (Fig. 12.20). Involvement is generally symmetric bilaterally, and the course of the disease can be followed by MRI. On radiographs, the characteristic abnormality is widespread soft-tissue calcification, particularly of intermuscular fascial planes between large proximal limb muscles (Figs. 12.21 and 12.22). There may also be subcutaneous calcifications similar to those in scleroderma (Fig. 12.23). Muscle atrophy, contractures, and chronic osteoporosis are findings late in the clinical course.

**FIGURE 12.21.** Dermatomyositis at the ankle with soft-tissue calcification.

**FIGURE 12.22.** Dermatomyositis at the knee with prominent soft-tissue calcification around the quadriceps muscles.

**FIGURE 12.23.** Polymyositis with soft-tissue calcification (*arrow*) involving the index finger.

## Overlap Syndromes

Patients may have rheumatic diseases with clinical features that overlap those of several of the more well-defined rheumatoid diseases, particularly at the beginning or end of the clinical course. The radiographic features of disease may also overlap so that an individual case may show combinations of features of rheumatoid arthritis, scleroderma, SLE, and dermatomyositis. These overlap syndromes may also be called *mixed connective tissue disease.*

## ■ SPONDYLOARTHROPATHY

The spondyloarthropathies are a heterogeneous group of interrelated conditions. Musculoskeletal manifestations common to these diseases include spinal involvement, especially of the SI joints, enthesopathy, and asymmetric peripheral arthritis of the lower limbs. Additional common features are genetic predisposition; extra-articular manifestations in the skin, gut, urogenital tract, or eyes; negative serum RF; and an association with HLA-B27. These conditions have in the past been called *rheumatoid variants* to distinguish them from rheumatoid arthritis and *seronegative spondyloarthropathy* to reflect the negative serum RF.

### Ankylosing Spondylitis

Ankylosing spondylitis is a chronic inflammatory disease of the spine and SI joints. The etiology is unknown, but there is a genetic component; 90% to 95% of white patients with classic ankylosing spondylitis have HLA-B27 (compared with 9% of all white patients). Symptomatic disease affects approximately 1% of the general population; the prevalence of severe disease is approximately 0.1%. The typical onset is insidious lower back pain and stiffness in adolescent men. In the severe classic form, there is gross ankylosis and deformity of the spine; in mild forms, there may be only occasional arthralgias. In most cases, ankylosing spondylitis is a benign, self-limited, and undiagnosed disease with absent or minimal radiographic changes. The overall sex distribution is probably equal, but men generally have severe, progressive disease, whereas women have mild, self-limited disease.

A

B

**FIGURE 12.24.** Ankylosing spondylitis. **A:** AP radiograph of the lumbar spine shows that the SI joints and the posterior elements of the spine (*arrow*) are ankylosed. **B:** Lateral radiograph of the lumbar spine shows squaring (*arrows*) of the anterior aspects of the lumbar vertebral bodies and ankylosis of the posterior elements.

**FIGURE 12.25.** Ankylosing spondylitis of the cervical spine. Lateral radiograph shows syndesmophytes (*arrow*) bridging C2 through C4 vertebral bodies.

Ankylosing spondylitis begins in the lumbosacral region and ascends to the cervical spine. Radiographically, the involved vertebral bodies become squared off by erosions from inflammation in the prevertebral soft tissues (Fig. 12.24). The facet joints become inflamed and then fused, and syndesmophytes—ossifications in and

**FIGURE 12.27.** Ankylosing spondylitis with symmetric, inflammatory arthritis of the hips, ankylosis of the SI joints, and hyperostosis at the ischial rami.

around the periphery of the annulus fibrosus—form at multiple contiguous levels, eventually leading to a spine that looks like bamboo (Figs. 12.25 and 12.26). Back pain diminishes or disappears as the spine fuses, but the fused spine becomes osteoporotic, fragile, and subject to insufficiency fractures. In the pelvis, the SI joints become symmetrically blurred, sclerotic, and fused (Fig. 12.27). Early in this process, the SI joints have subchondral granulation tissue, and the joint cartilage becomes replaced by fibrous tissue. Ankylosis follows the formation of new cartilage and bone in the joint space.

Approximately 20% of patients with ankylosing spondylitis present initially with peripheral polyarthritis, and, ultimately, approximately 35% will have peripheral disease. This peripheral

**FIGURE 12.26.** Ankylosing spondylitis with syndesmophytes and ossification of the posterior ligamentous structures. The SI joints have fused.

**FIGURE 12.28.** Ankylosing spondylitis with traumatic cervical spine fracture at C5–6 (*arrow*).

polyarthritis is similar to rheumatoid arthritis in clinical manifestations, radiographic appearance, and pathophysiology, but the distribution of disease tends to be different. Feet, ankles, knees, hips, and shoulders are typically involved in an asymmetric fashion; the hands are usually spared. Permanent stiffness or bony ankylosis is likely. Peripheral polyarthritis may precede, coincide with, or follow the onset of spinal manifestations.

MRI has proved more sensitive than radiography in the early detection of sacroiliitis. T1-weighted fat suppression with gadolinium administration and fast inversion recovery are superior to T1- and T2-weighted images. MRI findings of sacroiliitis include abnormal cartilage signal intensity, erosions, increased intensity in the joint, and subchondral bone marrow edema. MRI may also be able to distinguish sacroiliitis due to spondyloarthropathy from septic arthritis of the SI joint.

One major orthopedic complication of ankylosing spondylitis is increased biomechanical fragility of the spine. Syndesmophytes bridging the vertebral bodies and ankylosis of the posterior elements result in a stiff spine that cannot move or dissipate traumatic forces. Bony remodeling of an ankylosed spine does not improve its biomechanical strength as a unit. When patients with ankylosing spondylitis are involved in falls or other accidents, fractures and fracture dislocations of the spine are common (Fig. 12.28). These fractures may progress to nonunion.

**FIGURE 12.29.** Reactive arthritis with sacroiliitis, greater on the left than the right (*arrow*).

## Reactive Arthritis

Reactive arthritis is an acute inflammatory arthritis that follows an infection elsewhere in the body, but infectious organisms cannot be cultured from the joint fluid or synovium. The pathogenesis of the disease is thought to be immunologic in nature, with a genetic predisposition. After gastrointestinal infections by *Shigella*, *Salmonella*, *Yersinia*, or *Campylobacter*, or a genitourinary infection with *Chlamydia*, approximately 1% to 4% of patients develop reactive arthritis. Although the triad of peripheral arthritis, conjunctivitis, and urethritis has been classically associated with reactive arthritis, the current definition generally includes cases of arthritis that occur within 2 months of an episode of venereal infection or epidemic dysentery. The classic triad is present in only one third of cases of reactive arthritis. The diagnosis may be difficult to make because there is no definite laboratory test, and the dysenteric or venereal episode may be mild or silent. There is a marked male predominance of at least 5:1. The typical age of onset is 15 to 40 years. HLA-B27 is present in 70% to 80% of cases, and the serum RF is negative. Clinically, reactive arthritis is an asymmetric lower extremity oligoarthritis manifested by sausage digits, heel pain and swelling, low back pain, and SI joint tenderness. Early clinical signs include effusion, periarticular edema, bursitis, and tendinitis. Fluffy periostitis, enthesopathy, paravertebral comma-shaped ossification, and asymmetric sacroiliitis often develop. Bone density is preserved in chronic disease.

Radiographic abnormalities develop in 60% to 80% of cases, with involvement of synovial joints, symphyses, and entheses. The disease has a predilection for the foot—especially the great toe, ankles, knees, and SI joints—and manifestations are rarely seen above the level of the umbilicus. Bony erosions combined with bony proliferation characterize an asymmetric arthritis. Erosions first appear at the joint margins and may progress to involve the subchondral bone in the central portion of the articulation. Bony proliferation may take the form of periostitis (linear or fluffy), calcification and ossification at entheses, and intra-articular bone production with bony ankylosis. Additional abnormalities may include fusiform soft-tissue swelling, effusions, regional or periarticular osteoporosis, and symmetric and concentric joint space narrowing.

Sacroiliitis is the most common manifestation. The incidence of sacroiliitis increases with the chronicity of the disease, rising from 5% to 10% of cases at onset to perhaps 75% after several years. Sacroiliitis is evident on radiographs as blurring and eburnation of the adjacent sacral and iliac articular surfaces, initially worse on the iliac side (Fig. 12.29). Bilateral changes are typical, and these may be symmetric or asymmetric.

Spinal involvement in reactive arthritis is much less frequent than in ankylosing spondylitis or psoriasis. Asymmetric paravertebral ossification about the lower three thoracic and upper three lumbar vertebrae in reactive arthritis is indistinguishable from the corresponding changes in psoriatic spondylitis. These ossifications are thought to result from inflammatory changes in the paravertebral connective tissue that lead to calcification and ossification. Unlike ankylosing spondylitis, squaring of the vertebral bodies, facet joint erosion, sclerosis, and osseous fusion are unusual in reactive arthritis.

## Psoriatic Arthritis

Psoriasis is a common skin disease characterized by dry, pink, scaly, nonpruritic lesions with a genetic predisposition. As many as 5% of patients with psoriasis have an associated arthritis. The onset and clinical course of skin lesions and arthritis are generally asynchronous and independent, but 80% to 85% have skin involvement first. There is some evidence that psoriatic arthritis may be a form of reactive arthritis incited by streptococcal and staphylococcal infection of psoriatic plaques and affected nails. HLA-B27 is

**FIGURE 12.30.** Psoriatic arthritis with "sausage digit" swelling, erosions (*long arrow*), and periostitis (*short arrow*) of the index finger.

**FIGURE 12.31.** Psoriatic arthritis with interdigitating erosions (pencil-in-cup appearance).

found in 60% to 80% of patients with psoriatic spondylitis but in only 20% of patients with psoriatic peripheral arthritis. Serum RF is absent. Psoriatic arthritis has five patterns of clinical presentation: (a) asymmetric oligoarthritis, seen in more than 50% of cases; (b) polyarthritis with predominantly DIP joint involvement, the classic presentation, which is seen in 5% to 19%; (c) symmetric seronegative polyarthritis simulating rheumatoid arthritis, seen in up to 25%; (d) sacroiliitis and spondylitis resembling ankylosing spondylitis, seen in 20% to 40%; and (e) arthritis mutilans with resorption of phalanges, seen in 5%. Individual patients may change from one clinical pattern to another. Two thirds of patients have an insidious onset, whereas one third have an acute onset mimicking gout or septic arthritis. The age of onset is 35 to 45 years, and there is no sex predominance.

The predominant radiologic abnormalities are found asymmetrically in the upper extremities and result from a synovitis that is similar in pathophysiology to rheumatoid arthritis. The distribution of articular involvement in the hands tends to be distal, commonly the DIP joints of the fingers, and usually accompanies fingernail involvement. Soft-tissue swelling of the digits tends to be of the "sausage" variety, in which the entire digit is swollen, not just the joints (Fig. 12.30). Dramatic joint space loss to the point of erosion and resorption of the articulating ends of bones may occur. Pencil-in-cup erosions (Fig. 12.31) and periosteal bony excrescences (Fig. 12.32) are other typical findings. The arthritis is highly erosive and in the hands or feet may lead to *arthritis mutilans*, which is severe resorptive arthritis of the phalanges (Figs. 12.33 and 12.34). In the spine, irregular, asymmetric paravertebral excrescences of the bone appear; these may be quite bulky and merge with the underlying vertebral bodies and disks (see Fig. 11.20). The changes in the spine and SI joints in psoriatic arthritis tend to be more marked than in reactive arthritis, but they are often indistinguishable. Sacroiliitis may progress to ankylosis.

## Enteropathic Spondyloarthropathy

Patients with inflammatory bowel disease (Crohn disease, ulcerative colitis) may have spondyloarthropathy associated with their disease. The prevalence of articular disease in patients with ulcerative colitis is approximately 10% to 15%; occasionally, it precedes the gastrointestinal disease. Common articular manifestations include peripheral joint arthralgias, soft-tissue swelling, and periarticular osteoporosis; less common manifestations include erosive changes

**FIGURE 12.32.** Psoriatic arthritis with inflammatory periostitis.

**FIGURE 12.33.** Psoriatic arthritis involving the foot. The IP joint of the great toe is severely eroded, as are the DIP joints of the third through fifth toes.

similar to rheumatoid arthritis. The peripheral arthritis may wax and wane in tandem with exacerbations and remissions in the bowel disease. Sacroiliitis and spondylitis resembling or identical to ankylosing spondylitis may also occur in ulcerative colitis. Up to 20%

**FIGURE 12.34.** Arthritis mutilans presentation of psoriatic arthritis in the hand and wrist. The DIP and PIP joints of all of the fingers are severely involved. There is pancompartmental involvement of the wrist, with erosions and mature periosteal bone.

**FIGURE 12.35.** Unilateral inflammatory sacroiliitis in a patient with inflammatory bowel disease. Axial CT scan shows erosions of the left SI joint (*arrows*).

of patients with Crohn disease may have bilateral sacroiliitis, and 25% of these develop ankylosing spondylitis. The sacroiliitis and spondylitis tend to be progressive and not particularly related to the bowel disease (Fig. 12.35). Certain dysenteric infections are associated with reactive arthritis, as discussed earlier in this chapter.

## Differential Diagnosis

Although the spondyloarthropathies have common features, it is frequently possible to distinguish one from the other in individual patients (Table 12.1). The manifestations of ankylosing spondylitis are usually severe in the spine and SI joints and less severe in the peripheral joints. The manifestations of psoriatic arthritis are usually severe in the small peripheral joints and less severe in the large peripheral joints, spine, or SI joints. The manifestations of reactive arthritis are usually mild and rarely involve the upper body. When disease is mild and radiographic findings are minimal, it may be difficult to recognize a specific form of spondyloarthropathy.

## ◼ JUVENILE IDIOPATHIC ARTHRITIS

Juvenile idiopathic arthritis is a heterogeneous group of idiopathic inflammatory joint conditions that have in common (1) involvement for 6 weeks or more and (2) onset before 16 years of age. This classification by the International League for Rheumatology (Table 12.2) has replaced older classifications of "juvenile rheumatoid arthritis" and "juvenile chronic arthritis." The radiologic findings in juvenile idiopathic arthritis reflect the effect of a chronic inflammatory arthritis on a growing skeleton and are generally not specific for a particular clinical entity. The radiologic features include synovitis, soft-tissue swelling, osteoporosis, periostitis, erosions, ankylosis, and growth disturbances (Fig. 12.36). The earlier the age of onset, the more severe the findings. Not all findings are likely to be present together, but combinations of these findings may point to the diagnosis. The disease may remit in adulthood, but permanent muscle wasting, growth deformities from epiphyseal overgrowth and early growth plate closure, loss of function from ankylosis and joint contractures, and secondary osteoarthritis are common sequelae (Fig. 12.37). Compared with

**TABLE 12.1**   **Distinguishing Features of Spondyloarthropathy**

| Feature | Ankylosing Spondylitis | Reactive Arthritis | Psoriatic Arthritis |
|---|---|---|---|
| Clinical setting | Low back pain, adolescents | Following dysenteric or venereal infection | Psoriasis |
| Sex predominance | Male (classic disease) | Male | None |
| Joint distribution | SI, entire spine | SI, lumbar spine, feet | Hands, feet, thoracolumbar spine |
| Severity of involvement | Severe ankylosis | Mild | Severe erosions |
| SI joint involvement | Bilateral, symmetric sacroiliitis invariably leading to ankylosis | Bilateral, asymmetric sacroiliitis | Bilateral, asymmetric sacroiliitis may progress to ankylosis |
| Type of phytes | Delicate syndesmophytes | Paravertebral ossification | Paravertebral ossification |

**TABLE 12.2**   **Frequency of Clinical Types of Juvenile Idiopathic Arthritis**

| Clinical Type | Frequency (%) |
|---|---|
| Systemic arthritis | 9 |
| Oligoarthritis (one to four joints) | 45 |
| Persistent | |
| Extended | |
| Polyarthritis (five or more joints) | |
| Seronegative | 21 |
| Seropositive | 2 |
| Enthesis-related arthritis | 10 |
| Psoriatic arthritis | 13 |

*Source*: Johnson K, Gardner-Medwin J. Childhood arthritis: Classification and radiology. *Clin Radiol.* 2002;57(1):47–58.

A                B

**FIGURE 12.36.**   Juvenile idiopathic arthritis in the hands. **A:** Left side shows the bones are osteopenic. Soft-tissue swelling is evident at all of the joints. Periostitis is present (*arrow*). The articular margins of the bones are eroded and small. **B:** Right side shows similar findings.

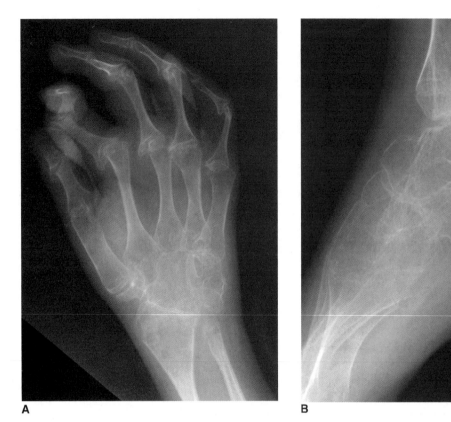

**FIGURE 12.37.** Sequelae of juvenile idiopathic arthritis in a young adult. **A:** The hand has short bones whose growth plates fused prematurely. **B:** Intra-articular tarsal fusions are present; the bones are osteoporotic.

radiography, MRI and sonography are more sensitive imaging indicators of disease activity and can demonstrate synovitis, erosions, and articular cartilage status. MRI can also demonstrate bone marrow edema.

**FIGURE 12.38.** Juvenile idiopathic arthritis involving the hips. Radiograph shows diffuse joint space narrowing, secondary dysplasia, and superimposed degenerative changes.

Symmetric involvement occurs in the systemic arthritis, seronegative and seropositive polyarthritis, and extended oligoarthritis forms of juvenile idiopathic arthritis. Typical sites of involvement may include the MCP and IP joints of the hand, the wrist, elbow, hip (Fig. 12.38), knee, ankle, foot, and cervical spine. In the hand, common findings include soft-tissue swelling, osteoporosis, bony ankylosis, periostitis, growth disturbances, epiphyseal compression fractures, and joint subluxation. Asymmetric involvement occurs in the persistent oligoarthritis, enthesis-related arthritis, and psoriatic arthritis forms of juvenile idiopathic arthritis. Unlike adult forms of inflammatory arthritis, monarticular onset in a knee appears to be a common presentation for all forms of juvenile idiopathic arthritis (Fig. 12.39).

## SEPTIC ARTHRITIS

Septic arthritis is usually caused by nongonococcal bacteria in small children or elderly adults. Infections of joints usually follow hematogenous spread of organisms to the synovium from a preexisting infection in a remote site. Less commonly, adjacent osteomyelitis extends into a joint, or, rarely, a penetrating wound introduces organisms. The most common infecting organism in adults is *Staphylococcus aureus*. The most common organism in infants is beta-hemolytic *Streptococcus* and in preschool-aged children, *Haemophilus influenzae*. In patients with a chronic underlying disease such as diabetes or alcoholism, Gram-negative bacteria are a common cause of septic arthritis in those with concurrent genitourinary tract infections, and *Streptococcus pneumoniae* is a common cause in those with concurrent lung infections. Other risk

A    B

**FIGURE 12.39.** Juvenile idiopathic arthritis in a 4 year old. Effusion is evident, but the disease is of too recent onset to have caused developmental effects. The appearance is nonspecific. **A:** Lateral radiograph. **B:** AP radiograph.

factors for septic arthritis include rheumatoid arthritis, SLE, total joint replacement, and old age.

From the initial site of inflammation and microabscess formation in the synovium, the infection may spread to the joint space, bones, and soft tissues. Proteolytic enzymes released into the joint space by synovial cells and activated PMNs destroy the ground substance and then the collagen framework of the articular cartilage. Destruction of the joint takes only a few days. The usual clinical presentation is the abrupt onset of pain in a swollen, tender, inflamed joint. Nonspecific physical and laboratory signs of local and systemic infection may be present, but a preexisting source of infection is not always obvious. The diagnosis is made by arthrocentesis; injection of contrast medium under fluoroscopy can confirm intra-articular needle placement when necessary. The joint fluid is opaque, with a cell count of more than 100,000 WBC/mm³, a differential with more than 85% PMNs, and a glucose level that is at least 50 mg/dL less than the concurrent serum level. Cultures of the fluid are almost always positive, and blood cultures are positive in 50% of cases. The knee is the most common site. On radiographs, acute septic arthritis is evident as soft-tissue swelling and effusion. Juxta-articular osteoporosis develops, and within 7 to 10 days, the articular cartilage is gone, and the joint space is narrowed. Findings in young children may be subtle, and sonography (to look for effusion) or MRI (to look for effusion and osteomyelitis) may be helpful (Fig. 12.40). Prolonged antibiotic treatment and surgical drainage are often required, but the joint is usually destroyed despite treatment. Secondary degenerative changes ultimately develop.

Gonococcal arthritis occurs among sexually active young adults, especially women (80% of cases), and is the most common infectious arthritis in this age group. Preexisting HIV infection is a risk factor. Hematogenous dissemination of the organism causes fever and arthralgias, typically evident 2 weeks after the initial infection. Polyarticular and asymmetric involvement is usual, and there is a predilection for the knees, wrists, and ankles. Arthrocentesis fluid cultures are positive in fewer than 25% of cases, but the response to antibiotics is rapid, and the outcome is good in nearly all cases. Radiographs may show only joint effusion and soft-tissue swelling.

**FIGURE 12.40.** Septic arthritis in a child. Axial T2-weighted fat-suppressed MRI shows large left hip effusion distending the capsule (*arrow*) and subluxating the femoral head (H).

# ◼ MISCELLANEOUS

## Granulomatous Synovitis

Tuberculosis, atypical mycobacteria, and fungi may spread to the joints, resulting in a granulomatous synovial infection that requires synovial biopsy or joint aspiration for diagnosis. These are chronic, insidiously destructive processes. In the usual situation, the underlying infection is in the lung, the process is monarticular, and there is osteomyelitis adjacent to the involved joint. On radiographs, osteopenia is prominent, and osteolysis with little or no reactive bone formation is characteristic (Fig. 12.41). A large joint effusion may be present. These infections have become progressively less rare in the United States since the beginning of the HIV epidemic (see Chapter 16).

## Viral Synovitis

Viral synovitis (toxic synovitis) is transient and self-limited in nearly all cases. The synovitis may be caused by direct viral infection of the synovium or by the deposition of immune complexes in the synovium as a systemic viremia is cleared. The viruses associated with arthritis include hepatitis B, rubella, enterovirus, adenovirus, varicella-zoster, Epstein-Barr, cytomegalovirus, and herpes simplex. No specific treatment is available or necessary, but aspiration of the joint may be indicated in children to exclude bacterial infection.

## Lyme Disease

Lyme disease is an inflammatory multisystem disease that follows infection by the spirochete *Borrelia burgdorferi*. The vector is the deer tick, an insect endemic to forested areas of the United States, Europe, and Australia. Clinical findings in the acute infection include a rash and flulike syndrome. Months later, multisystem involvement may become apparent. In the musculoskeletal system, arthralgias of sudden onset and short duration appear, sometimes migratory and recurrent. One or more joints may be involved, most frequently the large joints, but also the temporomandibular and SI joints and the hands and feet. The radiographic appearance is nonspecific and may include peripheral enthesopathy and periostitis. Occasionally, a chronic inflammatory oligoarthritis that resembles rheumatoid arthritis develops, particularly in the knees.

**FIGURE 12.41.** Tuberculous arthritis. Radiograph of the thumb shows destruction of the MCP joint (*arrow*) with osteoporosis and minimal reactive bone formation.

## SOURCES AND READINGS

Arnett FC, Edworthy SM, Bloch DA, et al. The American Rheumatism Association 1987 revised criteria for the classification of rheumatoid arthritis. *Arthritis Rheum.* 1988;31:315–324.

Brower AC. *Arthritis in Black and White.* 2nd Ed. Philadelphia, PA: WB Saunders; 1997.

eMedicine. http://emedicine.medscape.com.

Firestein GS, Budd RC, Harris ED Jr, et al. *Kelley's Textbook of Rheumatology.* 8th Ed. Philadelphia, PA: Saunders; 2008.

Forrester DM, Brown JC. *The Radiology of Joint Disease.* 3rd Ed. Philadelphia, PA: WB Saunders; 1987.

Griffin LY. *Essentials of Musculoskeletal Care.* 3rd Ed. Rosemont, IL: American Academy of Orthopedics; 2005.

Jacobson JA. *Fundamentals of Musculoskeletal Ultrasound.* Philadelphia, PA: Saunders; 2007.

Johnson K, Gardner-Medwin J. Childhood arthritis: Classification and radiology. *Clin Radiol.* 2002;57(1):47–58.

Koopman WJ, Boulware DW, Heudebert G. *Clinical Primer of Rheumatology.* Philadelphia, PA: Lippincott Williams & Wilkins; 2003.

Koopman WJ, Moreland LW, eds. *Arthritis and Allied Conditions: A Textbook of Rheumatology.* 15th Ed. Philadelphia, PA: Lippincott Williams & Wilkins; 2004.

Martino F, Silvestri E, Grassi W, Garlaschi G. *Musculoskeletal Sonography: Technique, Anatomy, Semeiotics and Pathological Findings in Rheumatic Diseases.* Berlin: Springer; 2007.

Oostveen JC, van de Laar MA. Magnetic resonance imaging in rheumatic disorders of the spine and sacroiliac joints. *Semin Arthritis Rheum.* 2000;30:52–69.

Resnick D, ed. *Diagnosis of Bone and Joint Disorders.* 4th Ed. Philadelphia, PA: Saunders; 2002.

Sommer OJ, Kladosek A, Weiler V, Czembirek H, Boeck M, Stiskal M. Rheumatoid arthritis: A practical guide to state-of-the-art imaging, image interpretation, and clinical implications. *Radiographics.* 2005; 25:381–398.

Sugimoto H, Takeda A, Hyodoh K. Early-stage rheumatoid arthritis: Prospective study of the effectiveness of MR imaging for diagnosis. *Radiology.* 2000;216:569–575.

# 13 Noninflammatory Joint Disease

This chapter covers joint diseases that have predominantly noninflammatory features on radiographs.

## OSTEOARTHRITIS

Osteoarthritis (degenerative joint disease) is a form of joint disease characterized by degenerative changes involving synovial joints. Osteoarthritis can be divided into primary and secondary types, but the division is artificial: The underlying cause is evident in secondary osteoarthritis but not in primary or idiopathic osteoarthritis. The distinction has some practical value in understanding the process and planning clinical management. Osteoarthritis is the most common form of arthritis. Its prevalence increases with age, so that osteoarthritis is nearly ubiquitous in patients older than 65 years of age. Up to 45 years of age, it is more prevalent in men; from 45 to 55 years of age, the prevalence is equal; and after 55 years of age, it is more prevalent in women. The most common presentation of osteoarthritis is joint pain and limitation of activity. Laboratory tests are used to eliminate other forms of arthritis as clinical possibilities.

### Primary Osteoarthritis

The early morphologic abnormality in primary osteoarthritis is fibrillation of the articular cartilage. The surface develops fibril-like projections and becomes irregular. Underlying this morphologic change is disruption at the molecular level of the superficial armor-plate layer and collagen framework, resulting in progressive loss of proteoglycans from the ground substance and collagen from the framework. Chondrocytes increase protein synthesis, presumably in response to the continuing loss of structural components. Progressive erosion and formation of fissures in the surface eventually expose the subchondral bone. The initial event that incites fibrillation of the cartilage surface is unknown; some forms of primary osteoarthritis may result from an initial alteration in articular cartilage physiology.

Radiographic findings do not appear in osteoarthritis until articular cartilage loss results in secondary adaptive changes in bone. These findings include uneven loss of articular space, subchondral sclerosis, osteophytes, and subchondral cysts (Fig. 13.1); the absence of osteoporosis, ankylosis, and erosions is characteristic. Osteophytes tend to be largest in the plane of motion; therefore, osteophytes at the distal interphalangeal (DIP) and proximal interphalangeal (PIP) joints are best seen on the lateral view. In the hand and wrist, primary osteoarthritis typically affects the DIP and PIP joints and the basal joints of the thumb (Fig. 13.2). The basal joints of the thumb are composed of the first carpometacarpal (CMC) joint and the scaphoid-trapezium-trapezoid joints. Isolated degenerative involvement at this specific site is virtually diagnostic of primary osteoarthritis. The first metatarsophalangeal (MTP) joint, hips and knees, and the cervical and lumbar spine are also common sites of involvement. The metacarpophalangeal (MCP) joints, wrist, elbow, shoulder, and ankle are typically spared. The severity of radiographic changes does not necessarily correlate with the severity of symptoms.

In the knee, the characteristic distribution of involvement is in the medial compartment and, to a less severe degree, the patellofemoral compartment. Joint space narrowing, subchondral sclerosis, osteophytes, and subchondral cysts are typical findings (Fig. 13.3). Occasionally, more severe involvement of the lateral or patellofemoral compartments occurs. Angular deformities and joint space narrowing are best demonstrated on standing views. Because the severity of involvement of the anterior and posterior portions of the femoral cartilage is typically uneven, the amount of joint space narrowing may vary between radiographs with the knee in extension and flexion. On MRI, early osteoarthritis is evident as abnormal high signal in articular cartilage on T2-weighted MRI. When isolated to the patella, this condition is called *chondromalacia patellae* (Fig. 13.4). Fibrillation of the cartilage surface, thinning of the cartilage, and frank loss of cartilage may be seen in progressively more severe cases. Subchondral

**FIGURE 13.1.** Osteoarthritis at the first CMC and scaphotrapezial joints with narrowing of the articular spaces, osteophyte formation, subchondral sclerosis, and subluxation.

bone edema at sites of cartilage loss, osteophyte formation, loose bodies, and effusions may be present in established osteoarthritis (Figs. 13.5–13.7).

In the hip, loss of articular space is usually found along the superior (horizontal) portion of the joint (Fig. 13.8). Less commonly, the medial joint space is narrowed. Osteophyte formation in the femoral head often forms a collar of bone around the femoral neck at the margin of the articular surface, usually seen best on frog lateral views. As with the knee, uneven involvement of the articular cartilage results in varying amounts of joint space narrowing from position to position. Mapping cartilage thickness with fluoroscopically positioned spot radiographs or cartilage-specific imaging parameters on MRI can be helpful in planning rotational osteotomies for treatment.

Osteoarthritis of the synovial joints of the spine may be the predominant feature of degenerative spine disease or may occur in association with other features such as degenerative disk disease, previous trauma, scoliosis, kyphosis, or vertebral anomalies. The common sites of synovial joint osteoarthritis are the lower cervical and lower lumbar spine. The atlantoaxial joint is also synovial and may be affected. The pathologic process is identical to that of other synovial joints, leading to joint space narrowing, subchondral sclerosis, and osteophytes. Loss of articular cartilage may allow subluxation or excessive motion; bony hypertrophy may reduce motion. Osteophytes and ligamentous thickening may lead to nerve root involvement. These findings are best demonstrated by CT (Fig. 13.9).

Osteoarthritis of the acromioclavicular joint is a common finding on shoulder imaging. On radiographs, osteophytes may be seen. On MRI, osteophytes and hypertrophy of the joint are typical, often with subchondral edema in the distal clavicle and acromion and fluid in the joint (Fig. 13.10).

Inflammatory (erosive) osteoarthritis is a condition in which an acute synovitis accompanies primary osteoarthritis. Although joint degeneration always has some component of synovial inflammation because of the presence of joint debris and cartilage breakdown products, the inflammation dominates the clinical presentation in erosive osteoarthritis. Radiographs show the degenerative features and distribution of primary osteoarthritis,

**A**

**B**

**FIGURE 13.2.** Osteoarthritis at the DIP joints of the fingers. **A:** PA radiograph. **B:** Lateral radiograph.

**A**

**B**

**FIGURE 13.3.** Osteoarthritis with asymmetric joint space narrowing, osteophytes, and subchondral sclerosis.
**A:** Right knee. **B:** Left knee.

but the acute synovitis causes inflammatory erosions, uniform joint space narrowing, and sometimes ankylosis (Fig. 13.11). A characteristic "seagull" appearance may be seen on PA radiographs at the interphalangeal (IP) joints of the fingers, corresponding to central erosions and bony hypertrophy. The typical age at onset

is in the fifth or sixth decade, and women are affected far more frequently than men. The inflammation usually subsides within a few months to a couple of years, leaving the degenerative changes. In the hand, erosive osteoarthritis characteristically affects the DIP and PIP joints and the basal joints of the thumb, as does nonerosive primary osteoarthritis.

## Secondary Osteoarthritis

Secondary degenerative changes in the joints result from three major factors: an abnormality of the articular cartilage, loss of subchondral bony support beneath normal articular cartilage, and abnormal alignment and mechanical stress. Any condition with one of these features may lead to permanent, progressive osteoarthritis. Secondary osteoarthritis may follow inflammatory arthritis if the inflammatory process has caused permanent cartilage damage and is quiescent long enough for the degenerative changes to develop. Mechanical trauma may injure the articular cartilage, which has a limited ability for repair. A fibrocartilage scar may replace damaged areas of hyaline cartilage. Joint debris, loose bodies, or displaced meniscal fragments within a joint may erode the articular cartilage. Osteochondral loose bodies derive nutrition from synovial fluid and may grow. Healthy cartilage wears prematurely when its underlying bony support is lost. For example, collapse of the subchondral bone of the femoral head after osteonecrosis leads rapidly to secondary degeneration. Less obvious changes in the subchondral bone due to repetitive subclinical trauma may also lead to osteoarthritis. An abnormally aligned joint or a joint that is subject to mechanical disadvantage or abnormal stresses may wear prematurely. Posttraumatic osteoarthritis may follow malunion of long-bone fractures, imperfectly reduced intra-articular fractures (Fig. 13.12), or posttraumatic joint instability. Many forms of

**FIGURE 13.4.** Chondromalacia patellae with effusion as well as fissured and fibrillated patellar cartilage (*arrow*) shown on axial T2-weighted, fat-saturated MRI.

A

B

C

**FIGURE 13.5.** Osteoarthritis. **A:** Coronal T1-weighted MRI shows cartilage loss and meniscal extrusion (*arrow*) in the medial compartment. Medial and lateral compartments are involved by osteophytes. **B:** Sagittal T2-weighted fat suppressed MRI shows patellofemoral compartment osteophytes (*arrow*) and cartilage loss. **C:** Sagittal T2-weighted fat suppressed MRI through the medial compartment shows effusion, cartilage loss, osteophytes, and degenerative posterior horn medial meniscal tear (*arrow*).

**FIGURE 13.6.** Patellofemoral osteoarthritis. Axial gradient echo MRI shows loss of cartilage from the lateral facet of the patella and the patellofemoral groove (*arrows*). Osteophytes are present on both sides of the patellofemoral joint and the posterior margin of the lateral condyle. An effusion is present.

**FIGURE 13.7.** Osteoarthritis of the knee with large, calcified intraarticular bodies in a popliteal cyst.

**FIGURE 13.8.** Osteoarthritis of the hip with advanced joint space asymmetric narrowing and prominent osteophytes.

**FIGURE 13.9.** Lumbar facet osteoarthritis on CT scan. Osteophytes extend into the lateral recesses bilaterally, causing nerve root compression.

developmental and acquired bone and joint dysplasia lead to early osteoarthritis, including developmental dysplasia of the hip (Fig. 13.13), Legg-Calvé-Perthes disease, and multiple epiphyseal dysplasia. The premature wear-out resulting from the abnormal joint geometry worsens in a vicious cycle of progressive malalignment, mechanical disadvantage, and abnormal stress.

## Femoroacetabular Impingement

Femoroacetabular impingement designates a spectrum of developmental or acquired conditions of the hip in which a morphologic mismatch between the femoral head and the acetabulum hip may lead to mechanical impingement of the acetabular rim on the femoral neck at the extremes of motion, restricting range of

**A**

**B**

**FIGURE 13.10.** Osteoarthritis of the acromioclavicular joint. **A:** Axial T2-weighted fat suppressed MRI shows subchondral edema in the clavicle and acromion (*arrows*). **B:** Oblique coronal T1-weighted MRI shows hypertrophy of the acromioclavicular joint (*arrow*) with mass effect on the supraspinatus muscle.

A

B

**FIGURE 13.11.** Inflammatory osteoarthritis with erosions and osteophytes at the PIP joints and the first CMC joint. **A:** Lateral radiograph. **B:** PA radiograph.

**FIGURE 13.12.** Posttraumatic osteoarthritis 12 years after acetabular fracture.

**FIGURE 13.13.** Secondary osteoarthritis in the left pseudoacetabulum (*short arrow*) in a 20-year-old woman with untreated DDH. The native acetabulum (*long arrow*) is empty.

**FIGURE 13.14.** Femoroacetabular impingement with reactive bone changes at the femoral neck (*arrows*). **A:** AP radiograph. **B:** Frog lateral radiograph.

motion, causing pain, and leading to acetabular labral pathology and degenerative changes. In the cam type of femoroacetabular impingement, the morphology of the femoral head and neck is abnormal as a result of conditions such as previous trauma, slipped capital femoral epiphysis, or Legg-Perthes disease. In the pincer type of femoroacetabular impingement, the morphology of the acetabulum is abnormal as a result of conditions such as acetabular retroversion or protrusio acetabuli. Patients who may be anatomically predisposed to femoroacetabular impingement may be asymptomatic if they do not engage in activities that require

**FIGURE 13.15.** Rotator cuff impingement. **A:** Oblique coronal T1-weighted MRI shows osteoarthritis of the acromioclavicular joint with hypertrophy (*arrow*) and mass effect on the supraspinatus muscle. **B:** Oblique sagittal T1-weighted MRI shows anterior hooking (*arrow*) of the acromion process.

**FIGURE 13.16.** Neuropathic osteoarthropathy. Sagittal T1-weighted MRI of the foot shows swelling, disorganization, and edema of the midfoot.

**FIGURE 13.17.** Neuropathic shoulder joint in a patient with syringomyelia.

extreme ranges of motion, such as ballet or yoga. Radiologic features of femoroacetabular impingement include reactive changes in the femoral neck (Fig. 13.14) and evidence of abnormal femoral or acetabular morphology.

## Subacromial Impingement

Subacromial impingement syndrome of the shoulder refers to trapping of the rotator cuff between the top of the humerus and the undersurface of the coracoacromial arch. The coracoid process, the coracoacromial ligament, and the acromion process form the coracoacromial arch. A downward-projecting bony excrescence or degenerative hypertrophy of the acromioclavicular joint is commonly associated with impingement syndrome (Fig. 13.15). However, impingement syndrome is considered to be a clinical rather than a radiologic diagnosis. Other conditions that may impinge on the rotator cuff include congenital, developmental, or acquired variations in the size and shape of structures around the coracoacromial arch, including the acromion and the coracoid. Other types of shoulder impingement include posterior superior glenoid impingement and subcoracoid impingement.

## Neuropathic Osteoarthropathy

Neuropathic joints (Charcot joints) have lost proprioception and deep pain sensation. With continued use of the joint, relaxation and hypotonia of the supporting structures lead to malalignment and recurrent injury. Rapidly progressive erosion of the articular cartilage, reactive subchondral sclerosis, fractures, and fragmentation of the subchondral bone result in a disorganized joint. The presence of joint debris induces synovitis and chronic effusion. The damage and derangement may occur over a period of days

to weeks with relatively little symptomatology. Both lower motor neuron (peripheral) and upper motor neuron (central) lesions may result in neuropathic osteoarthropathy. Diabetic neuropathy is the most common lower motor neuron lesion causing neuropathic osteoarthropathy; other causes include alcoholism, tuberculosis, amyloidosis, leprosy, peripheral nerve trauma, steroids, and congenital indifference to pain. Syringomyelia is the most common upper motor neuron lesion; other causes include meningomyelocele, trauma, multiple sclerosis, tabes dorsalis (syphilis), and cord compression.

Neuropathic osteoarthropathy occurs in 0.1% of all diabetics and in 5.0% of those with diabetic neuropathy. Diabetic peripheral neuropathy causes loss of pain sensation and proprioception, leading to exceptional wear and tear without patient awareness of injury. The most frequent site of involvement is the foot (80%), especially the tarsometatarsal, intertarsal, and MTP joints; involvement may be unilateral or bilateral. Tarsal-metatarsal fracture dislocation (Lisfranc fracture dislocation) may occur spontaneously or with minimal trauma. Extensive sclerosis, osteophytosis, fractures, bony fragmentation, subluxation, dislocation, bony debris, effusion, and subchondral cysts are common findings. Chronic osteomyelitis is also relatively common in the diabetic foot, and the possible combination of neuropathic osteoarthropathy with infection can pose a diagnostic dilemma (Fig. 13.16). MRI with gadolinium enhancement may be helpful in this circumstance.

Neuropathic osteoarthropathy occurs in 25% of patients with syringomyelia. The joint changes are usually in the upper extremity (80%), and they may be atrophic rather than proliferative. Acute resorption of the articulating ends of the bone without evidence of repair, gross soft-tissue swelling, and bony debris in the soft tissues are common findings. This process may mimic destruction from tumor or infection. The most commonly involved joint is the shoulder (Fig. 13.17).

| TABLE 13.1 | Crystal Deposition Diseases of Joints |
|---|---|
| Crystal | Associated Clinical Conditions |
| CPPD | Chondrocalcinosis |
|  | Pseudogout |
|  | Pyrophosphate arthropathy |
| Calcium hydroxyapatite | Asymptomatic calcification |
|  | Calcific tendonitis, bursitis, and periarthritis |
|  | Calcific tendonitis, bursitis, and periarthritis |
|  | Chronic destructive joint disease |
| Monosodium urate monohydrate | Hyperuricemia |
|  | Gouty arthritis |
|  | Tophaceous gout |

# ■ CRYSTAL-ASSOCIATED DISEASES

Crystal-associated joint diseases are pathologic conditions that occur in the presence of crystals. The crystals contribute to tissue damage, but the causal relationship between crystals and tissue damage is not well understood. Crystals precipitate from the extracellular fluid space into the articular tissues, where they accumulate. Deposits of crystals may then be shed episodically into the joint space. Clearance of crystals from the joint space and articular cartilage is poor because these structures are avascular, alymphatic, and largely devoid of scavenger cells. The presence of particles alters the mechanical properties of the tissues, tending to make them less elastic. Articular cartilage is particularly vulnerable to damage and ultimately undergoes degenerative changes. Large crystalline particles in the joint space can cause direct abrasive damage to the articular surfaces. Small particles can cause damage by biophysical and biochemical interactions with cell membranes and macromolecules and may also provoke an acute synovitis. Although the precise mechanisms mediating acute synovial inflammation are incompletely understood, different mechanisms appear to be activated by different crystals. These crystal-induced inflammatory reactions tend to have a sudden onset and a rapid, self-limited course. The sudden onset is probably related to the abrupt shedding of crystals into the joint space from a deposit in the articular tissues.

Crystal deposition diseases have three clinical presentations: (a) an asymptomatic state in which crystals can be detected, (b) an inflammatory arthritis, and (c) a chronic destructive arthropathy. The particular diseases are defined by the presence of characteristic crystals within affected joints. Aspiration of the joint during an acute inflammatory episode may yield material in which the associated crystal can be demonstrated. The three types of crystals that are commonly associated with joint diseases are calcium pyrophosphate dihydrate (CPPD), calcium hydroxyapatite, and monosodium urate monohydrate (Table 13.1).

## Calcium Pyrophosphate Dihydrate Crystal Deposition Disease

CPPD crystal deposition disease is a polyarticular arthritis with deposition of CPPD crystals in articular tissues. Its initial presentation may be monoarticular. The definitive clinical diagnosis requires the identification of CPPD crystals from joint fluid, but the radiologic findings can be diagnostic. CPPD deposition disease has been associated with hyperparathyroidism, hemochromatosis, aging, and osteoarthritis. It has been weakly associated with hypothyroidism, ochronosis, Paget disease, Wilson disease, acromegaly, diabetes, and gout. CPPD crystal deposition disease has three manifestations: chondrocalcinosis, crystal-induced synovitis, and pyrophosphate arthropathy (Table 13.2).

CPPD crystals are generated locally in the articular tissues, where asymptomatic deposits may accumulate in cartilage, joint capsules, intervertebral disks, tendons, and ligaments. In cartilage, these deposits may be evident radiographically as chondrocalcinosis. Chondrocalcinosis is most common in the knees, wrists, elbows, and hips, and is found in both fibrocartilage and hyaline cartilage. Chondrocalcinosis in the menisci has high signal intensity that can mimic a meniscal tear on MRI. Chondrocalcinosis in the hyaline cartilage appears as linear or punctate areas of low signal intensity, which becomes more noticeable on gradient recalled echo (GRE) sequence because of the blooming artifact.

Shedding of crystals into the joint space after rupture of a deposit causes an acute, self-limited, crystal-induced synovitis. This acute synovitis is clinically similar to acute gouty arthritis and has been known as *pseudogout*. As with gouty arthritis, acute episodes of inflammatory synovitis may recur intermittently. During an acute episode, CPPD crystals can be recovered by joint aspiration and identified by polarized light microscopy or more definitive physical means. Uncommonly, these episodes can run together into a subacute or chronic crystal synovitis that resembles rheumatoid arthritis, except that the large joints of the limbs tend to be involved rather than the small ones of the hands and feet.

Pyrophosphate arthropathy is the degenerative result of structural joint damage caused by chronic CPPD crystal deposition and irreversible destruction of the articular cartilage. The degenerative changes can be identical to osteoarthritis, but the distribution of involvement is different. In the hand, the MCP joints are characteristically involved. In the wrist, the radiocarpal joint is characteristically involved. In severe cases, the process causes gross scapholunate dissociation in association with degenerative radiocarpal changes. The scaphoid and lunate separate, and the capitate migrates proximally into the resulting gap. This syndrome is called *scapholunate advanced collapse*, or *SLAC*, wrist (Figs. 13.18 and 13.19). The SLAC wrist usually includes pancompartmental degenerative involvement. The shoulder (glenohumeral), knee (especially patellofemoral), elbow, ankle, and foot (talonavicular) are the other common sites of involvement (Fig. 13.20). Chondrocalcinosis need not be present, and is absent if there is no remaining cartilage. Isolated severe involvement of the patellofemoral compartment of the

| TABLE 13.2 | Clinical Syndromes of CPPD Deposition Disease |
|---|---|

Asymptomatic chondrocalcinosis

Crystal synovitis
  Acute, intermittent (pseudogout)
  Subacute or chronic (resembles rheumatoid arthritis)

Pyrophosphate arthropathy (resembles osteoarthritis)
  Without attacks of pseudogout
  With intermittent attacks of pseudogout
  Neuropathic-like (resembles neuropathic osteoarthropathy)

**FIGURE 13.18.** Pyrophosphate arthropathy with SLAC wrist. Chondrocalcinosis involves the triangular fibrocartilage complex (*arrow*).

knee or selective radiocarpal involvement of the wrist is virtually diagnostic of pyrophosphate arthropathy. Pyrophosphate arthropathy is often, but not necessarily, combined with acute episodes of crystal-induced synovitis. Very severe degenerative changes may lead to an appearance that resembles neuropathic osteoarthropathy.

## Hydroxyapatite Deposition Disease

Hydroxyapatite deposition disease is a heterogeneous group of conditions that have in common the abnormal presence of amorphous hydroxyapatite (basic calcium phosphate) crystals in the soft

tissues. Ion contaminants such as carbonate, magnesium, fluoride, and chloride are present. It is probably the result of multiple causes, and there may be more than one mechanism of deposition. The radiologic manifestations of hydroxyapatite deposition disease are similar to other crystal-associated conditions: asymptomatic deposits, acute crystal-induced synovitis, and chronic destructive arthropathy. Unlike CPPD deposition disease, hydroxyapatite deposition disease typically involves the tendons, ligaments, and joint capsules rather than the articular cartilage and subchondral bone.

Deposits of hydroxyapatite in the soft tissues appear on radiographs as dense, homogeneous, sharply marginated, and amorphous calcifications. They may have linear, angular, or round shapes, and unlike chondrocalcinosis, the calcifications do not conform to hyaline or fibrocartilage structures. Occasionally, these deposits may mimic mineralized osteoid tumor matrix, which they may resemble. The soft-tissue calcifications of immune-mediated connective tissue diseases such as scleroderma, polymyositis, and dermatomyositis are also in the form of hydroxyapatite, but the clinical condition of hydroxyapatite deposition disease is different from these. Hydroxyapatite deposition disease is thought to be a process of abnormal mineral metabolism, possibly systemic but perhaps localized only to the sites of tissue damage; the cause and pathogenesis are not understood. These deposits may occur in periarticular soft tissues as well as tendons, ligaments, capsules, entheses, and bursae (Figs. 13.21–13.24). A minority of patients with hydroxyapatite deposits have symptoms. Metastatic soft-tissue deposits of hydroxyapatite around joints (periarticular calcinosis, tumoral calcinosis) may be found in patients on dialysis for chronic renal failure (Fig. 13.25). Because the crystals are often aqueous suspensions (milk of calcium), CT and upright radiographs may demonstrate fluid-sediment levels. The calcification is difficult to detect on most MRI sequences, except for gradient-recalled echo sequences, because the calcified collections are of low signal and isointense to the involved tendons. MRI may show muscle and soft-tissue edema associated with the calcifications.

Recurrent episodes of calcific tendonitis or calcific bursitis are commonly associated with hydroxyapatite deposits. Most

**A**    **B**    **C**

**FIGURE 13.19.** CPPD hand on MRI. **A:** PA radiograph shows joint space narrowing (*arrows*) at the index and middle MCP joints. **B:** Coronal T2-weighted MRI with fat suppression shows high signal (*arrows*) at the index and middle MCP joints. **C:** Coronal T1-weighted MRI with fat suppression following injection of gadolinium shows enhancement (*arrows*) at the index and middle MCP joints.

**FIGURE 13.20.** Pyrophosphate arthropathy of the glenohumeral joint with prominent humeral osteophyte.

**FIGURE 13.22.** Hydroxyapatite deposit (*arrow*) in the rotator cuff shown on axial GRE MRI.

patients are adults in their 40s and 50s and present with acute pain, swelling, and tenderness. Symptoms respond rapidly to a non-steroidal anti-inflammatory agent. The shoulder, commonly the supraspinatus tendon, is a common site of involvement. Tendons may atrophy and rupture, but it is unclear whether the deposits initially caused the local tissue damage or preexisting tissue damage allowed the deposits to accumulate. The deposits around the shoulder are bilateral in approximately half of cases and may migrate to

contiguous structures. After clinical resolution, the deposits may disappear. The process is usually monoarticular, but multiple joints may be involved at the same time or successively. Other common sites of involvement include the long head of the biceps tendon, the extensors of the wrist, the myotendinous attachments along the linea aspera (thigh adductors) and at the medial border of the proximal tibia (pes anserinus), the olecranon bursa, the trochanteric bursa, and the ischial bursa.

**FIGURE 13.21.** Calcium hydroxyapatite deposit in the supraspinatus tendon of the rotator cuff (*arrow*).

**FIGURE 13.23.** Hydroxyapatite deposition in the acetabular labrum (*arrow*).

**FIGURE 13.24.** Calcific retrocalcaneal bursitis.

Hydroxyapatite crystals have been associated with a chronic destructive arthritis similar to osteoarthritis or CPPD deposition disease. This situation is relatively uncommon and most often occurs in the setting of renal failure and hyperparathyroidism (Fig. 13.26). Mixtures of crystals may be recovered from such joints, including CPPD and hydroxyapatite.

## Gout

Gout is defined by the presence of hyperuricemia (serum uric acid concentration >7 mg/dL). Hyperuricemia may be idiopathic or secondary to known conditions, including excess ingestion (in protein), intrinsic overproduction, or reduced renal secretion. There is a familial incidence that appears to be controlled by multiple genes. Specific mutations with biochemical defects in purine metabolism leading to hyperuricemia have been found in a few cases. Gout is associated with obesity, diabetes, hyperlipidemia, hypertension, atherosclerosis, alcohol consumption, acute illness, and pregnancy. There is a negative association with rheumatoid arthritis. The prevalence of the symptomatic forms of gout, gouty arthritis, and tophaceous gout has declined dramatically with the increasing use of drugs that control hyperuricemia. Gouty arthritis is similar to other crystal-related joint diseases, whereas tophaceous gout has the radiology of a metabolic deposition disease (discussed in "Metabolic Deposition Disease").

Gouty arthritis is the articular disease associated with monosodium urate monohydrate, the crystalline form in which uric acid is precipitated from solution into the soft tissues. The age of peak onset of gouty arthritis is 50 years, and it develops only after decades of sustained hyperuricemia. Gouty arthritis commonly presents as an acute crystal-induced synovitis that tends to be recurrent and episodic. Radiographs may show only fusiform soft-tissue swelling unless there are concurrent features of tophaceous gout. Shedding of monosodium urate crystals into the synovial fluid or synovial tissues apparently causes the acute synovitis, provoking an inflammatory response. A chronic destructive arthropathy may also develop. Approximately 90% of cases occur in men. The manifestations of gouty arthritis are generally peripheral, in the hands or feet. Gouty arthritis has a predilection for the joints of the lower extremity, especially the first MTP joint (podagra), intertarsal joints, ankle, and knee. The first MTP joint is the most common site of initial involvement; the great toe is the site of 70% of attacks. Involvement of the hands, wrists, and elbows may occur later in the clinical course. The limb girdles and axial skeleton are typically spared. The acute episode usually responds quickly and dramatically to colchicine or a nonsteroidal anti-inflammatory agent.

**FIGURE 13.25.** Periarticular calcinosis in patient on hemodialysis for chronic renal failure. **A:** Radiograph shows calcium deposits around the hip (*long arrow*) and gluteal musculature (*short arrow*). **B:** Axial CT scan shows fluid-fluid levels (*arrow*) within the calcium deposits.

**FIGURE 13.26.** Hydroxyapatite arthropathy. Hip shows destructive changes in the femoral head and acetabulum. Note the medial acetabular protrusion (protrusio acetabuli).

# ■ METABOLIC DEPOSITION DISEASE

Metabolic deposition diseases involving the joints, in which the body accumulates a substance it cannot excrete or metabolize, include tophaceous gout, multicentric reticulohistiocytosis, and amyloidosis. Except for gout, these types of joint disease are relatively uncommon. If focal, masslike deposits are located in the musculoskeletal system, the result is a clinically indolent disease with randomly distributed, slowly enlarging, space-occupying deposits.

## Tophaceous Gout

Unlike the other crystal-induced joint conditions, gout may present with the radiologic features of a metabolic deposition disease. Deposits of monosodium urate crystals are called *tophi*. The development of tophi requires decades of sustained hyperuricemia and is related to the degree and duration of hyperuricemia. Control of hyperuricemia by drugs has reduced the incidence of tophi in people with gout from more than 50% in the 1950s to approximately 3% currently. Deposits near the joints and tendons cause a lumpy-bumpy appearance. These localized areas of swelling may cause the slow development of pressure erosions on adjacent bone. Such erosions have well-defined sclerotic margins. A shell of new bone may attempt to encompass the deposit, leaving an overhanging edge (Figs. 13.27–13.30). The articular spaces may be preserved until late in the disease. Tophaceous gout may occur in combination with episodes of gouty arthritis.

## Multicentric Reticulohistiocytosis

In the rare condition of multicentric reticulohistiocytosis, lipid-containing macrophages are deposited in the soft tissues around joints and tendons in random distribution. Skin nodules are common. As with gout and other metabolic deposition diseases,

**FIGURE 13.27.** Tophaceous gout with overhanging edges and chronic erosions of the first, fourth, and fifth MTP joints. The adjacent articular space in the first MTP joint is preserved.

**FIGURE 13.28.** Tophaceous gout involving the hand. PA radiograph shows lumpy-bumpy soft-tissue swelling and chronic, focal bone erosions.

**FIGURE 13.29.** Tophaceous gout involving the carpus. Coronal T1-weighted MRI shows multiple low signal masses eroding the carpal bones.

**FIGURE 13.31.** Multicentric reticulohistiocytosis. The soft tissues are thickened, and there are chronic erosions with overhanging edges.

normal bone density and normal joint spaces are associated with intraosseous and juxta-articular accumulations. Bone erosions with sclerotic margins and overhanging edges are typical (Fig. 13.31), but sometimes a destructive arthritis ensues (arthritis mutilans). The origin of the abnormal lipid is unknown. In approximately 28% of cases, multicentric reticulohistiocytosis appears to be caused by a paraneoplastic disorder related to an underlying malignancy.

## Amyloid Arthropathy

Amyloidosis is the result of several different underlying diseases in which a characteristic proteinaceous material accumulates in the body. The joint findings of amyloidosis in chronic renal dialysis patients have been well documented. Hemodialysis clears beta-immunoglobulins poorly from the blood. As these proteins accumulate in the body, they polymerize into beta-pleated sheets

and become deposited in subcutaneous tissues, around joints, and occasionally in parenchymal organs. In addition to periarticular masses, a chronic symmetric arthropathy may also result, with clinical features similar to those of rheumatoid arthritis. Compression of the median nerve may result from deposition of amyloid in the carpal tunnel. Contractures and soft-tissue swelling are common, and severe constitutional symptoms may be present. Amyloidosis has variable MRI appearance: low signal on both T1-weighted and T2-weighted images (corresponding to fibrous tissue, amyloid deposits, or both), low signal on T1-weighted images, with high signal on T2-weighted images (corresponding to fluid), and high signal on both T1-weighted and T2-weighted images (corresponding to fatty component) (Fig. 13.32).

## ■ MISCELLANEOUS JOINT CONDITIONS
### Pigmented Villonodular Synovitis

Pigmented villonodular synovitis (PVNS) is a benign neoplasm (rather than an inflammatory condition) of the synovium that usually presents as recurrent monoarticular hemorrhagic effusions in adults. It may have localized or diffuse involvement of the joint. The localized variety is typically represented by a focal nodular mass projecting into a joint. Common locations include the knee or hip, but any synovial tissue may be involved. Chronic, erosive changes from thickened, nodular synovial proliferation may be seen on radiographs. Localized osteoporosis is common. Arthritic changes such as joint space narrowing and osteophytes are generally absent. Arthrography shows multiple nodular filling defects. MRI shows effusion and multiple low-signal synovial masses (Fig. 13.33). The lesions are pigmented on gross examination because of hemosiderin deposition from repeated bleeding.

The extra-articular counterpart of PVNS, which is histologically identical, is called *giant cell tumor of the tendon sheath*. This

**FIGURE 13.30.** Tophaceous gout involving the midfoot. Sagittal CT reformatted image shows multiple erosions with fragmentation.

**FIGURE 13.32.** Amyloid arthropathy. **A:** Radiograph of the shoulder shows cartilage space loss and remodeling of the glenohumeral joint. **B:** Axial GRE MRI shows synovial masses (*arrows*) and degenerative changes.

lesion presents most commonly as a painless soft-tissue mass in the hand, located along a tendon sheath. On radiographs, soft-tissue swelling may be seen. On MRI, a soft-tissue mass with low to intermediate signal intensity on T1-weighted images and

heterogeneous high signal intensity on T2-weighted images is typical (Fig. 13.34). Enhancement after gadolinium injection may be seen on T1-weighted images. Giant cell tumor of the tendon sheath is not related to giant cell tumor of bone.

**FIGURE 13.33.** Diffuse PVNS of the hip. **A:** Coronal T1 MRI shows bulky low signal synovial masses around the left hip with femoral head erosions. **B:** Axial GRE MRI shows blooming dark signal around the left hip.

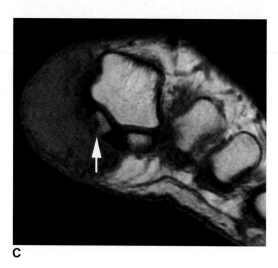

**FIGURE 13.34.** Giant cell tumor of tendon sheath. **A:** AP radiograph shows a focal soft-tissue mass along the medial aspect of the first metatarsal head. **B:** Axial T2-weighted fat suppressed MRI shows lobulated morphology and high signal within the lesion. **C:** Coronal T1-weighted MRI shows low signal within the mass. The mass erodes the medial sesamoid (*arrow*).

## Synovial Chondromatosis

Synovial chondromatosis (synovial osteochondromatosis, synovial chondrometaplasia) is a condition characterized by the presence of multiple, benign cartilaginous nodules in the synovium. They may be loose within the joint or attached to the synovium. They may be calcified, ossified, or neither. When a synovial chondromatosis is not calcified, MRI examination shows a confluent soft-tissue mass of high signal intensity on T2-weighted images within the joint. The mass may have foci of low signal on both T1-weighted and T2-weighted images (Figs. 13.35 and 13.36). Synovial chondromatosis appears to be a reactive process rather than a neoplastic or degenerative one and can be distinguished histologically from secondary synovial chondrometaplasia, in which pieces of bone or cartilage from trauma or osteoarthritis become embedded in the synovium and stimulate a secondary cartilaginous metaplasia. Because synovial chondromatosis may cause a mechanical destructive osteoarthritis, it may coexist with secondary synovial chondrometaplasia. Men are affected more than women by a ratio of 2:1, and the peak age of presentation is in the 40s.

## Synovial Hemangiomatosis

Synovial hemangiomatosis is an unusual condition in which the joint capsule is involved by hemangiomas. Hemangiomatosis results in intracapsular soft-tissue masses that may cause extrinsic erosion of bone similar to those seen in PVNS or synovial chondromatosis. On radiographs, effusion, phleboliths, and erosions are seen. On arthrography or CT arthrography, synovial masses are seen. On MRI, the vascular nature of the lesion may be evident, with low signal on T1-weighted MRI, high signal on T2-weighted MRI, and enhancement on T1-weighted MRI after gadolinium injection. Repeated hemarthrosis is a potential complication.

## Baker Cyst

A Baker cyst is a common synovial cyst that is located in the popliteal fossa. A Baker cyst results from distention of the gastrocnemius-semimembranosus bursa by fluid from the knee joint. The fluid enters through a slitlike communication with the posteromedial aspect of the knee capsule—just above the joint

**FIGURE 13.35.** Synovial chondromatosis of the elbow. Axial T1-weighted fat suppressed MRI with intra-articular gadolinium shows synovial chondromas.

**FIGURE 13.36.** Synovial chondromatosis (*arrows*) of the shoulder. Oblique sagittal T2-weighted MRI shows multiple small synovial chondromas filling the subdeltoid subacromial bursa.

line—between the tendons of the medial head of the gastrocnemius and semimembranosus muscles. Baker cysts may be associated with any condition in which there is a knee effusion, including various forms of arthritis and various types of internal derangements. The most common complication of Baker cyst is rupture or dissection of fluid into the adjacent gastrocnemius muscle belly, often resulting in a

pseudothrombophlebitis syndrome that mimics deep venous thrombosis of the calf. On MRI, a ruptured Baker cyst may be recognized by the presence of fluid extending from a Baker cyst or the site of a Baker cyst into the belly of the medial gastrocnemius muscle or the adjacent calf or thigh muscles (Fig. 13.37). A coexistent deep venous thrombosis may be present.

**A**

**B**

**FIGURE 13.37.** Ruptured Baker cyst. **A:** Axial T2-weighted fat suppressed MRI at the level of the joint line shows a decompressed Baker cyst (*arrow*). **B:** Axial image through the distal thigh shows fluid (*arrow*) tracking along the medial head of the gastrocnemius muscle.

**A**

**B**

**FIGURE 13.38.** Osteolysis of the distal clavicle (different patients). **A:** Radiograph shows subchondral erosions (*arrow*). **B:** Oblique coronal T2-weighted MRI shows erosions and marrow edema.

## Posttraumatic Osteolysis of the Distal Clavicle

Posttraumatic osteolysis of the distal clavicle is a painful condition that may result from previous acromioclavicular joint dislocation or repetitive microtrauma. On radiographs, posttraumatic osteolysis is evident as cortical irregularity of the distal clavicle with cystlike erosions of subchondral bone, osteopenia, and soft-tissue swelling (Fig. 13.38). Sometimes, aggressive osteolysis of the entire distal clavicle may be seen. On MRI, bone marrow edema in the distal clavicle without marrow edema in the acromion process is characteristic. Soft-tissue swelling, periarticular erosions, and periostitis may also be present.

## ■ DEGENERATIVE FOOT CONDITIONS
## Flatfoot (Pes Planus)

Acquired flatfoot in adults (pes planus) is a common condition in which the medial longitudinal arch collapses during standing. The medial longitudinal arch consists of the bones along the medial side of the foot (calcaneus, talus, navicular, first cuneiform, and first metatarsal) and the plantar fascia that helps maintain their position like a bowstring. The tibialis posterior muscle is a dynamic stabilizer of the arch that inserts on the navicular, the keystone of the arch. On the weight-bearing lateral radiograph, the talus, navicular, first cuneiform, and first metatarsal should be oriented in a straight line (Fig. 13.39). If the midfoot is convex dorsally, a cavus foot is present. Flatfoot is characterized by sagging of the midfoot below this hypothetical line at either the talonavicular joint or the navicular-cuneiform joint, indicating loss of the medial arch. An additional radiologic feature of flatfoot may be superimposition of the metatarsal bases, indicating loss of the transverse arch. On the weight-bearing AP radiograph, the metatarsals may appear splayed, and the talocalcaneal angle may be widened. If the medial longitudinal arch is restored to its normal alignment on non–weight-bearing radiographs, the flat foot is said to be flexible. The most common cause of flatfoot is hereditary, and the majority of the 15% to 20% of the adult U.S. population with flatfoot is asymptomatic. Patients with developmentally hypermobile joints—such as those with Marfan syndrome, Ehlers-Danlos syndrome, or Down syndrome—often have flexible flatfoot. Flexible flatfoot is also common among those with acquired hypermobile joints in conditions such as systemic lupus erythematosus. Rigid flatfoot may result from conditions such as heel cord contractures and tarsal coalitions.

## Calcaneus

Calcaneal spurs are common enthesopathic changes involving the insertions of the plantar aponeurosis and the Achilles tendon. They may become symptomatic through pressure and inflammation of adjacent soft tissues and bursae. Posttraumatic ossification is also common at these sites.

A Haglund deformity is a prominence of the posterior superior margin of the calcaneus that becomes symptomatic because of impingement of improperly fitted footwear.

Plantar fasciitis is an inflammatory condition involving the calcaneal origin of the medial cord of the plantar aponeurosis. The sole of the foot is typically painful with weight-bearing or athletic activity. A bony spur may develop at the plantar aspect of the calcaneus. On MRI, the plantar aponeurosis may be thickened at its origin and show increased signal on both T1-weighted and T2-weighted images (Fig. 13.40). Surrounding edema may also be present in the soft tissues and occasionally in the adjacent calcaneal tuberosity.

## Great Toe

A bunion (hallux valgus, metatarsus primus varus) is a symptomatic complex of deformities characterized by a bony prominence

**FIGURE 13.39.** Foot alignment on weight-bearing lateral radiographs. **A:** Cavus foot with a convex midfoot. **B:** Normal foot in which the axes of the talus, navicular, medial cuneiform, and first metatarsal are collinear. **C:** Flatfoot with sagging between the navicular and medial cuneiform results in a concave midfoot. **D:** Flatfoot with sagging between the talus and navicular, and overlap of the metatarsal bases.

at the medial aspect of the first MTP joint. It consists of lateral deviation of the great toe (hallux valgus), medial deviation of the first metatarsal (metatarsus primus varus), soft-tissue contractures of the great toe flexors, and secondary degenerative change at the first MTP joint. Progressive soft-tissue contracture pulls like a bowstring to increase the deformity. A bunion can be recognized on weight-bearing AP radiographs of the foot by varus deviation of

**FIGURE 13.40.** Plantar fasciitis. Sagittal T2-weighted fat suppressed MRI shows high signal at the calcaneal origin of the medial cord of the plantar aponeurosis (*arrow*).

the first metatarsal and valgus deviation of the great toe. The degree of uncovering of the articular surface of the first metatarsal head by the proximal phalanx of the great toe depends on the severity of the hallux valgus. Together, these deformities result in lateral subluxation of the sesamoids relative to the head of the first metatarsal (Fig. 13.41). In severe cases, the second toe may override the great toe because of the hallux valgus.

*Hallux rigidus* and *hallux limitus* refer to osteoarthritis at the first MTP joint with stiffness and limitation of motion. There is typically a prominent dorsal osteophyte at the distal articular surface of the first metatarsal.

## Lesser Toes

Deformities of the lesser toes are usually caused by contractures of the flexor or extensor tendons of the foot. A claw toe deformity is hyperextension of the MTP joint and flexion of the IP joints. A hammer toe deformity is flexion at the PIP joint, usually with hyperextension at the MTP joint (it may be similar to a claw toe deformity) (Fig. 13.42). A mallet toe deformity is DIP flexion. These various toe deformities are generally treated surgically with resection arthroplasty or arthrodesis. Rather than lengthening the tendons, these procedures shorten the bones so that the tendons are at the correct relative length. A bunionette deformity is a bony prominence on the lateral side of the fifth metatarsal head. When symptomatic, there may be overlying soft-tissue swelling.

## ■ INTERVERTEBRAL DISK DEGENERATION

Intervertebral disk degeneration commonly coexists with osteoarthritis of the synovial joints of the spine. The biomechanical loads on the spine are shared among the intervertebral disk joints, the various fibrous articulations, and the synovial joints, so that the

A

B

**FIGURE 13.41.** Bunion deformity (hallux valgus, metatarsus primus varus). **A:** AP weight-bearing radiograph of the foot shows varus deformity of the first metatarsal combined with valgus deformity of the great toe. Note the overriding of the second toe over the great toe and lateral subluxation of the lateral sesamoid (*arrow*), relative to the head of the first metatarsal. **B:** Coronal T1-weighted MRI through the head of the first metatarsal shows lateral subluxation of the sesamoids (*arrow*) with degenerative change.

A

B

**FIGURE 13.42.** Hammer toes. **A, B:** AP and lateral radiographs show PIP joint flexion deformities of the lesser toes.

**FIGURE 13.43.** Discogenic sclerosis in the lower lumbar spine, with loss of disk height, shown on sagittal CT reformatted image.

**FIGURE 13.44.** Degenerative lumbar disk herniation. Sagittal T2-weighted MRI shows degenerative disk disease (low signal) at L4–5 and L5–S1. The L4–5 disk has herniated posteriorly (*long arrow*). Note normal disk height and normal hydration (high signal) of the nucleus pulposus at L3–4 and L2–3 (*short arrows*).

integrity of each component is dependent on the others. There is some evidence that primary degeneration of the cartilaginous end plates, through which water diffuses to the disk, leads to dehydration of both the nucleus pulposus and the annulus fibrosus. Dehydration of the nucleus pulposus can be demonstrated by MRI in young adults and is perhaps an early consequence of aging. The normal nucleus pulposus has high signal on T2-weighted MRI; if it is dehydrated, it has low signal. Congenital factors as well as abnormalities such as scoliosis and spondylolysis may contribute. The loss of hydration results in decreased tissue resiliency and is greatest in the nucleus pulposus. The normal hydraulic distribution of stresses over the entire articular surface is lost, and secondary tears and degeneration of the annulus fibrosus may result. Adaptive changes eventually involve the bones. The radiographic result is moderate to severe loss of intervertebral disk height, gas in the intervertebral disk, and well-defined sclerosis of the adjacent vertebral body end plates (Fig. 13.43). This condition of disk degeneration is called *intervertebral osteochondrosis*. Breakdown of the attachment of the outer (Sharpey) fibers of the annulus fibrosus to the vertebral rim allows circumferential displacement (bulging) of the disk. Osteophytes grow at the attachments of the annulus fibrosus and the anterior longitudinal ligament to the vertebral body. This degenerative process with osteophyte formation is called *spondylosis deformans*. Tears through the annulus fibrosus allow fragments of the disk to protrude into the substance of the annulus and herniate through it. Herniated disk fragments may impinge on neural structures, often nerve roots, and cause symptoms. Circumferential disk bulges may narrow the spinal canal. CT and MRI may demonstrate degenerative changes and disk pathology (Fig. 13.44), but the correlation of radiologic findings with symptoms is not consistent. The facet and costovertebral joints may be secondarily involved from altered biomechanics caused by disk degeneration.

Senile kyphosis occurs in the thoracic spine of older patients. It is related to mechanical failure of the anterior aspect of the intervertebral disk, leading to loss of disk height anteriorly, secondary vertebral sclerosis, and sometimes ankylosis. Osteoporotic kyphosis is a different (but sometimes coexisting) process involving insufficiency fractures of the anterior aspects of osteoporotic vertebral bodies (see Chapter 15).

# ◼ DIFFUSE IDIOPATHIC SKELETAL HYPEROSTOSIS

Diffuse idiopathic skeletal hyperostosis (DISH) (ankylosing hyperostosis of the spine, Forestier disease) is a radiographically defined condition characterized by ossification of the soft tissues at the attachments of muscles, ligaments, and tendons to bone. DISH appears to represent an ossifying diathesis or bone-forming tendency of unknown etiology that increases in incidence with age.

DISH is common in older adults, more frequently men, and the symptoms are often back stiffness and pain. The precise definition of DISH is still evolving. Resnick and Niwayama give the following criteria for spinal involvement in DISH: (a) flowing calcification and ossification along the anterolateral aspect of at least four contiguous vertebral bodies, (b) relative preservation of disk height in the involved vertebral body segments and absence of extensive radiographic changes of degenerative disk disease (gas in the disk space or vertebral body sclerosis), and (c) absence of facet joint ankylosis and sacroiliac joint erosion, sclerosis, or intra-articular osseous fusion. These criteria distinguish DISH from spondylosis deformans, intervertebral osteochondrosis, and ankylosing spondylitis. There are no associated laboratory abnormalities. Bone density remains normal. Extraspinal manifestations of DISH are exceedingly common in older patients. Ossification at the insertion of tendons may be seen throughout the extremities (Fig. 13.45). In the pelvis, whiskering bone proliferation is common along sites

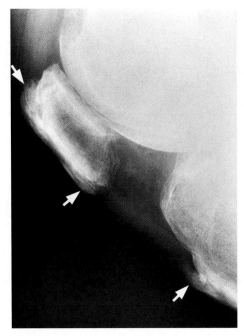

**FIGURE 13.45.** DISH with ossified entheses at the quadriceps and infrapatellar tendons (*arrows*).

**FIGURE 13.46.** DISH involving cervical spine.

A

B

**FIGURE 13.47.** Fracture (*arrows*) at the thoracolumbar junction in a patient with DISH. **A:** Lateral radiograph. **B:** Sagittal CT reformatted image.

where muscles and ligaments attach. Para-articular bone growths correspond to ossification at the attachments of joint capsules. For practical purposes, the diagnosis of DISH can be made radiographically when there is excessive enthesal ossification in the absence of other conditions known to cause such ossification (e.g., spondyloarthropathy or previous trauma).

Extra-articular bony ankylosis is very common in the thoracic spine and somewhat less common in the cervical and lumbar regions (Fig. 13.46). Extra-articular ankylosis of the spine makes the spine stiff. Despite the increase in bone mass, the spine may be more fragile biomechanically when subjected to trauma. The lack of motion and the loss of the energy-absorbing function of the intervertebral disks and ligaments contribute to its decreased ability to absorb loading. Fractures and fracture dislocations of the spine may be catastrophic (Fig. 13.47).

A                                                B

**FIGURE 13.48.** Baastrup disease (different patients). **A:** Lateral radiograph shows hyperostosis of the spinous processes with kissing spines (*arrow*). **B:** Sagittal CT reformation shows kissing spines (*arrow*).

## ■ BAASTRUP DISEASE

Baastrup disease (osteoarthrosis interspinalis) is a degenerative condition described in the lumbar spine in which there is hyperostosis of the spinous processes leading to remodeling and joint formation between adjacent spinous processes (Fig. 13.48). The condition has also been described as *kissing spines*. The relationship of Baastrup disease to chronic low back pain is uncertain.

## SOURCES AND READINGS

Brandt KD, Doherty M, Lohmander LS, eds. *Osteoarthritis*. 2nd Ed. New York, NY: Oxford University Press; 2003.

Brower AC. *Arthritis in Black and White*. 2nd Ed. Philadelphia, PA: WB Saunders; 1997.

eMedicine. http://emedicine.medscape.com.

Firestein GS, Budd RC, Harris ED Jr, McInnes IB, Ruddy S, Sergent JS. *Kelley's Textbook of Rheumatology*. 8th Ed. Philadelphia, PA: Saunders; 2008.

Forrester DM, Brown JC. *The Radiology of Joint Disease*. 3rd Ed. Philadelphia, PA: WB Saunders; 1987.

Griffin LY. *Essentials of Musculoskeletal Care*. 3rd Ed. Rosemont, IL: American Academy of Orthopedics; 2005.

Helms CA, Major NM, Anderson MW, et al. *Musculoskeletal MRI*. 2nd Ed. Philadelphia, PA: WB Saunders; 2009.

Koopman WJ, Boulware DW, Heudebert G. *Clinical Primer of Rheumatology*. Philadelphia, PA: Lippincott Williams & Wilkins; 2003.

Koopman WJ, Moreland LW, eds. *Arthritis and Allied Conditions: A Textbook of Rheumatology*. 15th Ed. Philadelphia, PA: Lippincott Williams & Wilkins; 2004.

McGonagle D, Gibbon W, Emery P. Classification of inflammatory arthritis by enthesitis. *Lancet*. 1998;352:1137–1140.

Moskowitz RW, Altman RD, Hochberg MC, Buckwalter JA, Goldberg VM, eds. *Osteoarthritis: Diagnosis and Medical/Surgical Management*. 4th Ed. Philadelphia, PA: Lippincott Williams & Wilkins; 2006.

Olivieri I, Barozzi L, Padula A. Enthesiopathy: Clinical manifestations, imaging and treatment. *Bailliere Clin Rheum*. 1998;12:665–681.

Resnick D, ed. *Diagnosis of Bone and Joint Disorders*. 4th Ed. Philadelphia, PA: Saunders; 2002.

Resnick D, Niwayama G. Entheses and enthesopathy. Anatomical, pathological, and radiological correlation. *Radiology*. 1983;146:1–9.

Wortmann RL, Schumacher R, Becker MA, Ryan LM. *Crystal-Induced Arthropathies: Gout, Pseudogout and Apatite-Associated Syndromes*. New York, NY: Taylor & Francis; 2006.

# PART IV

# Miscellaneous Topics

# 14 Developmental and Congenital Conditions

T his chapter describes the radiology of many developmental and congenital conditions that affect the musculoskeletal system. Some of these conditions may not present until adolescence or adulthood.

## SKELETAL MATURATION

The skeleton develops and matures with a consistent and irreversible sequence of changes in osseous size and contour. Particular features in the contours of developing bones are useful maturational landmarks in the sequence of ossification. These features are used to estimate skeletal age. The most practical method is to use the radiographic atlas of Greulich and Pyle.

This atlas contains radiographs of the left hand and wrist in boys and girls of different ages—correlated with their chronologic age—from the neonate to the skeletally mature. A radiograph of the left hand and wrist of the individual patient is compared to these standards, and a best match is found. Each chronologic age has a mean bone age and a standard deviation in bone age. The radiologic report of the bone age should include the bone age itself as well as the standard deviation in the bone age for the patient's chronologic age.

Greulich and Pyle's atlas is based on radiographs of healthy children of northern European ancestry from Cleveland, Ohio, whose families were incidentally above average in economic and educational status. These children were followed between 1931 and 1942 as part of a longitudinal long-term investigation of human growth and development. This project produced atlases of skeletal development of the hand and wrist, the knee, and the foot and ankle. The applicability of these atlases to individuals from other ethnic and socioeconomic populations is uncertain.

## HERITABLE CONNECTIVE TISSUE DISORDERS

### Osteogenesis Imperfecta

Osteogenesis imperfecta is a group of inborn connective tissue disorders characterized by radiographically decreased bone density. The underlying problem is one of abnormal collagen synthesis, in which a variety of different molecular defects in collagen produces a continuous spectrum of phenotypes. In the skeleton, the bone matrix is deficient, resulting in thin, osteoporotic, and fragile bones that are subject to repeated insufficiency fractures and consequent deformity (Fig. 14.1). The condition is heritable, but cases are often sporadic. In general, there are autosomal-recessive severe forms that present at birth and autosomal-dominant forms that present later and have a mild course. The condition ranges from severe, congenital involvement with multiple fractures in utero and perinatal death to mild, late manifestations in adulthood. The severe forms account for 10% of cases; the less severe forms account for the remaining 90%. The incidence of osteogenesis imperfecta is 1 per 20,000 to 60,000 live births. Associated clinical features—with variable expression— include blue sclerae (90%); thin, translucent skin; hypermobile, lax peripheral joints; abnormal teeth (dentinogenesis imperfecta); and deafness (fragile otic bones).

**A**    **B**

**FIGURE 14.1.** Osteogenesis imperfecta. **A:** Radiograph of forearm shows osteoporosis, bowing deformity, and healing insufficiency fractures of different ages. **B:** Lower extremities show similar findings along with popcorn epiphyses.

**FIGURE 14.2.** Marfan syndrome. Radiograph of the hand shows arachnodactyly. Hypermobility is present at the carpus, with overlap of the proximal and distal carpal rows.

## Other Disorders

Marfan syndrome, homocystinuria, and Ehlers-Danlos syndrome are heterogeneous groups of heritable connective tissue disorders with musculoskeletal manifestations. Marfan syndrome is associated with excessive height, long spidery digits (arachnodactyly), hypermobile joints, and scoliosis (Fig. 14.2). Ocular and cardiovascular abnormalities dominate the clinical picture. Accumulation of amino acid metabolites in homocystinuria interferes with collagen cross linking, leading to fragile bones, scoliosis, and excessive length of long bones. Ehlers-Danlos syndrome is associated with fragile skin and hypermobile joints.

## ■ SCLEROSING DYSPLASIAS

The sclerosing skeletal dysplasias are a heterogeneous group of conditions characterized radiographically by dense bones.

## Osteopetrosis

Osteopetrosis is a group of heritable diseases characterized by reduced bone resorption from osteoclast failure. Many genetic defects may cause osteoclast failure, each having different underlying biochemical and histopathologic abnormalities. One form is associated with renal tubular acidosis and rickets. The final common effect is that bone remodels incompletely or not at all. There are three major clinical groups: infantile-malignant autosomal recessive, which is fatal within the first few years of life (in

**FIGURE 14.3.** Osteopetrosis, autosomal recessive type (infantile). **A:** Radiograph of the forearm shows dense bones lacking a medullary space. **B:** Radiograph of femurs shows club-shaped metaphyses.

the absence of effective therapy); intermediate autosomal recessive, which appears during the first decade of life but does not follow a malignant course; and autosomal dominant (Albers-Schönberg disease or marble bones), which has a normal life expectancy but many orthopedic problems. The infantile variant has clinical

**FIGURE 14.4.** Osteopetrosis, incidental adult presentation. Note the sandwich appearance of the vertebrae.

manifestations that correlate with the lack of marrow development (anemia and thrombocytopenia) and the lack of enlargement of bony remodeling (small cranial foramina result in cranial nerve dysfunction, hydrocephalus, convulsions, and mental retardation). Radiographs show uniformly dense bones with no medullary space, broadened metaphyses (Erlenmeyer flask deformity), and bone-within-a-bone appearance at the tarsals, carpals, phalanges, vertebrae, and iliac wings (Fig. 14.3). Transverse insufficiency fractures occur often. Medical treatments involve high-dose calcitriol to stimulate osteoclast differentiation and bone marrow transplantation to provide monocytic osteoclast precursors. The intermediate and autosomal-dominant forms have mild manifestations that include anemia, cranial nerve palsies, and orthopedic problems. The fragility of osteopetrotic bone and its inability to remodel in response to stress result in repeated insufficiency fractures. Coxa vara, long-bone bowing, hip and knee degenerative arthritis, and mandibular and long-bone osteomyelitis may also occur. Even milder forms of osteopetrosis may be asymptomatic and discovered incidentally on radiographs (Fig. 14.4).

## Osteopoikilosis

Osteopoikilosis (spotted bones, osteopathia condensans disseminata) is an uncommon osteosclerotic dysplasia with sporadic and familial occurrence. Symptoms are generally absent or mild, and its discovery is frequently incidental. The condition is defined by the presence of numerous small, well-defined, homogeneous ovoid or circular foci of increased radiodensity clustered in periarticular

A

B

**FIGURE 14.5.** Osteopoikilosis. **A:** AP radiograph. **B:** CT scan.

osseous regions. The distribution is symmetric, typically involving the epiphyses and metaphyses of long bones, as well as the carpus, tarsus, scapula, and pelvis (Fig. 14.5). The lesions may increase or decrease in size or number. They are histologically identical to bone

**FIGURE 14.6.** Osteopathia striata.

islands but have no clinical significance unless mistaken for other lesions.

## Osteopathia Striata

Osteopathia striata (Voorhoeve disease) is a rare condition whose transmission is probably autosomal dominant. The condition is defined by the presence of linear, regular bands of increased radiodensity extending from the metaphyses to the diaphyses of tubular bones and the pelvis (Fig. 14.6). Osteopathia striata is usually bilateral, and it is unusual for it to involve the small bones of hands or feet, skull or face, or spine. The cause and pathogenesis are unknown. Clinical manifestations are usually absent, although facial deformity has been described. Discovery is usually incidental.

## Melorheostosis

Melorheostosis is a rare, nonhereditary condition that presents in childhood with extremity pain, limitation of motion, and intermittent joint swelling. Growth disturbances, soft-tissue involvement, and increasing muscle contractures due to tendon and ligament shortening may result in considerable deformity and disability. The condition is commonly limited to a single limb, usually lower. Radiologically, there is extensive periosteal or endosteal cortical hyperostosis with bony excrescences extending along the length of the bone, giving it a wavy contour that has been likened to wax dripping down a candle (Figs. 14.7 and 14.8). Endosteal hyperostosis may fill the medullary cavity, but periosteal and endosteal hyperostosis usually do not occur together. The radiologic appearance is characteristic. The cause and pathogenesis are unknown; the bony excrescences are histologically normal bone.

**FIGURE 14.7.** Melorheostosis involving the fourth and fifth rays of the hand.

# ◼ CONGENITAL DWARFISM

Dwarfism is the condition of being disproportionately undersized. Skeletal dysplasias with dwarfism are legion. Dozens of specific types are listed in the International Nomenclature of Constitutional Diseases of Bone as revised in 1983 by the European Society of Pediatric Radiology. For most of these conditions, there are only a handful of reported cases. Many conditions are lethal, none are reversible, and most are not defined on a radiologic basis. The distinction among the dysplasias with dwarfism often requires detailed genetic, biochemical, histochemical, and histopathologic analysis.

## Achondroplasia

Achondroplasia is the most common type of dwarfism and has a classic radiologic appearance. Achondroplasia is the result of a generalized defect in enchondral bone formation, leading to underdevelopment of the portions of bones that grow by this mechanism. The result is a symmetric short-limbed dwarfism in which the proximal segments of the extremities are disproportionately short (rhizomelic micromelia). Because periosteal bone growth is unaffected, the shafts of the long bones are of normal diameter. The fingers are short and stubby. The skull base, formed by enchondral bone formation, is abnormally short and has a small foramen magnum. The calvaria, formed by intramembranous bone formation, is appropriately large for the intracranial contents, giving the head a characteristic brachycephaly with frontal bossing and a small face (Fig. 14.9). The spinal canal is narrow in both anteroposterior and lateral dimensions, but the trunk length is nearly normal. There is

**FIGURE 14.8.** Melorheostosis involving the foot shown on axial CT scan.

an exaggerated lumbar lordosis with prominent buttocks. These abnormalities are usually evident at birth and become more apparent with age. Achondroplasia has autosomal-dominant genetic transmission, but most cases are sporadic. The classic form is heterozygous, has no associated congenital defects, and is compatible with a normal life span. Complications of congenital spinal stenosis are common in adulthood (Fig. 14.10). The homozygous condition is lethal in infancy and has a radiologic appearance identical to thanatophoric dwarfism. Thanatophoric ("death-bringing") dwarfism is the most common lethal bone dysplasia.

## Other Types

Other types of dwarfism may be characterized and classified by the predominant location of disproportionate shortening. Mesomelic micromelia refers to shortening of the forearms and lower legs. Examples of mesomelic dwarfism include camptomelic dwarfism and dyschondrosteosis of the Nievergelt and Langer types. Acromelic micromelia refers to shortening of the hands and feet. Examples of acromelic dwarfism include asphyxiating thoracic dystrophy (Jeune syndrome), chondroectodermal dysplasia (Ellis-van Creveld syndrome), and pyknodysostosis. Many of these dysplasias are amenable to prenatal diagnosis with obstetric sonography, reducing even further the role of radiography.

# ◼ MISCELLANEOUS GENERALIZED CONDITIONS

## Neurofibromatosis

Neurofibromatosis is one of the heritable phakomatoses, characterized by multisystem involvement of hamartomas involving all three germ cell layers. Neurofibromatosis has autosomal-dominant transmission. There are multiple subtypes. Major musculoskeletal manifestations include scoliosis, mesodermal dysplasia, and

**FIGURE 14.9.** Achondroplasia. **A:** The base of the skull is short and the face is small. **B:** The bones are disproportionately short and the fingers appear stubby. **C:** The femurs are short and thick.

neurofibromas (Fig. 14.11). Although the scoliosis may be gently curving and identical to idiopathic scoliosis, occasionally a sharply angulated dysplastic thoracic kyphoscoliosis is present and virtually diagnostic. Mesodermal dysplasia may result in focally abnormal or deficient bone formation. Orthopedic complications in neurofibro-

matosis include bowing, pathologic fracture, pseudoarthrosis, and defective fracture healing (Fig. 14.12). The tibia is a characteristic site for pseudoarthrosis; repeated failures to heal after treatment often lead to amputation. Neurofibromas may erode adjacent bones and present as soft-tissue masses.

**FIGURE 14.10.** Achondroplasia in adult with spinal stenosis in the lumbar region. Laminectomy has been performed at all levels.

**FIGURE 14.12.** Neurofibromatosis with pseudoarthrosis (*arrow*) of the tibia in a child. A telescoping rod has been placed for mechanical support.

## Cerebral Palsy

Cerebral palsy can result in generalized or focal neuromuscular disease in which secondary bone changes and complications are seen. These changes are the result of abnormal stresses on the growing skeleton from muscular spasm, weakness, atrophy, and imbalance. When the normal skeleton remodels in response to abnormal stress, dysplastic changes in the bones and joints may result. Long bones often appear overtubulated (narrow shaft, broad epiphysis). Hip dysplasia secondary to chronic, spastic dislocation is common. Spasm of the thigh adductor muscles positions the femoral head on the lateral acetabular rim, resulting in deformity, subluxation, and, ultimately, hip dislocation (Fig. 14.13). Scoliosis, soft-tissue atrophy, and flexion or extension contractures may be found. Foot deformities of various kinds are common. Similar developmental changes are seen in conditions such as arthrogryposis, muscular dystrophy, peripheral nerve palsy, and polio.

## Muscular Dystrophy

Muscular dystrophy comprises a heterogenous group of genetic diseases characterized by progressive atrophy of skeletal muscle. Depending on the particular genetic defect and its expression, age of onset, anatomic distribution, severity, rate of progression, and pattern of inheritance vary among the different types of muscular dystrophy, dozens of which have been described. Radiologic features of muscular dystrophy in the musculoskeletal system include fatty replacement of muscles, usually symmetric and diffuse (Fig. 14.14), and, if the onset is during skeletal maturation, dysplastic bone changes. Multisystem manifestations may also be present in some forms of muscular dystrophy.

**FIGURE 14.11.** Neurofibromatosis in an adult. **A:** Axial T1 MRI shows multiple lobulated soft-tissue mass in and around the right buttock with dysplastic underlying bone and muscle atrophy. **B:** Axial T2 MRI shows high signal within the masses.

**FIGURE 14.13.** Adult with DDH resulting from cerebral palsy and chronic hip dislocation without weight-bearing.

## Arthrogryposis Multiplex Congenita

Arthrogryposis multiplex congenita is an uncommon nonhereditary congenital disorder that manifests with deformed joints, dislocations, and muscle wasting (Fig. 14.15). The deformities are widespread and bilateral and usually cause severe disabilities, but the patient's life span is often normal. Frequent deformities include clubfoot (talipes equinovarus, present in 75% of cases), flexion

**FIGURE 14.15.** Arthrogryposis with poor muscle development and recurvatum deformity (anterior to left; *arrow* points to cartilaginous patella).

deformity of the knee (60%), flexion deformity of the hip (40%), and dislocation of the hip with resultant dysplasia (40%).

## Down Syndrome

Generalized ligamentous laxity in Down syndrome (also called trisomy 21) may be manifested by atlantoaxial (C1–2) subluxation (Fig. 14.16), recurrent patellar dislocation, pes planus

**FIGURE 14.14.** Limb girdle muscular dystrophy in an adult. Oblique coronal T1-weighted MRI shows fatty replacement of all of the shoulder muscles.

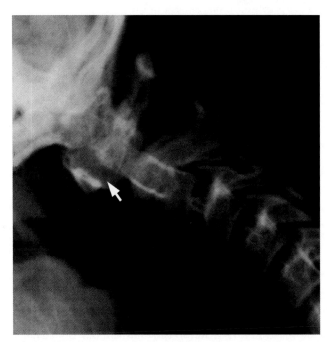

**FIGURE 14.16.** Down syndrome with atlantoaxial subluxation (*arrow*).

**FIGURE 14.17.** Charcot-Marie-Tooth disease in a young adult with cavus foot, hammertoe deformities, and muscle atrophy.

**FIGURE 14.18.** Multiple epiphyseal dysplasia (dysplasia epiphysealis multiplex).

(flatfoot deformity), and voluntary, painless hip dislocation. The iliac wings may have a flared appearance. The significance of atlantoaxial subluxation with respect to participation in sports is controversial.

## Charcot-Marie-Tooth Disease

Charcot-Marie-Tooth disease (also called hereditary motor and sensory neuropathy, hereditary sensorimotor neuropathy, or peroneal muscular atrophy) is a collection of heritable neuropathies that present with predominant involvement of the lower extremities in late childhood or early adulthood. Foot drop, cavus foot (Fig. 14.17), hammertoe deformities, and muscle atrophy in the peroneal nerve distribution, and scoliosis are common features, but the upper extremities may also be involved. The multiple types of this disease are distinguishable by specific chromosomal abnormalities.

## ◼ MISCELLANEOUS LOCALIZED CONDITIONS

### Multiple Epiphyseal Dysplasia

Multiple epiphyseal dysplasia (dysplasia epiphysealis multiplex, Fairbank disease) is the most common of a heterogeneous group of disorders characterized by abnormal growth and development of epiphyses at multiple sites. Multiple epiphyseal dysplasia has autosomal-dominant transmission. The primary defect involves an abnormality in the biochemical composition of the ground substance produced by the epiphyseal chondrocytes, resulting in delayed and disorderly ossification, joint incongruity, and secondary degenerative change. After onset in early childhood, the variable clinical manifestations include articular pain, gait disturbances, short stature, and involvement of multiple sites. Radiographically, the secondary ossification centers occur late and are irregular in morphology. After skeletal maturity, the epiphyses remain irregular and abnormal in shape, tending to be flattened and squared off (Fig. 14.18). Early osteoarthritis is a common sequela.

## Cleidocranial Dysplasia

The cardinal features of cleidocranial dysplasia (cleidocranial dysostosis) are absence of a portion of the clavicles and poor ossification of the skull with wormian bones and hypoplastic paranasal and mastoid sinuses. Sometimes, there may be total absence of the clavicles (Fig. 14.19). Other dysplastic features may be present throughout the skeleton, including hypoplastic limb girdles, dysplastic long bones with narrow diaphyses and expanded ends, and spina bifida occulta at multiple levels. Cleidocranial dysplasia is an autosomal-dominant condition with high penetrance.

## Radioulnar Synostosis

Radioulnar synostosis is an anomaly of longitudinal segmentation in which the proximal radioulnar joint space fails to form (Fig. 14.20). It occurs both sporadically and familially and is bilateral in approximately 60% of cases. It may also be seen in a variety of other developmental syndromes and can be acquired from conditions such as infantile cortical hyperostosis or infection. Patients

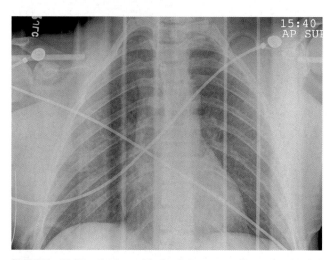

**FIGURE 14.19.** Cleidocranial dysplasia. AP Radiograph obtained because of trauma incidentally shows complete absence of both clavicles.

**FIGURE 14.21.** Bilateral proximal focal femoral deficiency.

**FIGURE 14.20.** Radioulnar synostosis.

have functional impairment of ability to pronate and supinate the forearm.

## Proximal Focal Femoral Deficiency

Proximal focal femoral deficiency is a spectrum of bony deficiencies of the proximal femur, ranging from shortening and varus deformity of the shaft to aplasia of the femoral head, neck, and proximal shaft. Dysplastic changes in the acetabulum correlate with the degree of femoral head deformity or hypoplasia. It is congenital but

not heritable; the cause is unknown. The condition can be bilateral (Fig. 14.21).

## Tibia Vara

Tibia vara (also called Blount disease) is a growth disorder of the medial portion of the proximal tibial growth plate that results in a varus deformity. The causes of tibia vara are thought to be multifactorial, but the end result appears to be an injury to the medial growth plate, slowing its growth, leading to the varus deformity from

**A**

**B**

**FIGURE 14.22.** Tibia vara. **A:** AP radiograph at age 3 years. **B:** AP radiograph at age 7 years.

**FIGURE 14.23.** Partial supernumerary digit between fourth and fifth rays.

continued normal growth on the lateral side of the growth plate. On radiographs, beaking, irregularity, and distortion of the metaphysis are seen along with the varus deformity at the growth plate (Fig. 14.22).

## Digital Anomalies

Anomalies of the fingers or toes may be sporadic or inherited and may be either isolated or associated with a congenital syndrome. Syndactyly is congenital fusion of two or more digits. The fusion

may be soft tissue or osseous tissue and either partial or complete. The most common situation is a soft-tissue web between two fingers. Polydactyly is the presence of supernumerary digits, either partial (Fig. 14.23) or complete (Fig. 14.24). Symphalangia is congenital fusion of one phalanx to another in the same digit, presumably from failure of the intervening joint to develop. Although other deformities of the appendage may be present, symphalangia is common in the small toes and generally has no significance. Hyperphalangia is the presence of extra phalanges in the longitudinal axis of a digit. It is seen almost exclusively as a triphalangeal thumb.

## Carpal Coalition

Carpal coalitions are relatively common anomalies in which two or more carpal bones fail to segment during development, resulting in a congenital fusion (Fig. 14.25). The fusion can be bony, cartilaginous, or fibrous. Carpal coalitions are usually isolated anomalies that involve bones of the same row. The most common coalition is between the lunate and triquetrum. These coalitions are often of no clinical significance, although some patients with carpal coalition may complain of pain.

## Tarsal Coalition

Tarsal coalition is an abnormal bony or fibrous articulation between two tarsal bones. The condition is congenital and appears to result from lack of segmentation rather than from fusion of a fully developed joint. Most coalitions are either between the calcaneus and the navicular or between the calcaneus and the talus. Talocalcaneal coalitions usually involve the middle facet. Coalitions are bilateral in approximately 20% of cases. Coalitions cause the foot to lose some of its normal mobility, leading to a painful flatfoot. The coalition may be fibrous, cartilaginous, or osseous. Typically, the coalition is cartilaginous but becomes ossified as the skeleton matures; with ossification come rigidity and the onset of symptoms. Special views

**FIGURE 14.24.** Polydactyly of the foot shown on T1-weighted MRI.

**FIGURE 14.25.** Carpal coalition (lunate and triquetrum).

**A**                                                                                                     **B**

**FIGURE 14.26.** Tarsal coalition. **A:** Lateral radiograph shows C-sign (*arrowheads*) of talocalcaneal coalition. **B:** Coronal CT reconstruction shows fusion of the middle subtalar facet (*arrow*).

and conventional tomography or CT may be necessary to identify the presence and precise site of coalition. An indirect sign of a coalition between the calcaneus and the talus is talar beaking. A talar beak is a bony spur from the anterior superior aspect of the talus consequent to limited subtalar motion, hypoplasia of the head of the talus, and dorsal subluxation of the navicular bone. A talar beak may occur in any condition that causes abnormal talonavicular motion. The C-sign may be evident on lateral views when a middle facet

coalition is present. The dome of the talus forms the top of the C, the coalition forms the middle, and the sustentaculum forms the bottom (Fig. 14.26). CT is an excellent method for identifying and characterizing tarsal coalitions. CT is most accurate when scanning or image reformations are obtained in axial, coronal, and sagittal planes (Fig. 14.27). MRI is also an excellent method for diagnosing tarsal coalitions (Fig. 14.28) and can demonstrate coalitions before they are ossified.

**FIGURE 14.27.** Tarsal coalition. Axial CT scan shows calcaneonavicular (*long arrow*) and middle subtalar facet (*short arrow*) coalitions.

**FIGURE 14.28.** Calcaneonavicular coalition (*arrow*) on sagittal T1-weighted MRI.

A                                          B

**FIGURE 14.29.** Os acromiale syndrome. T2 MRI shows bone marrow edema in the distal clavicle (*short arrow*) and in an os acromiale (long arrow). **A:** Axial; **B:** Sagittal.

## Muscle Anomalies

Muscle anatomy in the extremities is variable; sometimes accessory muscles or anomalous muscle attachments may become clinically important. Vascular or neurologic entrapment syndromes may be caused by anomalous muscle attachments at various locations, or by anomalous relationships between muscles and neurovascular structures. For example, an anomalous attachment of the gastrocnemius may result in entrapment of the popliteal artery, and an accessory anconeus may result in entrapment of the ulnar nerve. On MRI or CT, the abnormal anatomy may be demonstrated, and in the case of nerve entrapment, denervation atrophy may be seen in the innervated muscle groups.

Accessory muscles of the ankle are commonly seen on radiologic examinations. The most common anomalous muscle of the ankle seen on radiography is the accessory soleus muscle. Other accessory muscles that may be seen on ankle MRI include peroneus quartus, flexor digitorum accessorius longus, and peroneocalcaneus internus muscles. Correct identification of the accessory muscles of the ankle is based on their relationship to the flexor retinaculum and tarsal tunnel and their origin and insertion. Proper recognition of these muscles prevents misdiagnosis as a soft-tissue mass. Additionally, they can be a cause of neuropathy or ankle impingement or may serve as donor tendon in ankle surgery.

## Accessory Ossicles

The most common variations in skeletal anatomy are small extra bones in various locations, generally called accessory ossicles. Accessory ossicles may be distinguished from acute fracture fragments by their rounded shape and complete cortex without discontinuities. Many accessory ossicles are simply sesamoid bones, occurring where tendons cross over bony prominences. Other accessory ossicles may result from variations in skeletal maturation and ossification, and some ossicles may actually be the sequela of remote trauma, unfused fracture fragments, or heterotopic bone.

Accessory ossicles are sometimes associated with symptoms; for example, an os acromiale (accessory ossicle resulting from unfused ossification center of the acromial apophysis) may contribute to shoulder pain, or *os acromiale syndrome*. Radiographs show the presence of an os acomiale; MRI shows bone marrow edema within the os acromiale itself (Fig. 14.29).

In the presence of an os trigonum (accessory ossicle resulting from unfused ossification center of posterior talar process), extreme plantar flexion in activities such as ballet may cause compression and entrapment of the posterior ankle soft tissues between the posterior lip of the tibia and the calcaneus. This condition may be called posterior ankle impingement syndrome or *os trigonum syndrome*, although impingement may occur without the presence of an os trigonum. On imaging, radiographs may show the accessory ossicle, MRI may show edema involving the ossicle or surrounding soft tissues (Fig. 14.30), and radionuclide bone scan may show abnormal activity.

## ◼ LIMB LENGTH AND ROTATIONAL DISCREPANCY

Limb length discrepancy (also called anisomelia) is usually a clinical problem only in the lower limbs, where it may result in abnormal gait and scoliosis. Lower-limb length discrepancy is often the result of undergrowth of one limb due to trauma (especially trauma to the growth plate) or disease. Angular deformity of the limb also results in shortening. Overgrowth of a limb is common in hyperemic states such as those accompanying fractures or inflammatory bone or joint disease. The presence and amount of leg length discrepancy can be assessed by a scanogram.

**FIGURE 14.30.** Accessory ossicle with posterior ankle impingement syndrome. **A:** Sagittal T1-weighted MRI shows a large os trigonum (*arrow*). **B:** Sagittal T2-weighted fat suppressed MRI shows edema in the soft tissues (*arrow*) around the os trigonum and in the adjacent calcaneus.

The radiographic scanogram is a view of both ankles, knees, and hips taken in separate exposures with the X-ray tube centered at the level of the joints; a radiopaque measuring stick is radiographed with the limbs. This allows the length of each femur and tibia to be measured. The computed scanogram using CT is more precise than the radiographic scanogram because it eliminates the effects of magnification and geometric distortion inherent in stan-

dard radiographic techniques and allows precise measurements on the workstation. The usual landmarks for measurement in children are the top of the femoral head, the bottom of the medial femoral condyle, and the tibial plafond.

The normal femoral neck is anteverted (externally rotated) relative to the femoral condyles at the knee. The normal tibia has external torsion (external rotation) of the ankle mortise relative

**FIGURE 14.31.** Limb length and rotation evaluation by CT. **A:** Scanogram shows malunion of left femur fracture with locked IM rod. The right femur measures 1 cm longer than the left. **B:** Axial scans through the hips and knees allow measurement of femoral anteversion. There is 15 degrees of anteversion of the femoral neck on the right (normal) and 23 degrees of retroversion on the left (abnormal), resulting in a discrepancy of 38 degrees.

to the tibial condyles at the knee. Developmental or posttraumatic abnormalities in lower limb rotation may lead to problems with gait. The degree of femoral neck anteversion and tibial torsion may be measured by obtaining CT slices through the hips, knees, and ankles (Fig. 14.31). The right and left sides should be compared with each other, and the discrepancy should be reported.

# ■ HIP CONDITIONS

Three distinct chronic conditions of the hip occur in children; each affects a different age group (Table 14.1).

## Developmental Dysplasia of the Hip

In developmental dysplasia of the hip (DDH), an abnormally lax joint capsule allows the femoral head to fall out of the acetabulum shortly before or after birth, leading to congenital or postnatal deformation of an initially normal structure. The causes of this condition are multifactorial and appear to be related to the effects of restricted movement in the womb and of maternal hormones on the fetus. Restricted fetal movement during the third trimester resulting from conditions such as breech presentation or oligohydramnios may partially or completely dislocate the hip. The maternal hormones (e.g., estrogen) that relax the ligaments of the pelvis and facilitate childbirth also affect the fetus by increasing the laxity of the ligaments and joint capsules. This effect is particularly evident in female fetuses and may account for the 6:1 female preponderance of DDH. This condition has a familial tendency perhaps related to an inherited abnormality in estrogen metabolism.

Both the femoral head and the acetabulum must be present and articulating with each other for a normal hip to form. If contact is absent, adaptive changes occur in both structures. DDH is the result of abnormal mechanical stresses caused by abnormal position of the femoral head. If the hip dislocates, the pressure of the femoral head on the rapidly growing, pliable chondroosseous pelvis produces a false acetabulum (pseudoacetabulum). The native acetabulum becomes flattened and dish shaped—rather than cup shaped—and fills with fibrofatty debris. The earlier in life the dislocation occurs, the greater the adaptive abnormalities are. If the hip subluxates, the pressure of the femoral head against the acetabular labrum causes the labrum to deform. The labrum can become completely inverted into the acetabulum; in this situation, it is called a limbus. Remodeling of the ilium as growth proceeds in the presence of subluxation is seen radiographically as a shallow, steep acetabulum. A pseudoacetabulum may eventually form. The abnormal position of the femur may cause secondary changes in the capsule and iliopsoas mechanism. The longer the abnormal position persists, the more fixed the abnormalities become. If the femoral head can be relocated and held in the normal position, normal development can often be reestablished.

DDH is best diagnosed clinically in the neonatal period. The capsule and iliopsoas mechanism are lax enough for the hip to be easily dislocated and relocated; this is felt as a characteristic click or clunk by the examiner. Clinical examination becomes more difficult as the baby grows older because contractures and progressive deformity make it difficult to relocate a partially or completely dislocated hip.

Sonography is useful and has the advantage of immediate correlation with physical examination (Fig. 14.32). Most sonographers image the infant hip in the coronal plane, the so-called standard imaging plane of Graf. The key features to observe on this image are the location of the femoral head relative to the acetabulum, the shape of the femoral head (round), the size and ossification of the femoral head (Is one side lagging in development?), the bony acetabulum, and the coverage of the femoral head by the bony acetabulum. The bony acetabulum is assessed by measurement of the alpha angle, the angle between the lateral cortex of the ilium and the acetabular roof (60 degrees or greater is normal). The bony coverage of the femoral head is expressed as a percentage but can also be described by qualitative terms such as "good," "adequate," or "deficient."

In the neonate, radiographs in suspected DDH are unreliable because of the paucity of skeletal ossification. After 1 month of age, the AP radiograph becomes more reliable (Fig. 14.33). Each hip is divided into quadrants by drawing a horizontal baseline through the triradiate cartilages (Hilgenreiner horizontal line) and a perpendicular line through the most lateral ossified margin of the roof of the acetabulum (Perkins line) (Fig. 14.34). The normal location of the femoral head is in the lower inner quadrant (down and in). A dislocated femoral head is in the upper outer quadrant (up and out), and a subluxated femoral head is in the lower outer quadrant (down and out). The angle between the acetabulum and the horizontal baseline should be less than 40 degrees in a newborn, 33 degrees in a 6-month-old child, and 30 degrees in a 1-year-old child. In the normal hip, a smooth curve can be drawn along the inferior margin of the superior pubic ramus and the medial femoral cortex (Shenton line). Other findings include a shallow acetabulum, development of a false acetabulum, and delayed ossification of the involved capital femoral epiphysis. CT may be necessary to confirm anatomic relocation of the hips once the patient has been placed in a cast. MRI may be used to evaluate problematic cases (Fig. 14.35). The long-term sequela of untreated DDH is early degenerative arthritis.

## Legg-Calvé-Perthes Disease

Legg-Calvé-Perthes disease is idiopathic osteonecrosis of the capital femoral epiphysis in a skeletally immature child. Boys are affected more often than girls by a 4:1 ratio. The mean age of onset is 7 years, and the range is 2 to 13 years. In 20% of cases, the condition

| TABLE 14.1 | Pediatric Hip Disease | | |
|---|---|---|---|
| Disease | Peak Age of Diagnosis | Sex Predominance | Bilaterality (%) |
| DDH | Neonates | Girls (6:1) | 25 |
| Legg-Calvé-Perthes disease | 7 years | Boys (5:1) | 10–20 |
| SCFE | Girls 11 years, boys 14 years | Boys (2.5:1) | 20–35 |

**FIGURE 14.32.** Neonatal hip at 3 weeks of age (head to left, feet to right). **A, B:** Sonogram of the right hip is normal. The femoral head is normally located, and there is greater than 50% bony coverage of the head. The alpha angle was measured at 61 degrees. **C, D:** Sonogram of the left hip shows acetabular dysplasia. The femoral head is normally located, but there is only 33% bony coverage of the head. The alpha angle was measured at 50 degrees. *H,* femoral head; *A,* acetabular roof.

is bilateral. The bone age of affected children is usually 1 to 3 years behind their chronologic age. Interruption of the blood supply to the femoral head leads to partial or total osteonecrosis. Both enchondral ossification of the capital femoral epiphysis and activity at the growth plate stop. The articular cartilage, nourished by synovial fluid, continues to grow. If the disease is detected at this stage,

the ossific nucleus of the capital femoral epiphysis is smaller than normal, and overgrowth of the articular cartilage is apparent as joint space widening. The patient may be asymptomatic. Revascularization of the femoral head leads to centripetal ossification, usually from multiple sites that are not contiguous with the original ossific nucleus. This results in an appearance often described as fragmentation of

**FIGURE 14.33.** DDH in a 12-month-old infant. The right hip is dislocated; the left hip is normal. Note the short, steep acetabulum and delayed ossification of the right femoral head.

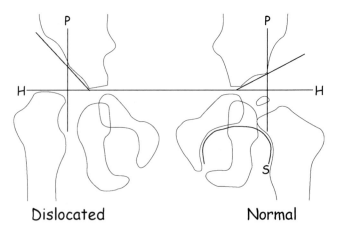

**FIGURE 14.34.** Radiologic diagnosis of DDH. *P*, Perkins line; *H*, Hilgenreiner horizontal line; *S*, Shenton line.

ossification. Apposition of new bone to the dead bone may increase the radiographic density of the head (Fig. 14.36). Resorption of subchondral bone may lead to subchondral fracture and the onset of clinical symptoms: hip pain and limp. MRI appears to be more sensitive in the detection of early changes of Legg-Calvé-Perthes disease. In addition to the morphologic changes that may be seen on radiographs, MRI may show marrow changes in the femoral head (Fig. 14.37). The severity of the clinical findings is highly variable and does not necessarily correlate with the radiographic findings. The end result is a short, thick femoral neck and an enlarged femoral head (coxa magna). Premature closure of the growth plate accentuates the deformity. Secondary osteoarthritis is a late complication.

The goal of therapy is to prevent the development of femoral head deformity and subsequent osteoarthritis. Centering of the femoral head within the acetabulum during the revascularization and reossification stages of healing presumably allows the acetabulum to act as a mold for the healing femoral head, averting the development of deformity. Acetabular coverage for the femoral head may be obtained by abduction of the femur relative to the acetabulum with a brace, varus osteotomy of the proximal femur, or osteotomy of the pelvis. Arthrography or MRI of the hip may be required to delineate the morphology of the unossified portion of the femoral head for surgical planning.

Osteonecrosis of the femoral head and other growing epiphyses may occur as a result of trauma or other disease. The pathophysiology and the gamut of radiologic findings are similar to those of Legg-Calvé-Perthes disease.

### Slipped Capital Femoral Epiphysis

A slipped capital femoral epiphysis (SCFE) is displacement of the femoral head relative to the femoral neck through the open growth plate in an adolescent. The head remains in the acetabulum as the neck progressively displaces anteriorly and superiorly (the head goes inferiorly and posteriorly). SCFE occurs in boys and girls of approximately the same skeletal age shortly before closure of the growth plate (chronologic age of approximately 11 years in girls and 14 years in boys). Boys are affected more often than girls by a ratio of 2.5:1.0. Many patients are overweight and have mildly delayed skeletal ages. Bilateral involvement is present in approximately half of the patients. The etiology is not known; the pathophysiology may be related to an endocrine process or a biomechanical problem. The slippage between the femoral head and neck occurs between the proliferative and hypertrophic zones of the growth cartilage. This

is different from a Salter type I fracture, which occurs between the hypertrophic and provisional calcification zones of the cartilage. SCFE may be a chronic, slow process that allows bony remodeling of both head and neck as the deformity progresses (Fig. 14.38), or it may be a relatively acute process (usually lasting <3 weeks), the presentation of which is like that of a stress fracture (Fig. 14.39). Mild cases may go undetected, but MRI appears to be more sensitive than radiographs for detecting SCFE. On MRI, abnormally increased signal within the region of the growth plate may be present on T2-weighted MRI (Fig. 14.40). SCFE is treated by stabilization of the head without attempt at anatomic reduction. Multiple pins fix the position of the head and promote closure of the growth plate. Dysplasia of the hip and early osteoarthritis may develop; osteonecrosis is a devastating complication that is more common in acute slips (see Fig. 14.39).

## ■ PREMATURE PHYSEAL CLOSURE

Premature closure of a growth plate results in an angular deformity if the closure is partial, and growth arrest if the closure is complete. Conditions that may cause premature closure include disuse, radiation, infection, tumor, vascular impairment, neural involvement, metabolic abnormality, frostbite, developmental,

**FIGURE 14.35.** MRI of DDH. Axial GRE MRI shows bilateral posterior dislocation of the femoral heads (*arrows*).

**FIGURE 14.36.** Legg-Calvé-Perthes disease of the right femoral head. **A:** At presentation, age 5 years, the right femoral head is large and misshapen. The femoral neck is short and broad. **B:** At age 6 years, the cartilaginous portion of the epiphysis is ossifying from multiple foci. **C:** At age 8 years, ossification of the epiphysis is complete; the head no longer fits into the acetabulum.

and iatrogenic. Disuse results in atrophy of muscle and other soft tissues and, if prolonged, of bone as well. Growth arrest lines are not uncommon (Fig. 14.41) and represent bone formation at the physis during a period of growth arrest. Rarely, the physis may close. Therapeutic radiation may inhibit or destroy physeal cartilage, resulting in closure; diagnostic radiation does not. Osteomyelitis involving the metaphysis may extend through the growth plate into the epiphysis, leading to closure. Benign tumors that involve the physis may lead to closure. Disruption of the epiphyseal blood supply may lead to closure. Neuromuscular conditions such as poliomyelitis, cerebral palsy, and congenital insensitivity to pain are associated with premature physeal closure; the mechanism is unknown. Metabolic abnormalities, including vitamin A toxicity and scurvy, may be associated with premature physeal closure. Cold injury may result in premature physeal closure, especially in the phalanges, from either direct injury to the chondrocytes or ischemic vascular changes. Surgery involving the growth plate may result in closure, including the placement of pins for fracture stabilization, curettage for nearby tumors, and debridement for infection. Immunosuppressive drugs may cause premature closure.

On radiographs, the growth plate is initially normal at the time of injury and only becomes abnormal in appearance as premature closure proceeds. If the closure involves the entire growth plate, then the growth plate disappears and the bone begins to remodel, leaving a short bone. If the closure is partial and asymmetric, continued growth in the open portion of the physis may lead to a progressive angular deformity as well as a short bone (Fig. 14.42). If the closure is partial and central, a coned epiphysis develops (Fig. 14.43).

# ■ OSTEOCHONDROSES

The osteochondroses are a varied group of acquired, localized conditions of childhood in which a disease process is superimposed on the growth process. Grouped together initially because

**FIGURE 14.37.** Legg-Calvé-Perthes disease. Coronal T1-weighted MRI shows abnormal signal and collapse of the right femoral epiphysis (*arrow*).

**FIGURE 14.38.** Chronic SCFE. **A:** AP radiograph shows abnormal left proximal femur. **B:** Frog-leg lateral radiograph.

**A**          **B**

**FIGURE 14.39.** SCFE in a 12-year-old male. **A:** Acute slip at presentation. **B:** Osteonecrosis with collapse of the femoral head, 6 months after the slip was reduced and fixed with pins.

of their radiographic appearance, these lesions are characterized by fragmentation and sclerosis of an epiphyseal or apophyseal ossification center in a child. These conditions have been described in a wide variety of locations, and most sites have eponyms associated with them. The eponyms in common usage are listed in Table 14.2. Avascular necrosis of the growing epiphysis is thought to be the predominant pathophysiology, and the underlying cause is thought to be repetitive microtrauma at a site with a tenuous blood supply. Fragmentation and collapse are followed by reossification as the blood supply is reestablished. On radiographs, the ossification center of the apophysis or epiphysis becomes dense and undergoes fragmentation, then reossification. Dysplastic change in the shape of the bone sometimes occurs, although it may

reconstitute itself. This process can be difficult to distinguish from the normal developmental variation in ossification of epiphyses and apophyses. The presence of pain in the appropriate age group and at the appropriate location should be established before making the diagnosis. Because healing is spontaneous in most cases, treatment is management of symptoms and modification of the aggravating activity.

**FIGURE 14.40.** Slipped capital femoral epiphysis. Coronal T2-weighted fat-suppressed MRI demonstrates slippage of the epiphysis on the left with increased signal (*arrow*) at the femoral growth plate.

**FIGURE 14.41.** Growth arrest lines. Ankle radiograph three months after surgery for proximal tibial osteomyelitis shows a growth arrest line (*arrow*) parallel to the distal tibial physis.

**FIGURE 14.42.** Premature closure of the growth plate following osteomyelitis. A well-developed bridge of bone (*arrow*) traverses the central portion of the physis.

## Osteochondritis Dissecans (Knee)

Osteochondritis dissecans is an osteochondrosis involving the knee, typically the non–weight-bearing lateral aspect of the medial femoral condyle in adolescents. (Osteochondrosis of the talar dome—

**FIGURE 14.43.** Multiple finger amputations and coned epiphyses in the hand from meningococcemia in infancy.

| TABLE 14.2 | Common Osteochondroses |
|---|---|
| Legg-Calvé-Perthes disease | Capital femoral epiphysis |
| Köhler disease | Tarsal navicular |
| Kienbock disease | Lunate |
| Osgood-Schlatter disease | Tibial tuberosity |
| Scheuermann disease | Vertebral ring apophyses |
| Freiberg infraction | Metatarsal head |
| Osteochondritis dissecans | Medial femoral condyle |
| Osteochondritis dissecans | Talar dome |
| Panner disease | Capitellum |
| Sever disease | Calcaneal apophysis |

a different condition—may also be called osteochondritis dissecans.) There is a male predominance of 3:1. The mechanism of injury is thought to be repetitive trauma transmitted to the subchondral bone through the articular cartilage that results in osteonecrosis and healing. The articular cartilage may be intact over the surface of the lesion, but if it is not, the fragment may become a loose body within the joint. On radiographs, osteochondritis dissecans may be recognized by the presence of a sclerotic lesion in the subchondral bone at the lateral surface of the medial femoral condyle (Fig. 14.44). If the osteochondral fragment has become displaced, a defect in the subchondral bone is seen. Depending on the severity of the lesion, MRI may show abnormal signal in the articular cartilage, abnormal signal in the marrow, or both. If a well-defined fragment is present, MRI may demonstrate whether the overlying cartilage is intact. Fluid signal surrounding the fragment on T2-weighted images indicates that it has become detached, although not necessarily displaced. In addition to the medial femoral condyle, other portions of the knee may be involved, including the lateral femoral condyle and the patella. Multiple sites may be involved in the same knee, and bilateral disease may be present in up to 25% of cases.

## Panner Disease (Capitellum)

Panner disease is osteochondrosis of the capitellum. Repetitive trauma is often the result of participation in throwing sports, such as baseball pitching. On radiographs, the condition is manifest by focal sclerosis and collapse in the capitellar ossification center (Fig. 14.45).

## Osgood-Schlatter Disease (Tibial Tubercle)

Osgood-Schlatter disease is osteochondrosis of the tibial tubercle from repetitive microtrauma, commonly the result of participation in jumping sports such as basketball. On radiographs, there is separation of small bone fragments from the developing ossification of the tibial tuberosity, with overlying soft-tissue swelling. After the acute stage, the soft-tissue swelling subsides and the fragments may remodel and coalesce to form a normal tibial tubercle, or ossific fragments may persist at the site.

## Sinding-Larsen-Johansson Disease (Patella)

Sinding-Larsen-Johansson disease is osteochondrosis of the distal pole of the patella that is similar to Osgood-Schlatter disease in that it also is thought to result from repetitive microtrauma, such as jumping sports. It is sometimes called jumper's knee and has

A

B

**FIGURE 14.44.** Osteochondritis dissecans. **A:** Knee radiograph shows lesion at the lateral aspect of the medial femoral condyle (*arrow*). **B:** Coronal T1-weighted MRI shows the lesion (*arrow*).

similar radiographic features, except that they occur at the inferior pole of the patella where the infrapatellar tendon attaches.

## Köhler Disease (Tarsal Navicular)

Köhler disease is osteochondrosis of the tarsal navicular. It occurs in boys between 3 and 5 years of age and in girls between 2 and 4 years of age. Radiographs show collapse and increased density of

the ossification center of the tarsal navicular, followed by patchy deossification and reossification. Localized inflammation, tenderness, and limpness characterize the clinical presentation. After reconstitution, sclerosis, dysplasia, and fragmentation of the tarsal navicular may persist (Fig. 14.46) and secondary degenerative changes may follow.

## Freiberg Infraction (Metatarsal Head)

Freiberg infraction is osteochondrosis of the metatarsal head, usually the second metatarsal. The condition most commonly affects adolescent girls. After reconstitution, residual overgrowth and articular irregularity may lead to secondary osteoarthritis (Fig. 14.47).

## ■ CONGENITAL FOOT DEFORMITIES

Most clinically evident deformities of the foot in the infant and child are flexible and mild and correct with growth or cause little or no handicap in adult life. The diagnosis of congenital foot deformities is accomplished principally by radiographs. Lateral and AP views should be obtained while weight bearing or, in the case of infants, with dorsiflexion stress simulating weight bearing. The hindfoot is comprised of the talus and calcaneus. In the normal foot, until approximately 2 years of age, the long axis of the talus and the long axis of the calcaneus form an angle (talocalcaneal angle) that is approximately 40 degrees on both lateral and AP radiographs (Fig. 14.48). If one considers the talus to be fixed in the ankle mortise, then abnormal varus (medial) alignment of the calcaneus relative to the talus reduces the talocalcaneal angle in the AP projection, and abnormal valgus (lateral) alignment increases it. Because of the geometric and ligamentous linkage between the talus and the calcaneus, changes in the talocalcaneal angles are approximately equal on both AP and lateral radiographs. Thus, on

**FIGURE 14.45.** Osteochondrosis of the capitellum (Panner disease) (*arrow*).

A

B

**FIGURE 14.46.** Residual features of Köhler disease in a teenager. **A:** Lateral radiograph shows sclerosis and dysplasia of the navicular (*arrow*). **B:** Coronal CT reformation shows sclerosis and fragmentation of the navicular.

AP and lateral radiographs, a small talocalcaneal angle (close to parallel, approximately 10 degrees or less) is called hindfoot varus, and a large talocalcaneal angle (approximately 70 degrees or more) is called hindfoot valgus. On AP radiographs, the first metatarsal should be aligned with the talus, and the fourth or fifth metatarsal should be aligned with the calcaneus. On lateral radiographs, the first metatarsal should be aligned with the talus. If the first metatarsal is angled plantar relative to the talus, the plantar arch is elevated

and the deformity is called a cavus arch or cavus foot. If the first metatarsal is angled dorsally relative to the talus, the plantar arch is flattened and the deformity is called pes planus or flatfoot. There is a wide range of normal variation in the alignment of the bones of the foot, and actually drawing and measuring any of these angles may give a misleading sense of accuracy and precision.

## Talipes Equinovarus

Talipes equinovarus, or congenital clubfoot, is a common abnormality with an incidence of 1 per 1,000 live births. The condition is bilateral in approximately half the cases and is three times more common in boys than in girls. When unilateral, it is usually the left foot that is abnormal. The deformity is believed to be caused by a combination of intrauterine and genetic factors. Clubfoot may also occur in association with arthrogryposis or meningomyelocele. The key radiologic finding is hindfoot varus (decreased talocalcaneal angle) combined with medial deviation and inversion of the forefoot (Fig. 14.49). The plantar arch is elevated. Clubfoot may be treated by serial manipulation and casting or by surgical release of the soft tissues and realignment of the foot.

## Metatarsus Adductus

Metatarsus adductus refers to a group of related foot deformities that produce incurvation of the forefoot. The incidence is approximately 1 per 1,000 live births. The most common of these is simple medial deviation of the forefoot relative to the hindfoot, without hindfoot abnormality. Less common varieties include inversion of the forefoot or combinations of medial deviation, inversion, and hindfoot valgus. Most cases are mild, supple deformities that resolve spontaneously; severe deformities may be rigid and require treatment. The condition is bilateral in 50% of cases.

**FIGURE 14.47.** Freiberg infraction of the second metatarsal head.

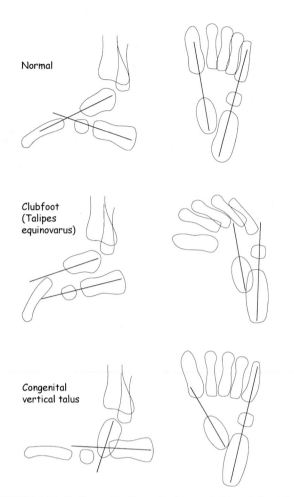

**FIGURE 14.48.** Radiographic diagnosis of congenital foot deformities.

## Congenital Vertical Talus

Congenital vertical talus is an unusual deformity characterized by hindfoot valgus (increased talocalcaneal angle) and dorsal dislocation of the navicular on the talus (Fig. 14.50). The plantar arch is flattened, and in severe cases, a rocker-bottom deformity (convex plantar surface of the foot) may result. Congenital vertical talus may occur in isolation or in association with neurofibromatosis, arthrogryposis, meningomyelocele, and other central nervous system and genetic syndromes.

## ■ SPINE CONDITIONS

### Idiopathic Scoliosis

Scoliosis is lateral spinal curvature in the coronal plane. By convention, it is named for the side that is convex so that right scoliosis is convex to the right. Known causes of scoliosis include congenital architectural imbalance; growth asymmetry; neoplastic, traumatic, or infectious damage; therapeutic irradiation; bone dysplasia; asymmetric neuromuscular control; leg length discrepancy; and reflexive splinting due to pain or nerve irritation. Approximately 85% to 90% of scoliosis cases are idiopathic. Idiopathic scoliosis is thought to have a genetic basis. In the United States, idiopathic scoliosis is usually found in children between 11 and 14 years of age during mandatory visual screening in schools. The prevalence of scoliosis is related to the severity of the curve (Table 14.3). Girls are much more likely to have severe or progressive curves. The classic curve is a painless, S-shaped curve that is convex to the right in the thoracic

A

B

**FIGURE 14.49.** Talipes equinovarus. **A, B:** Lateral and AP radiographs show a narrow talocalcaneal angle (*arrow* indicates talus).

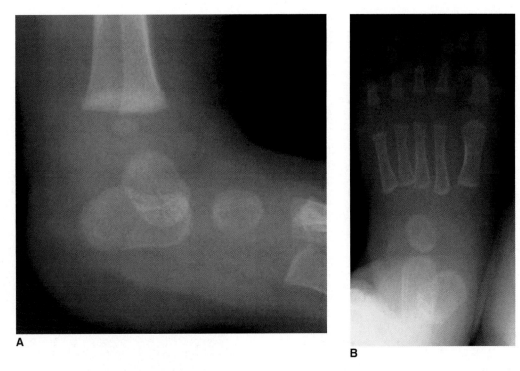

**FIGURE 14.50.** Congenital vertical talus. **A:** Lateral radiograph. **B:** AP radiograph.

region between T5 and T12 (Fig. 14.51). In addition to the more obvious abnormality of alignment of the entire spine in which the relations between vertebrae are abnormal, each individual vertebra in the region of the curves has an abnormal shape. A painful curve raises suspicion of an underlying lesion. Radiography is used to confirm the presence of scoliosis, to document its magnitude and extent, and to detect or exclude congenital or other abnormalities. Radiographs are made with the patient standing without shoes and should include the entire spine on a single long (3-ft) film; spot films and additional imaging modalities are used as needed. The standard of measurement is the Cobb method, but the variability of the method is 5 to 10 degrees. It is important to protect the breasts from radiation, particularly in girls, because the average patient followed for idiopathic scoliosis will have many examinations. Severe curves in the thoracic region interfere with the mechanics of respiration. The primary goal of treatment is the ultimate preservation of lung function. Scoliotic curves of 20 degrees or less are usually not treated. Modalities of treatment include rigid braces, electrical stimulation, and spinal fusion (see Chapter 17 for methods of surgical fusion).

| TABLE 14.3 | Prevalence of Idiopathic Scoliosis in the United States |
| --- | --- |
| Magnitude of Curve | Prevalence |
| ≥10 degrees | 25 per 1,000 |
| ≥20 degrees | 5 per 1,000 |
| ≥30 degrees | 1.5 per 1,000 |

***Source:*** Data from Kane WJ. Scoliosis prevalence: A call for a statement of terms. *Clin Orthop.* 1977;126:43–46.

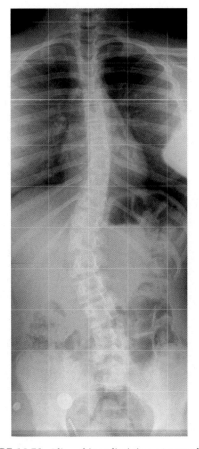

**FIGURE 14.51.** Idiopathic scoliosis in a 14-year-old girl.

**FIGURE 14.52.** Congenital scoliosis with multiple vertebral anomalies.

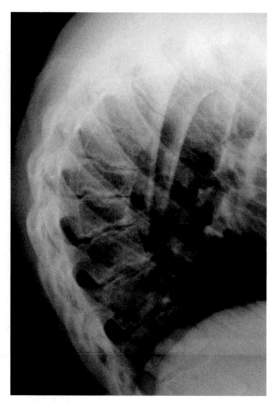

**FIGURE 14.54.** Scheuermann disease (juvenile kyphosis).

**FIGURE 14.53.** Vertebral anomalies in a 3-year-old girl with hemivertebrae (*arrowheads*) and a trapezoidal vertebra (*arrow*).

## Congenital Scoliosis

The obvious causes of congenital scoliosis relate to failure of normal formation of individual vertebrae. During the embryonic conversion of mesenchymal vertebrae to cartilaginous vertebrae before week 9 of development, each vertebral body becomes chondrified from two centers of chondrification on either side of the midline. If chondrification fails on only one side, an isolated hemivertebra results. If the centers of chondrification do not fuse at the same level (as they should) but fuse across levels instead, a trapezoidal vertebra results (Figs. 14.52 and 14.53). Each side of the neural arch also has its own center of chondrification, and similar failures of development or abnormal fusion result in anomalies. The most common vertebral anomalies causing congenital scoliosis include hemivertebrae, trapezoidal vertebrae, and unilateral neural arch fusions. Combinations of anomalies and multilevel involvement are frequent. Congenital scoliosis may also result from differences in growth potential between vertebrae and from congenital neurologic conditions that result in neuromuscular imbalance.

## Juvenile Kyphosis

Juvenile kyphosis is a term that is used to describe thoracic kyphosis exceeding 40 degrees in adolescents, as measured from the superior end plate of T3 or T4 to the inferior end plate of T12. Most cases are considered postural kyphosis and may simply represent the extremes of normal variation. Kyphosis is the only clinical and radiographic finding. Scheuermann disease (juvenile thoracic kyphosis) is diagnosed on radiographs by decreased disk space heights, increased AP diameter of the involved vertebral bodies, and irregularity of the end plates (Fig. 14.54). Anterior wedging of at least 5 degrees typically involves three or more consecutive vertebrae. The process is thought to result from fissures developing in the cartilaginous vertebral end plates through which material from the nucleus pulposus herniates. Fibrosis and reactive sclerosis outline these pockets (individually called Schmorl nodes). The loss of disk material results in kyphosis. Increased stress on the anterior portion of the vertebral bodies results in growth abnormality, leading to the wedge shape and the increased AP dimension. These are not compression fractures. An alternative explanation for Scheuermann disease is that the condition is an osteochondrosis of the vertebral ring apophyses.

## SOURCES AND READINGS

Davis LA, Hatt WS. Congenital abnormalities of the foot. *Radiology.* 1955;64:818–825.

Del Fattore A, Cappariello A, Teti A. Genetics, pathogenesis and complications of osteopetrosis. *Bone.* 2008;42(1):19–29. Epub 2007 Aug 30.

eMedicine. http://emedicine.medscape.com.

Freyschmidt J, Brossmann J, Weins J, Sternberg A. *Freyschmidt's "Köhler/Zimmer" Borderlands of Normal and Early Pathological Findings in Skeletal Radiography.* 5th Ed. Stuttgart: Thieme Medical Publishers; 2003.

Gilmore A, Thompson GH. Radiographic evaluation of children and adolescents with a spinal deformity. *Sem Musculoskelet Radiol.* 2000;4:349–359.

Greulich WW, Pyle SI. *Radiographic Atlas of Skeletal Development of the Hand and Wrist.* 2nd Ed. Stanford: Stanford University Press; 1959.

Harty MP, Hubbard AM. MR imaging of pediatric abnormalities in the ankle and foot. *Magn Reson Imaging Clin N Am.* 2001;9:579–602.

Hoerr NL, Pyle SI, Francis CC. *Radiographic Atlas of Skeletal Development of the Foot and Ankle. A Standard of Reference.* Springfield, IL: Charles C Thomas; 1962.

Jones KL, Smith DW, Fletcher J, eds. *Smith's Recognizable Patterns of Human Malformation.* Philadelphia, PA: WB Saunders; 1996.

Keats TE, Anderson MW. *Atlas of Normal Roentgen Variants that May Simulate Disease.* 8th Ed. Philadelphia, PA: Elsevier Health Sciences; 2006.

Kozlowski K, Beighton P. *Gamut Index of Skeletal Dysplasias: An Aid to Radiodiagnosis.* 3rd Ed. New York, NY: Springer-Verlag New York; 2001.

Lachman RS. *Taybi and Lachman's Radiology of Syndromes, Metabolic Disorders and Skeletal Dysplasias.* 5th Ed. Philadelphia, PA: Elsevier Health Sciences; 2006.

Loder RT, Aronsson DD, Weinstein SL, Breur GJ, Ganz R, Leunig M. Slipped capital femoral epiphysis. *Instr Course Lect.* 2008;57:473–98.

Lohman M, Kivisaari A, Vehmas T, et al. MRI in the assessment of growth arrest. *Pediatr Radiol.* 2002;32:41–45.

Lovell WW, Weinstein SL, Morrissy BT. *Lovell and Winter's Pediatric Orthopaedics.* 6th Ed. Philadelphia, PA: Lippincott Williams & Wilkins; 2005.

McAlister WH, Shackelford GD. Measurement of spinal curvatures. *Radiol Clin North Am.* 1975;13:113–121.

Oestreich AE. *Growth of the Pediatric Skeleton: A Primer for Radiologists.* New York, NY: Springer-Verlag; 2007.

Offiah AC, Hall CM. Radiological diagnosis of the constitutional disorders of bone. As easy as A, B, C? *Pediatr Radiolol.* 2003;33(3):153–161.

Pyle ST, Hoerr NL. *Radiographic Atlas of Skeletal Development of the Knee.* Springfield, IL: Charles C Thomas Publisher; 1955.

Royce PM, Steinmann B. *Connective Tissue and Its Heritable Disorders: Molecular, Genetic, and Medical Aspects.* New York, NY: Wiley-Liss; 2002.

Shapiro F. Epiphyseal disorders. *N Engl J Med.* 1987;317:1702–1710.

Slovis TL. *Caffey's Pediatric Diagnostic Imaging.* 11th Ed. Philadelphia, PA: Elsevier Health Sciences; 2007.

Staheli LT. Fundamentals of Pediatric Orthopedics. 4th Ed. Philadelphia, PA: Lippincott Williams & Wilkins; 2007.

Storer SK, Skaggs DL. Pearls and pitfalls in the evaluation of pediatric congenital and developmental disorders. *Instr Course Lect.* 2006;55:615–623.

Wheelees CR III, ed. *Wheeless' Textbook of Orthopaedics.* http://www.wheelessonline.com.

his chapter describes the radiology of many systemic, metabolic, and endocrine conditions that have bone or soft-tissue manifestations.

## OSTEOPOROSIS

Osteoporosis is the most common metabolic bone disease. Osteoporosis is characterized by generalized loss of mass from an otherwise normal bone. This loss of bone substance results in microarchitectural deterioration of the trabecular structure, increased bone fragility, and increased risk of fracture. Osteoporosis may be considered to be primary or secondary. Primary osteoporosis, also called *involutional osteoporosis*, is idiopathic in etiology. Secondary osteoporosis has a known, underlying etiology.

### Primary Osteoporosis (Involutional Osteoporosis)

More than 95% of adults with osteoporosis have involutional osteoporosis (also called *idiopathic* or *primary osteoporosis*). There are two main clinical types: (a) postmenopausal and (b) senile or age related. Postmenpausal osteoporosis is characterized by accelerated bone loss, mainly trabecular, and is caused by factors related to menopause. Age-related osteoporosis is characterized by slowly progressive bone loss, mainly cortical, and is caused by factors related to aging. The pathogenesis of osteoporosis is incompletely understood; it seems to involve not only excessive bone resorption but also impaired bone formation. Deteriorating bone strength results in increased vulnerability to traumatic and fatigue fractures. Most fractures of the spine, proximal femur, and distal radius in adults older than 50 years of age are associated with osteoporosis (see Chapter 1). In postmenopausal osteoporosis, vertebral crush fractures and distal radius fractures are the most common; in age-related osteoporosis, multiple vertebral wedge fractures and hip fractures are the most common. Fractures and the resulting loss of function are the major cause of morbidity and mortality in osteoporosis.

The prevalence of involutional osteoporosis in the United States is estimated at 28 million, or approximately 10% of the entire population. Risk factors for developing involutional osteoporosis include advancing age; female gender; white or Asian race; family history; thin, small bones; menopause; low dietary calcium; low dietary vitamin D; excessive alcohol, caffeine, and salt; smoking; and sedentary lifestyle. As the proportion and absolute numbers of the population in the United States older than 50 years of age increase, the prevalence of involutional osteoporosis may be expected to increase substantially.

The radiographic hallmark of osteoporosis is osteopenia, the increased radiolucency of bone. Osteopenia may not be recognizable on plain films until 30% to 50% of the bone mineral has been lost. A coarsened trabecular pattern results from the loss of smaller trabeculae, making the remaining ones more prominent. Linear, bandlike, or spotty radiolucent areas may also be seen. Cortical thinning can be a generalized, uniform, slowly progressive process (Fig. 15.1). Cortical bone loss may also be manifested by scalloped, endosteal erosions, intracortical radiolucent areas or striations (intracortical tunneling), or subperiosteal erosions. Vertebral deformities are related to insufficiency fractures of the end plates. These can have the form of biconcave depressions of contiguous superior and inferior end plates (so-called fish or codfish vertebrae, named for their resemblance to vertebrae in codfish), anterior wedge fractures, crush fractures of entire vertebral bodies, and increased thoracic kyphosis (dowager hump) (Figs. 15.2 and 15.3). The net result is progressive loss of stature.

### Bone Mineral Densitometry

Bone mineral densitometry (BMD) is the best noninvasive method for the diagnosis of osteoporosis in asymptomatic patients. BMD can also be used to estimate the risk of fracture and monitor patients receiving therapy for osteoporosis. The availability of effective therapies for osteoporosis—including estrogen, bisphosphonates, and other pharmacologic agents—has increased the usefulness of screening patients with various risk factors. The absolute

**FIGURE 15.1.** Osteoporosis of the hip with thin cortex and loss of trabecular bone in the neck.

**FIGURE 15.3.** Osteoporosis with multiple anterior wedge fractures in the thoracic spine.

amount of bone mineral is predictive of fracture risk. Radiographic measurement of BMD accurately and precisely assesses bone mineral content. Dual-photon absorptiometry (DPA) and dual-energy X-ray absorptiometry (DXA) use a dual-energy radionuclide and

**FIGURE 15.2.** Osteoporosis in the spine with central endplate depressions of the vertebral bodies at multiple levels.

X-ray source, respectively, to measure the bone density of the lumbar spine or hip. DPA and DXA measure the absorption of photons by the bone and provide a combined measurement of cortical and trabecular bone density. Quantitative CT measures the trabecular bone density in lumbar vertebral bodies by comparing the CT numbers of trabecular bone with the CT numbers of standardized solutions of calcium suspensions. Quantitative ultrasound measures the sound conduction in bone as a correlate of BMD. Broadband ultrasound attenuation has also been correlated with BMD as another method of quantitative ultrasound. Measures of BMD can be compared to populations matched for age, sex, and race to establish criteria for normality and abnormality. The relative risk of an osteoporotic fracture can also be estimated for various levels of BMD by comparing the incidence of fractures in large populations with BMD measurements. Because cortical and trabecular bone may not be involved to the same extent, methods that measure one or the other, or both, may not yield identical results.

DXA works on the physical principle that bone mineral (predominantly calcium) and soft tissue (predominantly fat and water) attenuate X-rays of high and low energy to different degrees. By measuring the differential absorption of X-rays of high and low energy, the absorption due to bone mineral alone can be determined, and from that, the absolute amount of bone mineral in the path of the X-rays can be calculated. Measuring the BMD at the spine and proximal femur (central measurement) is considered more useful clinically than measuring the BMD in the extremities (peripheral measurement). DXA provides measurements that reflect the BMD of trabecular and cortical bones together.

Clinical interpretation of the results of DXA is based on population statistics. An individual's BMD measurement from DXA

| TABLE 15.1 | WHO Diagnostic Criteria for Involutional Osteoporosis |
| --- | --- |
| Diagnosis | T-score |
| Normal | −1.0 or higher |
| Osteopenia | <−1.0 but >−2.5 |
| Osteoporosis | <−2.5 but without fractures |
| Established osteoporosis | <−2.5 with fractures |

The T-score is the number of standard deviations from the mean relative to a normal young adult population.

is compared with those of normal populations. The consensus criteria used for clinical diagnosis are those of the World Health Organization (WHO) (Table 15.1). According to WHO criteria, an individual's BMD is compared with those of a population of normal, young adults to derive a "T-score." The T-score is related to the number of standard deviations from the young, normal population mean the individual's measurement falls, so that a T-score of −2.0 would be 2 standard deviations below the mean of the young, normal population. Particular levels of bone mineral have been established as corresponding to the disease. A T-score of less than −1.0 but greater than −2.5 corresponds to a diagnosis of *osteopenia*. A T-score of less than −2.5 corresponds to a diagnosis of *osteoporosis*. If fractures are present in a patient with a T-score of less than −2.5, the diagnosis is *established osteoporosis*. The comparison of an individual's BMD to an age-matched population (the Z-score) is not used in WHO criteria. There is significant controversy regarding the particular normal, young adult populations on whom the T-scores are based with regard to sample size, gender, and race. The use of the terms *osteopenia* and *osteoporosis* may also lead to

**FIGURE 15.4.** DXA of the lumbar spine showing osteoporosis. **A:** Image shows regions of interest. **B:** Graphic shows bone mineral density relative to young-adult and age-matched reference populations. The T-score was −3.3, diagnostic of osteoporosis.

**FIGURE 15.5.** DXA of the hips showing osteopenia. **A:** Image shows regions of interest. **B:** Graphic shows bone mineral density relative to young-adult and age-matched reference populations. The T-score on the right was −2.0, and the T-score on the left was −2.2, both diagnostic of osteopenia.

**FIGURE 15.6.** DXA artifacts. **A:** Degenerative spine disease with endplate sclerosis and osteophytosis. **B:** Compression fracture at L1 and degenerative changes at L4. **C:** Laminectomy and posterolateral fusion at L4. **D:** Lumbar spine fusion with hardware.

confusion unless the context is clear; when these terms are used in conjunction with DXA, they should only refer to diagnoses according to WHO criteria.

In current practice, the DXA diagnosis of osteopenia and osteoporosis is based on BMD measurements of the lumbar spine and the proximal femur. In the spine, the frontal projection is used, and, ideally, an average of L1 through L4 is used to obtain the T-score (Fig. 15.4). If it is not possible to use L1 through L4, any two or three consecutive L1 through L4 vertebrae can be used. Use of a single vertebra is considered unreliable. In the hip, a region of the femoral neck is used (Fig. 15.5). The DXA report should include, as a minimum, a description of the basis of the measurement, the T-score, the relative fracture risk associated with the T-score, and the diagnosis according to WHO criteria.

Because DXA is a projection technique that measures the sum of the bone mineral between the X-ray source and the detector, disease or postsurgical conditions that increase or decrease the attenuation of the X-rays may compromise accuracy (Fig. 15.6). The most common condition leading to spurious BMD measurements (Table 15.2) is degenerative spine disease, in which sclerosis and osteophytes increase the BMD measurement. Similarly, diffuse idiopathic skeletal hyperostosis (DISH) may increase the BMD measurement. Other common conditions that affect DXA measurements include compression fractures, laminectomy, metal artifacts and bone graft from spine fusion, focal sclerotic lesions such as blastic metastases or Paget disease, and focal lytic lesions such as lytic metastases or multiple myeloma. Similar conditions may affect DXA measurements of BMD at the hip.

**TABLE 15.2**   **Common Potential Causes of Spurious BMD Measurements in the Spine**

Spuriously increased BMD measurement
  DJD
  DISH
  Spinal fusion
  Orthopedic hardware
  Compression fracture
  Blastic metastases
  Paget disease
Spuriously decreased BMD measurement
  Laminectomy
  Lytic metastases
  Multiple myeloma

## Secondary Osteoporosis

Secondary osteoporosis is the loss of bone mass from an otherwise normal bone as a result of a known cause. Secondary osteoporosis may manifest acutely or chronically, in a regional or systemic distribution. DXA and other methods for determining BMD may be applied to patients with chronic, systemic, secondary osteoporosis. DXA may be used to establish the diagnosis and to follow therapy. Common causes of secondary osteoporosis are listed in Table 15.3. More detailed descriptions of these conditions may be found in the appropriate portions of this book.

**TABLE 15.3**   **Some Causes of Secondary Osteoporosis in Adults**

Inherited
  Osteogenesis imperfecta
  Homocystinuria
  Marfan syndrome
Nutritional
  Malabsorption syndromes
  Chronic liver disease
  Alcoholism
  Calcium deficiency
Endocrine
  Hypogonadism
  Thyrotoxicosis
  Hypercortisolism
  Hyperparathyroidism
Drugs
  Corticosteroids
  Phenobarbital
  Synthroid
  Dilantin
Others
  Multiple myeloma
  Rheumatoid arthritis
  Acromegaly
  Mastocytosis

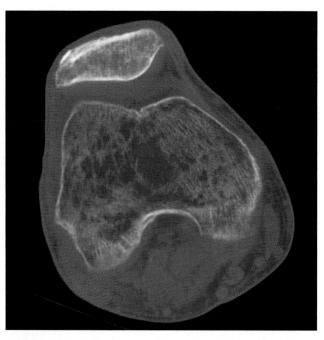

**FIGURE 15.7.** Acute osteoporosis, associated with a healing femoral shaft fracture, demonstrated on CT scan.

## Acute, Transient, Regional, and Migratory Osteoporosis

Acute osteoporosis accompanies fracture healing as a normal physiologic response to hyperemia. It may also accompany immobilization and disuse, both common features of healing fractures, as well as conditions such as reflex sympathetic dystrophy (also called *complex regional pain syndrome*). On radiographs, acute osteoporosis may be recognized in cancellous bone by subcortical resorption of trabeculae, resulting in subcortical lucency that parallels the cortical surface. On CT, the bone resorption tends to appear patchier (Fig. 15.7).

Transient regional osteoporosis typically presents with monoarticular joint symptoms. It is characterized by a rapidly developing osteoporosis affecting periarticular bone that is self-limited and reversible and has no definite inciting event. There are two clinical syndromes that occur in adults, both more common in men. The first clinical syndrome is transient osteoporosis of the hip. This presents with the rapid onset of severe hip pain without a precipitating event. It is usually unilateral, involving either the right or the left hip in men or usually the left hip in women. The pain is self-limited but aggravated by activity and regresses in 2 to 6 months without permanent sequelae. Imaging may show a rapidly developing periarticular osteoporosis, particularly in the femoral head, that returns to normal after the resolution of symptoms. MRI shows diffuse edema and hip effusion but no infarction. Bone scans show increased activity consistent with osteoporosis. The condition is thought to have a neurogenic origin, possibly related to reflex sympathetic dystrophy. The second clinical syndrome is regional migratory osteoporosis (Fig. 15.8). This usually involves the lower extremities of adults. Local pain and swelling develop rapidly, last up to 9 months, and then disappear only to be followed by the involvement of other regions months to years later. Within weeks of the onset of each episode, periarticular osteoporosis is evident. This condition may begin as transient osteoporosis of the hip.

**FIGURE 15.8.** Transient osteoporosis of the hip. Coronal T2-weighted MRI with fat suppression shows amorphous bone marrow edema (*arrow*) in the right proximal femur.

# ◼ DISEASES OF MINERAL METABOLISM

The skeleton is a metabolically active reservoir of calcium and phosphorus in the extracellular space. These minerals are maintained in tiny hydroxyapatite crystals that have in aggregate a vast surface area and are rapidly and freely exchanged into the extracellular fluid space. When necessary, the skeleton gives up calcium to maintain the correct serum levels. The ionic concentration of calcium is generally determined by the renal glomerular filtration rate, tubular reabsorption of calcium, and the formation and resorption of bone. The serum calcium level is tightly controlled by parathyroid hormone and 1,25-dihydroxyvitamin D. Calcium can be directly released from the hydroxyapatite crystal or liberated by osteoclastic destruction of bone. Bone formation and destruction are closely coupled in a healthy person.

## Hyperparathyroidism

Hyperparathyroidism stimulates osteoclastic resorption of bone. The excess parathyroid hormone can be a result of primary or secondary hyperparathyroidism. Primary hyperparathyroidism results in hypercalcemia and is caused by excess parathyroid hormone production from diffuse parathyroid hyperplasia or autonomously functioning parathyroid adenomas (single or multiple). Secondary hyperparathyroidism is a response to sustained hypocalcemia that is typically caused by chronic renal failure or gastrointestinal malabsorption. Patients with long-standing secondary hyperparathyroidism may develop relatively autonomous parathyroid function or tertiary hyperparathyroidism. Diagnosis of these disorders is made by clinical and laboratory findings, including direct measurement of serum calcium and parathyroid hormone levels.

Although radiographic changes may occur at many sites, they are best detected and monitored in the hands. Skeletal surveys of the whole body are generally unnecessary. Radiologic

**FIGURE 15.9.** Secondary hyperparathyroidism. Subperiosteal bone resorption is evident throughout the hand and more advanced on the radial aspect.

signs of hyperparathyroidism include bone resorption, brown tumors, bone sclerosis, and chondrocalcinosis. Bone resorption occurs at all surfaces, including subperiosteal, intracortical (along haversian systems), endosteal, trabecular, subchondral, and subligamentous locations. Subperiosteal bone resorption is virtually diagnostic of hyperparathyroidism. Seen best and most frequently along the radial aspect of the phalanges of the hands, especially the middle phalanges of the index and middle fingers, subperiosteal bone resorption may also be evident at the phalangeal tufts (Fig. 15.9). Bone resorption at other surfaces is nonspecific. Subchondral bone resorption may lead to articular disease (Fig. 15.10).

**FIGURE 15.10.** Hyperparathyroidism with sacroiliac joint bone resorption. Axial CT scan shows subchondral bone resorption and widening of the sacroiliac joints.

**A**

**B**

**FIGURE 15.11.** Brown tumor in hyperparathyroidism. **A:** AP radiograph shows osteoporosis and destructive lesion (*arrow*) in proximal humerus. Chondrocalcinosis is present (*arrowhead*). **B:** CT shows mass destroying cortex.

Brown tumors are focal areas of bone resorption where the bone has been replaced by fibrous tissue and osteoclasts (Fig. 15.11). Brown tumors may have the appearance of aggressive, focally destructive bone lesions such as metastases, but the associated presence of other radiographic changes of hyperparathyroid bone disease should clarify the situation. Brown tumors may be single or multiple in number and central, eccentric, or cortical in location (Figs. 15.12 and 15.13). Brown tumors heal by ossification (Fig. 15.14). Widespread sclerosis of bone in hyperparathyroidism occurs by an uncertain mechanism and may be prominent in the axial skeleton, especially the skull and spine. Widespread sclerosis is common in secondary hyperparathyroidism. When the spine is involved, horizontal bands of sclerosis in the vertebral bodies adjacent to the vertebral end plates may result in a rugger jersey appearance (Fig. 15.15). Chondrocalcinosis, or calcification of the

cartilage, is associated with the combination of primary hyperparathyroidism and calcium pyrophosphate dihydrate crystal deposition disease (see Chapter 13). This combination is found in 18% to 40% of primary hyperparathyroidism cases.

Sometimes, the distinction between primary and secondary hyperparathyroidism can be suggested. The following combination of findings is highly suggestive of primary hyperparathyroidism: subperiosteal bone resorption, bone resorption at other sites, bony sclerosis, and chondrocalcinosis. In secondary hyperparathyroidism, there is an increased frequency of vascular and soft-tissue calcification, more commonly and more widespread bone sclerosis, and a decreased frequency of chondrocalcinosis. Secondary hyperparathyroidism is common; primary hyperparathyroidism is uncommon.

## Rickets, Osteomalacia, and Renal Osteodystrophy

Rickets and osteomalacia are childhood and adult manifestations, respectively, of a systemic disease in which the calcification of osteoid is deficient. The final common pathway in both conditions is the lack of available calcium or phosphorus (or both) for mineralization of osteoid. In rickets, the predominant effect is on the growth plates; in osteomalacia, the predominant effect is on remodeling of the mature bone. When rickets or osteomalacia occurs in conjunction with chronic renal failure, the condition is called *renal osteodystrophy*.

Dietary deficiency of vitamin D, usually coupled with inadequate exposure to sunlight so that photochemical synthesis of vitamin D in the skin does not occur, results in reduced gastrointestinal calcium absorption, hypocalcemia, and secondary hyperparathyroidism to mobilize calcium from the skeleton. Pure vitamin D deficiency–induced rickets and osteomalacia

**FIGURE 15.12.** Secondary hyperparathyroidism with brown tumors (*arrows*) and bone resorption on CT.

A  B

**FIGURE 15.13.** Brown tumor of the proximal femur. **A:** AP radiograph shows a lytic lesion (*arrow*) in the intertrochanteric region of the proximal femur. **B:** Axial T1-weighted MRI with fat suppression following a gadolinium injection shows rim enhancement (*arrow*) in this cystic lesion.

are relatively rare in the United States except among immigrants, food faddists, the institutionalized elderly people, and patients on total parenteral nutrition. Other causes include failure of enzymatic conversion of 25-hydroxyvitamin D to its physiologically more active metabolite 1,25-dihydroxyvitamin D, end-organ insensitivity to 1,25-dihydroxyvitamin D, genetic and acquired renal tubular reabsorptive defects, and gastrointestinal malabsorption of dietary calcium or phosphorus. In the United States, gastrointestinal malabsorption from a variety of

etiologies is the most common cause of rickets and osteomalacia. Rickets and osteomalacia may occur in association with polyostotic fibrous dysplasia and neurofibromatosis and may also be caused by chronic use of anticonvulsant medications or aluminum-containing antacids.

In rickets, there is widening of the growth plate because of continued cartilage growth in the absence of normal mineralization and

**FIGURE 15.14.** Healing brown tumors involving the pelvis and proximal femurs (*arrows*).

**FIGURE 15.15.** Secondary hyperparathyroidism. Osteosclerosis with greater density at the endplates (rugger jersey spine).

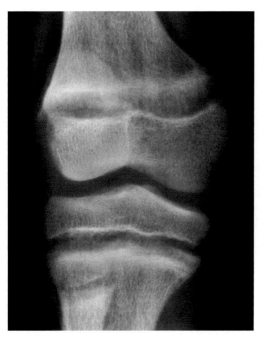

**FIGURE 15.16.** Renal osteodystrophy with thickened growth plates and irregular ossification at the interface with the metaphysis.

**FIGURE 15.18.** Osteomalacia with bowing deformity and Looser zones (*arrows*).

ossification (Fig. 15.16). Radiographic findings are most apparent in the most active regions of growth, and the uncalcified cartilage may become quite bulky. Frequent sites of radiographic abnormalities include the costochondral junctions of ribs, the distal femur, both ends of the tibia, the proximal humerus, the distal radius, and the ulna. Irregular, disorganized mineralization of the zone of provisional calcification creates a frayed appearance. Mechanical stress on the thickened growth plate may lead to widening, cupping, and bowing deformities. Bone texture (trabecular pattern) appears

**FIGURE 15.17.** Healing rickets.

coarsened, and there is delayed appearance of ossification centers. Rachitic bone is less resistant to bending and shearing loads, and stress fractures and bowing deformities are common. Transverse zones of lucency on the concave side of long bones, called *Milkman pseudofractures* or *Looser zones*, are focal collections of nonmineralized osteoid; they probably do not represent insufficiency injuries. After the initiation of successful treatment of rickets, the uncalcified osteoid calcifies, so that the zone of provisional calcification appears as a wide band that narrows the growth plate to its normal thickness (Fig. 15.17). Ossification of nonmineralized subperiosteal osteoid is apparent as new periosteal bone.

In osteomalacia, the radiologic findings are more subtle than in rickets because the adult skeleton is less metabolically active. Osteopenia is the predominant appearance, and it may be indistinguishable from osteoporosis unless Looser zones or bowing deformities are present (Fig. 15.18). Occasionally, the bone texture may be recognized as subtly coarsened. As in osteoporosis, the risk of fractures from falls escalates with deteriorating bone strength.

In renal osteodystrophy, skeletal abnormalities include the findings of rickets or osteomalacia, secondary hyperparathyroidism, osteoporosis, and soft-tissue and vascular calcifications (Fig. 15.19). In children, slipped capital femoral epiphysis is common. The extent of the abnormalities depends on the severity and duration of the disease. Advanced changes have become uncommon as the management of renal failure has improved. Articular conditions that are related to chronic renal failure include amyloidosis, periarticular calcinosis (hemodialysis-related tumoral calcinosis), and hydroxyapatite crystal synovitis. These conditions are detailed in Chapter 13.

## Idiopathic Tumoral Calcinosis

Idiopathic tumoral calcinosis is an uncommon disorder characterized by accumulations of calcium hydroxyapatite crystals in the

**FIGURE 15.19.** Renal osteodystrophy. AP radiograph of the foot shows a coarsened trabecular bone pattern, cortical thinning, osteopenia, and vascular calcification.

periarticular soft tissues with granulomatous reaction. An inborn error in phosphorus metabolism is thought to be the cause of these nonneoplastic lesions; approximately one third of reported cases are familial. The masses tend to grow slowly over many years to a large size; symptoms may be caused by their physical bulk. Most are discovered in the first or second decade of life. These accumulations are comprised of multiple globules of calcification separated by radiolucent bands. Fluid levels are usually present but may not be evident except on CT (Fig. 15.20). The lesions are frequently found in the normal location of bursae. The treatment is surgical, but local recurrences are not uncommon.

## ■ ENDOCRINE BONE DISEASE

### Hypercortisolism

Hypercortisolism, or Cushing syndrome, is a clinical manifestation of excessive amounts of glucocorticoids. *Cushing disease* refers to endogenous, spontaneous hypercortisolism caused by an autonomously functioning pituitary or adrenal lesion or by nonendocrine adrenocorticotropic hormone–producing tumors. More commonly, hypercortisolism results from treatment with high doses of synthetic cortisol-like corticosteroids such as prednisone. Hypercortisolism has three major effects on the musculoskeletal system: osteoporosis, osteonecrosis, and muscle wasting. The combination of osteoporosis of the axial skeleton and multifocal osteonecrosis of the appendicular skeleton is typical of hypercortisolism. However, both osteoporosis and osteonecrosis may have other causes.

Demineralization of bone is almost always present if hypercortisolism has been present for a sufficient period. Glucocorticoids inhibit the absorption of calcium from the intestine and increase renal calcium loss, leading to secondary hyperparathyroidism. Glucocorticoids also exert a direct stimulatory effect on osteoclasts.

**A**

**B**

**C**

**FIGURE 15.20.** Idiopathic tumoral calcinosis. **A, B:** AP and oblique foot radiographs show amorphous multilobular calcifications. **C:** Axial CT shows amorphous calcifications, some with sedimentation level (*arrow*).

At the same time, glucocorticoids inhibit osteoblastic activity by suppressing the collagen synthesis necessary for the formation of osseous matrix. The net result is continued generalized loss of bone that is prominent in the spine, pelvis, ribs, and cranial vault. In addition to osteopenia, there may be thinning of the cortex, loss of trabecular structure, intracortical tunneling, vertebral central endplate depressions, and insufficiency fractures. Insufficiency fractures characteristically heal with exuberant callus formation. Vertebral end plates may have a sclerotic appearance that results from a combination of insufficiency compressive microfractures and subsequent healing (Fig. 15.21). The osteoporosis of hypercortisolism is virtually indistinguishable from involutional osteoporosis. Osteoporosis may persist long after cortisol metabolism has been restored to normal or synthetic corticosteroid treatment has ended.

Focal regions of osteonecrosis may result from hypercortisolism, particularly when the hypercortisolism results from exogenous corticosteroids. Classic sites of involvement have been reported as the femoral and humeral heads, but radiographically occult infarctions of the marrow in the shafts of long bones are also common. Manifestations of corticosteroid-associated osteonecrosis may be delayed, possibly appearing months or years after the treatment has begun or ended (see Chapter 16). The mechanisms through which corticosteroid treatment results in focal osteonecrosis are unknown. Severe secondary arthropathy may occur as a consequence of osteonecrosis and mechanical collapse of the subchondral bone; the resulting loss of the bony support of the articular cartilage leads to excessive wear and osteoarthropathy. This is a particularly common problem in the femoral head.

Muscle wasting is frequent in hypercortisolism but may vary in severity from mild and virtually imperceptible to profound and obvious. In pronounced cases, it may simulate muscular dystrophy.

Hypercortisolism during skeletal immaturity suppresses growth, resulting in a short child with osteoporosis, truncal obesity, and delayed bone age. Growth resumes when the hypercortisolism is

corrected, but permanent stunting may occur. Osteonecrosis of a growing epiphyses may lead to abnormal development at the ends of bones and eventually results in the early development of degenerative osteoarthropathy.

## Acromegaly and Gigantism

Clinical acromegaly is caused by excess growth hormones in adults. The underlying cause in the majority of cases is a pituitary adenoma that produces growth hormone autonomously; however, extrapituitary growth hormone–secreting tumors as well as central and peripheral tumors that secrete growth hormone–releasing hormone may also cause acromegaly. Acromegaly has an equal incidence in men and women and has a mean age of diagnosis of 40 and 45 years, respectively. In younger patients, the onset tends to be rapid and often correlates with an aggressive tumor; in older patients, the onset may be slow and insidious with subtle changes occurring over a 5- to 10-year period. Clinical features of acromegaly are distinctive and include acromegalic facies, enlargement of the hands and feet, prognathism, and oily skin. Carpal tunnel syndrome, degenerative joint disease, hypertension, Raynaud phenomenon, and diabetes mellitus are commonly associated conditions. Many patients present with the signs and symptoms of a pituitary or hypothalamic mass rather than those of growth hormone excess. Definitive diagnosis is made by direct serum measurements of hormone levels.

Growth hormone activates sites of bone remodeling and may increase bone formation more than bone resorption. As a consequence, the bone mass may actually be elevated, with thickened cortex and increased trabecular bone volume. Periosteal bone formation at the insertions of tendons and ligaments and periarticular hypertrophy at the insertions of joint capsules contribute to the increase in the skeletal mass.

Growth hormone increases chondrocytic activity and leads to hypertrophy of the hyaline articular cartilage. This thickened cartilage lacks the normal biomechanical characteristics of articular cartilage and is vulnerable to fissuring, ulceration, denudation, and degeneration of the articular surface. Disordered joint mechanics and a brisk reparative process lead to widespread osteophytic growths, subchondral cyst formation, and eventually to acromegalic arthropathy. Superficially, the appearance of acromegalic arthropathy is similar to osteoarthritis, but the joint spaces tend to be widened rather than narrowed (Fig. 15.22). When the process is so advanced that the cartilage has completely disintegrated, the joint spaces are narrowed. The distribution of involvement usually includes the large joints and the lumbosacral spine, including sites normally spared by osteoarthritis such as the ankle and glenohumeral joint. Calcinosis, skin hypertrophy, and nonspecific synovitis may be associated.

Radiologic features of acromegaly include soft-tissue thickening; enlarged sella with destructive changes; prominent facial bones and occipital protuberance; enlarged, excessively pneumatized sinuses; increased vertebral body and intervertebral disk height; posterior vertebral scalloping; exaggerated thoracic kyphosis; hand and foot changes; and bony proliferation at entheses. Osteoporosis may occur late in the clinical course.

The rare condition of growth hormone excess during skeletal development causes gigantism. Growth hormone stimulates bone growth and leads to proportional enlargement. The most striking feature is extreme height with normal body proportions, but because the sites of bone and cartilage formation that are stimulated in acromegaly (when the growth plates are closed) are also

**FIGURE 15.21.** Hypercortisolism. Osteoporotic spine with advanced insufficiency fractures of all the vertebral bodies.

A                                                        B

**FIGURE 15.22.** Acromegaly with mature proliferative bone at the phalangeal tufts and the insertions of the joint capsules. The soft tissues are thick and the joint spaces are wide. **A:** PA radiograph. **B:** Lateral radiograph.

stimulated when the growth plates are open, features of acromegaly may be present. As with acromegaly, the most common cause of gigantism is an autonomously functioning pituitary adenoma. Unless treated, patients with gigantism develop progressively more striking features of acromegaly because the growth hormone excess continues after closure of the growth plates.

## Thyroid Disorders

Deficiency of thyroid hormone in the neonate results in mental retardation and developmental abnormalities. Bone maturation nearly stops, and dental development is delayed. Mass screening programs at birth for T4 and/or thyroid-stimulating hormone levels have made untreated congenital hypothyroidism rare. Knee films rather than hand films are more useful for bone age. In adult hypothyroidism, skeletal manifestations are mild, and typically, no radiographic features are evident.

Hyperthyroidism causes catabolism of protein and loss of connective tissue. Accelerated skeletal maturation occurs in children. In adults, increased bone turnover and remodeling lead to changes in bone mass and a rapidly progressive, generalized osteoporosis. Hypercalcemia, hypercalciuria, and elevated serum alkaline phosphatase levels may also be seen. Reestablishment of a euthyroid state is accompanied by partial recovery of bone mineral content. Myopathy is a common clinical feature of hyperthyroidism, and symptoms may simulate those of arthritis. Muscle wasting, especially in the proximal muscle groups, is common.

## Gonadal Disorders

Gonadal disorders may affect the skeleton through excessive or deficient levels of sex steroids. There are also syndromes that include both gonadal disorders and musculoskeletal dysmorphisms,

not necessarily related. Albright syndrome, for example, occurs predominantly in females and consists of precocious puberty, fibrous dysplasia of bone, and café au lait spots, but the fibrous dysplasia is not believed to have an endocrine basis. The skeletal manifestation of hypergonadism in a child is precocious growth and maturation. The epiphyseal ossification centers appear early, the long bones grow rapidly, and the growth plates close early. Although there is an initial precocious growth spurt, the early closure of the growth plates has the ultimate result of short stature, with a tall child becoming a short adult (Table 15.4). The morphology of the skeleton is normal.

Hypogonadism in the prepubertal child results in delayed adolescence and delayed skeletal maturation. Delayed closure of the epiphyses has the effect of prolonging longitudinal growth and results in unusually long and slender tubular bones of the extremities. There may be generalized osteoporosis and a lack of normal muscular development. In the adult, hypogonadism may be associated with osteoporosis and its complications.

| TABLE 15.4 | Some Endocrine Disorders Causing Abnormal Stature in Children |
|---|---|

Tall stature
  Gigantism
  Hypergonadism (tall child, short adult)
  Hyperthyroidism
  Hyperinsulinemic states
Short Stature
  Hypopituitarism
  Hypothyroidism
  Diabetes mellitus
  Hypercortisolism
  Somatomedin deficiency

**FIGURE 15.23.** Diabetic neuropathic arthropathy with rocker-bottom deformity. **A:** Lateral radiograph. **B:** AP radiograph.

## Diabetes Mellitus

Insulin deficiency in childhood results in decreased growth, often with generalized osteoporosis and short stature. Insulin-dependent diabetes mellitus in the adult may be accompanied by generalized osteoporosis, but only if obesity is absent. Calcification of the interdigital arteries of the foot is common in diabetics and uncommon in other conditions. Additional skeletal manifestations relate to complications. Diabetic foot disease, the condition of chronic ulceration and infection, is the result of peripheral neuropathy and vascular insufficiency. Sensory loss leads to unrecognized trauma, often minor but chronic and repetitive. Motor defects result in foot deformities that lead to unusual pressure points and weight-bearing areas. Gradual derangement of the normal foot architecture progresses in a vicious cycle (Figs. 15.23 and 15.24). Autonomic deficits and vascular disease contribute to impaired host defenses against infection. Trophic ulcers with secondary infection and cellulitis are common. The initial soft-tissue lesions typically occur at the first and fifth metatarsophalangeal

**FIGURE 15.24.** Diabetic neuropathic arthropathy. **A:** Sagittal T1-weighted MRI shows dorsal subluxation of the midfoot with fragmentation of tarsal bones (*arrow*). **B:** Sagittal T2-weighted MRI shows edema in the bones involved with the neuropathic joint, as well as in the adjacent soft tissues. A plantar ulceration is present with adjacent inflammatory change (*arrow*).

A

B

C

**FIGURE 15.25.** Diabetic osteomyelitis. **A:** Radiograph shows osteolysis and soft-tissue swelling at first metatarsal in a patient with previous toe amputations. **B:** Coronal T1-weighted MRI shows dark signal replacing the normal subcutaneous fat and marrow signal (*arrow*). **C:** Coronal T1-weighted fat-suppressed postgadolinium MRI shows enhancement in the first metatarsal (*arrow*) and surrounding soft tissues.

joints and at the calcaneus. On radiographs, one may find defects in the soft-tissue contour, loss of definition of tissue planes, and swelling. Contamination of bones and joints may lead to septic arthritis and osteomyelitis (Fig. 15.25). The typical findings of osteomyelitis may be absent in the diabetic foot because the blood supply is often inadequate for reactive bone formation and osteoporosis; therefore, great reliance may be placed on MRI for diagnosis. Peripheral arteriovenous fistulae may cause marked focal osteopenia or lysis of the bone. In a small proportion of cases, frank neuropathic osteoarthropathy (Charcot joint) develops (see Chapter 13). Diabetes is the most common cause of neuropathic osteoarthropathy. Certain soft-tissue conditions occur frequently in diabetics, including frozen shoulder, calcific tendinitis or bursitis, Dupuytren contracture, flexor tenosynovitis (trigger finger), and carpal tunnel syndrome. Skeletal muscle infarction may occur as a result of vascular insufficiency, particularly in the lower extremities. Acute muscle infarction may present as pain, tenderness, or swelling, similar to infection. On MRI, the condition is evident as diffuse enlargement and high signal on T2-weighted images in the regions of involvement (Fig. 15.26); these findings are not specific.

**FIGURE 15.26.** Diabetic myonecrosis. Coronal T2-weighted fat-suppressed MRI shows high signal in regions of myonecrosis (*arrow*).

# ◼ PAGET DISEASE

Paget disease (osteitis deformans) is a bone disease seen in middle-aged and elderly individuals. It is characterized by excessive and abnormal remodeling of the bone. Usually asymptomatic, Paget disease has a prevalence of 3% in the adult population older than 40 years of age. In most cases, involvement is polyostotic. Although any bone may be involved, the preponderance of cases involves the pelvis, spine, skull, femur, or tibia.

Current evidence suggests that development of Paget disease is an autosomal dominant trait with genetic heterogeneity and an as-yet undetermined relationship with paramyxoviral infection. The disease has active and quiescent (inactive) phases. The active phase begins with a focus of excessive osteoclastic activity that results in a localized area of osteolysis, where the bone is replaced by nonossified fibrovascular tissue. The demarcation between normal uninvolved bone and the area of osteolysis is typically quite sharp. Subsequently, the areas of osteolysis are filled in with the pagetoid bone, even as the osteoclastic activity continues. The pagetoid bone consists of layers of disorganized woven bone separated by resorption cavities and nonossified fibrovascular tissue. Bone is formed both endosteally and periosteally. The combination of osteoclastic and osteoblastic activities results in rapid remodeling and turnover of the bone. Eventually, for unknown reasons, the osteoclastic activity moderates, and after the osteolytic areas have filled with bone, the rate of bone turnover decreases. With the decrease in turnover, the bone enters the quiescent phase of Paget disease. Focal areas of pagetoid bone may be replaced by islands of lamellar bone, but haversian systems and remodeling along the lines of stress do not occur. Slow endosteal and periosteal apposition of the bone may continue to thicken the cortex and enlarge the bone, sometimes obscuring the marrow space on radiographs. The juxtaposition of the lamellar and woven bones yields a mosaic appearance on microscopy that is diagnostic of Paget disease.

**FIGURE 15.28.** Paget disease at the knee. Coronal T1-weighted MRI shows enlargement and the thick trabeculae.

The progression of the disease may be seen radiographically in a long bone (Fig. 15.27). The disease begins typically at an epiphysis and slowly advances at the rate of a few millimeters per year to involve the entire bone. The advancing edge of osteolysis is radiolucent, with a sharp transition between normal uninvolved bone and osteolysis. Behind the advancing osteolysis, the pagetoid bone is found. The pagetoid bone has a coarsened trabecular appearance with diminished cortical density. In the quiescent phase, the bone may become extremely dense, and the overall size may be enlarged. Because remodeling along the lines of stress does not occur, insufficiency fractures and deformity are not uncommon. On MRI, thickening of the cortex and trabeculae may be seen (Fig. 15.28); however, the marrow space remains normal.

In vertebral bodies, the periphery (cortex) is involved first, widening the body into a picture-frame appearance (Fig. 15.29).

**FIGURE 15.27.** Paget disease in a femur showing the lucent zone of osteolysis (*arrow*) advancing distally into the normal bone.

**FIGURE 15.29.** Paget disease with picture-frame vertebra appearance.

A

B

**FIGURE 15.30.** Ivory vertebra from Paget disease. **A:** Lateral radiograph shows sclerosis of the L1 vertebral body, obliterating the normal cortex and trabecular bone pattern. The process extends from the vertebral body into the pedicles. **B:** Axial CT shows increased density of the L1 vertebra with a disordered pattern of bone deposition.

Continued endosteal progression results in a dense, sclerotic body. Characteristically, Paget disease involves the entire vertebra, including the posterior elements (Fig. 15.30).

In the skull, the common region of involvement is the cranial vault. The osteolytic phase is called *osteoporosis circumscripta* and appears as a geographic, well-demarcated region of bone resorption that may be mistaken for a metastasis.

Focal radiodensities occur as the pagetoid bone is formed. In the quiescent phase, there is a radiodense cotton-wool appearance with a thickened vault (typically 2 to 3 cm thick but often thicker). Basilar invagination of the skull may follow because, despite its thickness, the pagetoid bone is weak. Radionuclide bone scan can be used to identify all sites of involvement (Fig. 15.31). Clinical monitoring is accomplished by

**FIGURE 15.31.** Paget disease in the femur. Radionuclide bone scan shows intense activity in the regions involved by Paget disease.

**FIGURE 15.32.** Insufficiency fractures (*arrows*) in Paget disease.

**FIGURE 15.33.** Paget sarcoma arising in the pelvis. **A:** Radiograph shows typical findings of Paget disease in the right hemipelvis and hip, with a medial region of destruction (*arrows*). **B:** CT shows destructive mass (*arrows*) and typical pagetoid changes in the remaining portion of the ilium.

measuring serum alkaline phosphatase levels and urinary hydroxy-proline levels, both of which are increased by osteoclastic activity. Although plain films can establish the initial diagnosis, they change too slowly and are too insensitive for clinical monitoring unless there is suspicion of a complication. Paget disease can be treated with agents that arrest the osteolytic process: bisphosphonates, which inhibit demineralization from the hydroxyapatite crystal, and calcitonin, which inhibits bone resorption.

Complications include insufficiency fractures and sarcomatous degeneration. Unless there is trauma, the insufficiency fractures are typically incomplete horizontal lucencies at the lateral cortex (Fig. 15.32). A complete fracture in the absence of trauma should raise suspicion of an underlying sarcoma. Sarcomatous degeneration of the pagetoid bone occurs rarely but is more likely in patients with extensive disease. Osteolysis is a dominant radiographic feature (Fig. 15.33).

The most important differential diagnosis for Paget disease is metastatic disease. Metastatic disease may bear a superficial resemblance to Paget disease but does not have the characteristic appearance of the pagetoid bone or the specific organization of active and quiescent phases in the long bones. Sometimes, the distinction is difficult to make. Although the distribution in the skeleton of Paget disease is similar to the distribution of metastatic disease, involvement of the ribs is rare in Paget disease and is common in metastases. Discovery of a metastasis within the pagetoid bone is a rare event.

## ■ NUTRITIONAL CONDITIONS

### Scurvy

Dietary vitamin C deficiency impairs the ability of the connective tissue to produce and maintain collagen. In a growing child, bone formation and cartilage proliferation cease, but mineralization and ossification of the preexisting cartilage proceed. Generalized osteoporosis and a ground-glass bone texture with cortical thinning are

seen (Fig. 15.34). There is widening and increased density of the zone of the provisional calcification. Large subperiosteal hemorrhages may occur, elevating the periosteum. Nutritional scurvy is quite rare in the United States.

## Chemical Toxicity

Chronic lead poisoning in children results in dense transverse lines across the growing metaphysis (Fig. 15.35). Lead interferes with the resorption of the primary spongiosa during growth. A new bone

**FIGURE 15.34.** Scurvy manifested by osteopenia and cortical thinning shown on radiograph of the lower limb.

**FIGURE 15.35.** Lead poisoning with characteristic dense transverse metaphyseal lines (*arrow*).

**FIGURE 15.36.** Skeletal fluorosis.

is laid down on top of the primary spongiosa, but because normal resorption of the primary spongiosa does not occur during the period of exposure, a dense line becomes evident on radiographs; lead is present in only minute amounts. Lead lines are a late manifestation of chronic lead poisoning and are best seen at the knee or distal radius, where growth is the most rapid. Lead toxicity has been reported after the retention of lead fragments after gunshot wounds. Chronic exposure to other heavy metals during growth, including phosphorus and bismuth, may result in transverse lines similar to those seen with chronic lead poisoning.

Fluorosis occurs after chronic ingestion of drinking water with endemic, excessive levels of fluoride (4 parts per million or greater), excessive industrial exposure, or excessive use of fluoride-containing medication. Radiographic findings include osteosclerosis and

hyperostosis involving the axial skeleton, periostitis and enthesopathy in the appendicular skeleton, and dental abnormalities (Fig. 15.36).

Aluminum toxicity may occur in the setting of dialysis for chronic renal failure. The clinical presentation is encephalopathy, myopathy, and bone pain. Radiographs may show rachitic or osteomalacic changes, but these may be impossible to distinguish from coexistent renal osteodystrophy.

## Drug Effects

Drugs with teratogenic effects on the musculoskeletal system include thalidomide, anticonvulsants, vitamin A and synthetic retinoids, alcohol, and folic acid antagonists. Many drugs

**FIGURE 15.37.** Bisphosphonate-related insufficiency fracture. **A:** Radiograph shows heaped up periosteal bone formation along the lateral subtrochanteric femoral cortex (*arrow*), corresponding to an incomplete insufficiency fracture. **B:** Subsequent radiograph shows catastrophic completion of the fracture.

**FIGURE 15.38.** Nephrogenic systemic fibrosis. Sagittal T1 MRI **(A)** and sagittal T2 MRI **(B)** show the equinus contracture of the foot. Fibrotic nodules (*short arrow*) are present in the plantar skin, with edema in the skin (*arrowheads*) and muscle compartments (*long arrow*).

may have nonteratogenic effects on the musculoskeletal system. Prostaglandin E, used in infants with ductus-dependent cyanotic congenital heart disease, is associated with cortical hyperostosis. Methotrexate in the setting of chemotherapy may cause osteoporosis and scurvylike changes in the bone. Other chemotherapeutic agents may be associated with inflammatory myositis. Phenyltoin and other anticonvulsants are associated with rachitic or osteomalacic changes in the bone.

High doses of vitamin D, sometimes used in the treatment of renal failure, are associated with metastatic calcification, osteoporosis, and osteosclerosis. The calcifications are often periarticular and may have a lobular morphology with fluid-fluid levels. Because similar findings are caused by renal osteodystrophy, hypervitaminosis D is usually not suspected until the clinical condition improves without corresponding radiographic improvement. Hypervitaminosis A, typically caused by excessive vitamin supplementation in infants and young children, causes soft-tissue swelling and cortical hyperostosis. Retinoids are commonly used to treat skin diseases. In patients in whom high doses are chronically administered, bone proliferation at joints and entheses may occur. These may cause orthopedic complications and may be associated with musculoskeletal pain.

Bisphosphonates are used to treat osteoporosis and other conditions associated with bone loss, such as multiple myeloma and lytic metastatic disease. These agents interfere with osteoclast action and bone turnover and are associated with increased bone mineral density measurements and decreased osteoporotic fracture frequency. In some patients, insufficiency fractures have been reported in the femoral shaft preceded by a characteristic triangular cortical bone reaction (Fig. 15.37).

Nephrogenic systemic fibrosis (NSF), also known as nephrogenic fibrosing dermopathy, occurs in patients with renal insufficiency who are exposed to gadolinium-based contrast agents during the course of MRI. Cutaneous changes of NSF include induration, thickening, hardening, and fibrotic nodules and plaques that may lead to contractures (Fig. 15.38). The nodules contain proliferations of dermal fibroblasts and dendritic cells, thickened bundles of collagen, elastic fibers, and deposits of mucin; gadolinium has been recovered in such tissue samples. Fibrosis may involve other organs. Patients with NSF have increased mortality and may have severe debility.

## ◼ MISCELLANEOUS CONDITIONS

### Sarcoidosis

Sarcoidosis is a multisystem disease of unknown etiology characterized by the presence of noncaseating granulomas. Although the predominant site of involvement is the pulmonary system, sarcoidosis may involve the joints in approximately 10% of cases. Sarcoidosis most often causes transient migratory polyarticular arthralgias without radiographic findings. A chronic granulomatous arthritis leading to chronic noncaseating granulomatous inflammation of the synovium develops in only a few patients. Granulomas within or adjacent to the bone may result in punched-out cortical erosions or central lytic lesions with nonaggressive features within the medullary cavity. Fingers and toes are the typical sites of involvement (Fig. 15.39). The characteristic appearance caused by the presence of multiple granulomatous lesions has been described as lacelike.

**FIGURE 15.39.** Sarcoidosis in the great toe with lacelike appearance.

**A**

**B**

**FIGURE 15.40.** Infantile cortical hyperostosis in a 5-month-old boy. **A:** Thick periosteal new bone is present along both tibias. **B:** Thick periosteal new bone is present along the mandible (*arrows*).

## Infantile Cortical Hyperostosis

Infantile cortical hyperostosis (Caffey disease) is a self-limited inflammatory condition of infants in which widespread, florid periostitis is seen at multiple sites, especially the mandible, ribs, clavicles, ulnas, and tibias (Fig. 15.40). Apposition of thick, mature periosteal new bone may be evident as tender, palpable lumpiness on clinical examination. The onset is usually around 2 months of age, but it is always before 5 months of age. Irritability and local inflammatory signs may be present. The affected bones remodel to a normal appearance over a period of months to years. The cause of infantile cortical hyperostosis is thought to be infectious or postinfectious, although this has not been shown conclusively. There is a familial tendency in some cases. The differential diagnosis includes accidental and intentional trauma and multifocal osteomyelitis. The absence of fractures helps exclude trauma, and the absence of joint effusions and bone destruction helps exclude osteomyelitis.

## Hypertrophic Osteoarthropathy

Hypertrophic osteoarthropathy is a combination of generalized periostitis and digital clubbing. In approximately 5% of cases, the condition is inherited and called *primary hypertrophic osteoarthropathy* or *pachydermoperiostosis*. In 95% of cases, hypertrophic osteoarthropathy is secondary to other—often pulmonary—diseases. Bronchogenic carcinoma is the most common cause of secondary hypertrophic osteoarthropathy, and approximately 5% of cases of bronchogenic carcinoma have secondary hypertrophic osteoarthropathy. Periostitis, the hallmark of this condition, is found in multiple sites, usually beginning in the diaphysis of the long bones and extending toward the metaphysis (Fig. 15.41). Increased vascular perfusion of the affected bones and overgrowth of vascular

connective tissues surrounding the bones, joints, and tendons appear to precede the periostitis. The clinical presentation is pain and swelling in the affected extremities. The pathogenesis of secondary hypertrophic osteoarthropathy is unknown; possibilities described in the literature include a humoral factor, a neurogenic mechanism, and hypervascularity.

**FIGURE 15.41.** Secondary hypertrophic osteoarthropathy (*arrows*) in a patient with lung cancer.

## SOURCES AND READINGS

Chew FS. Radiologic manifestations in the musculoskeletal system of miscellaneous endocrine disorders. *Radiol Clin North Am.* 1991;29:135–147.

Cummings SR, Melton LJ. Osteoporosis. I: Epidemiology and outcomes of osteoporotic fractures. *Lancet.* 2002;359(9319):1761–1767.

Curtiss PH, Clark WS, Herndon CH. Vertebral fractures resulting from prolonged cortisone and corticotropin therapy. *JAMA.* 1954;156:467–469.

Duque G, Troen BR. Understanding the mechanisms of senile osteoporosis: New facts for a major geriatric syndrome. *J Am Geriatrics Soc.* 2008;56(5):935–941.

eMedicine. http://emedicine.medscape.com.

Greenblatt RB, Nieburgs HW. Some endocrinologic aspects of retarded growth and dwarfism. *Med Clin North Am.* 1947;31:712–730.

Hudson TM. *Radiologic-Pathologic Correlation of Musculoskeletal Lesions.* Baltimore, MD: Williams & Wilkins; 1987:491–504.

Lawson JP. Drug-induced metabolic bone disorders. *Semin Musculoskeletal Radiol.* 2002;6(4):285–297.

Mankin HJ, Mankin CJ. Metabolic bone disease: A review and update. *Instr Course Lect.* 2008;57:575–593.

Naganathan V, Jones G, Nash P, et al. Vertebral fracture risk with long-term corticosteroid therapy: Prevalence and relation to age, bone density, and corticosteroid use. *Arch Intern Med.* 2000;160:2917–2922.

Olsen KM, Chew FS. Tumoral calcinosis: Pearls, polemics, and alternative possibilities. *Radiographics.* 2006; 26(3):871–885.

Resnick D. Disorders due to medications and other chemical agents. In: Resnick D, ed. *Diagnosis of Bone and Joint Disorders.* 4th Ed. Philadelphia, PA: WB Saunders; 2002:3423–3455.

Scheinfeld NS, Cowper S. Nephrogenic fibrosing dermopathy. emedicine.medscape.com/article/1097889-overview.

Siris ES, Miller PD, Barrett-Connor E, et al. Identification and fracture outcomes of undiagnosed low bone mineral density in postmenopausal women: Results from the National Osteoporosis Risk Assessment. *JAMA.* 2001;286:2815–2822.

States LJ. Imaging of metabolic bone disease and marrow disorders in children. *Radiol Clin North Am.* 2001;39(4):749–772.

Swislocki ALM, Barnett CA, Darnell P, et al. Hyperthyroidism: An underappreciated cause of diffuse bone disease. *Clin Nucl Med.* 1998;23:241–243.

Tan PL, Teh J. MRI of the diabetic foot: Differentiation of infection from neuropathic change. *Br J Radiol.* 2007; 80(959):939–948. Epub 2006 May 10.

Theodorou DJ, Theodorou SJ. Dual-energy x-ray absorptiometry in clinical practice: Application and interpretation of scans beyond the numbers. *Clin Imaging.* 2002;26(1):43–49.

# Infection and Marrow Disease

T his chapter describes the radiology of musculoskeletal infections, osteonecrosis and other marrow space disorders, and a few other skeletal conditions not covered elsewhere in this book.

## ACUTE OSTEOMYELITIS

Acute osteomyelitis is a pyogenic infection of bone that typically occurs in a child who presents with an acute, systemic febrile illness. The infection is usually carried into the bone by the nutrient artery from a preexisting remote site of infection. Branches of the nutrient artery extend into the metaphysis, where they loop back and enter large sinusoidal veins. Slowing of blood flow in these sinusoidal veins permits bacterial colonies to grow and spread into the adjacent marrow where small abscesses form. Thrombosis from minor mechanical trauma may be an associated factor. From the initial focus in the metaphysis, the acute suppurative inflammatory process may extend throughout the medullary cavity. Edema and the collection of pus increase the pressure within the closed space of the medullary cavity, leading to decreased blood flow, thrombosis, and necrosis. Osteoclasts separate dead bone from living bone. Enzymes elaborated by inflammatory cells dissolve the necrotic bone. Under pressure, pus exudes through the cortex into the subperiosteal space by way of haversian and Volkmann canals. The periosteum becomes elevated by pus, stripping away the periosteal blood supply and leading to cortical osteonecrosis. Infection may penetrate the periosteum and extend into the soft tissues (Figs. 16.1–16.3). Where there is capsular investment of the metaphyseal cortex, the joint may become infected. Reactive periosteal bone forms a shell around the infection, called the *involucrum* (Fig. 16.4). The central, devitalized bone is called the *sequestrum*. Defects in the involucrum, called *cloaca*, may permit drainage of pus or extrusion of sequestra through fistulas. Hyperemia causes osteoporosis in the limb. Because the metaphyseal arteries do not penetrate the growth plate, the epiphysis is initially spared, but the infection may extend contiguously into the

epiphysis, damaging the growth plate in the process. A solitary bone lesion that crosses the epiphyseal plate from the metaphyseal side is usually osteomyelitis. The common causative organism is *Staphylococcus aureus.*

Multifocal osteomyelitis is rare except in neonates. Because the nutrient vessels penetrate the epiphysis in neonates, early involvement of the epiphysis and growth plate is common, with extension into the joint. Effusion may be the only early radiographic clue to the presence of infection. Subsequent bony reaction is exuberant, with periosteal reaction often involving the entire bone. Fistula formation is rare. The organisms that commonly cause multifocal osteomyelitis in neonates are β-hemolytic *Streptococcus* and *Escherichia coli*. When infection is monostotic, *S. aureus* may also be a causative organism.

Adults at risk for hematogenous osteomyelitis include patients who are debilitated or immunocompromised, elderly patients with genitourinary tract infections, patients with peripheral vascular insufficiency (especially diabetes), and intravenous drug abusers. Pathogens may also be implanted directly into the bone during trauma or surgery. Osteomyelitis does not occur in otherwise healthy adults. An antecedent history of trauma is common, and the bones of the hands and feet are commonly involved (Figs. 16.5 and 16.6). The feet are particularly vulnerable to infection as a complication of peripheral vascular disease. In adults, the initial location of infection is epiphyseal and subchondral because the nutrient artery loops into the sinusoidal veins at the ends of the bones. The common organism is *Staphylococcus*, unless the patient is immunocompromised. Contiguous spread of infection may involve the diaphysis, adjacent soft tissues, and joints. Fistula formation is frequent. Periosteal reaction may be minimal, especially in the feet. Because the periosteum is tightly applied, penetration of pus into the soft tissues is common, but subperiosteal collections are not. Multiple foci of infection do not occur.

Radiographic changes occur relatively late in acute osteomyelitis. Soft-tissue swelling with obliteration of fat planes may be seen 3 days after onset, at which time pus has already penetrated

A                                    B

**FIGURE 16.1.** Acute osteomyelitis in the humeral metaphysis. **A:** Radiograph shows destruction (*arrowhead*) and involucrum (*arrow*). **B:** Coronal T2-weighted MRI shows marrow edema and subperiosteal pus (*arrow*).
*Source*: From Chew FS, Schulze ES, Mattia AR. Osteomyelitis. *AJR*. 1994;162:942, with permission.

the cortex. Periosteal reaction and osteolysis may not be evident on radiographs until 5 to 7 days in children and 10 to 14 days in adults. If the suspected site contains fatty marrow, CT can reveal marrow infiltration by fluid and pus early in the course of osteomyelitis, before bone destruction is detectable. CT extends the radiographic ability to define sequestra, soft-tissue abscesses, sinus tracts, intramedullary and soft tissue gas, bone destruction, and reactive bone.

MRI is highly sensitive and specific in distinguishing between osteomyelitis and adjacent soft-tissue infection, even in the presence of previous surgery, fracture, or chronic osteomyelitis. Early marrow edema is evident well before other imaging studies become abnormal, and subperiosteal or soft-tissue collections of pus can be identified early. The key finding on MRI is abnormal signal within the marrow, low signal on T1-weighted images, and high signal on T2-weighted images. Enhancement is generally seen after gadolinium injection on T1-weighted images. Abscesses have high signal on T2-weighted images with rim enhancement after gadolinium injection on T1-weighted images.

The radionuclide bone scan is typically positive within 24 hours of onset, and a normal bone scan at this time eliminates osteomyelitis as a diagnostic possibility. Foci of acute osteomyelitis appear as areas of intense activity because of the hyperemia and reactive osteoblastic activity. Reactive hyperemia and osteoblastic activity are more extensive than the actual infected area. Devitalized, avascular areas of bone may appear as focal areas of decreased or absent activity, but the surrounding bone always has increased tracer uptake. Previous surgery, trauma, and other bone disease may complicate the interpretation of positive bone scans.

Additional problem-solving imaging tools in suspected osteomyelitis are nuclear scans with labeled leukocytes or with gallium. Both of these radiopharmaceuticals localize at sites of WBC aggregation, such as collections of pus, but both may require delayed imaging 24 to 72 hours after injection. The gallium scan may be particularly useful in following the course of treatment to confirm healing and obviate concern about possible chronic osteomyelitis.

Treatment of bacterial osteomyelitis with systemic antibiotics is effective when begun early. If there is pus formation and bone necrosis, the pus must be drained and the necrotic bone removed. Acute osteomyelitis may be complicated by chronic osteomyelitis.

**FIGURE 16.2.** Osteomyelitis in the femur. Axial T1-weighted fat-suppressed post-gadolinium MRI shows enhancement in the marrow and surrounding soft tissues, with a layer of periosteal reaction (involucrum) (*arrow*).

# ■ CHRONIC OSTEOMYELITIS

Chronic osteomyelitis may exist many years after acute osteomyelitis, even if the acute infection was treated appropriately. Systemic antibiotics are ineffective against organisms sequestered in necrotic

**FIGURE 16.3.** Osteomyelitis in a child. **A:** Radiograph of the femur shows a lytic lesion in the distal metaphysis (*long arrow*). Periosteal reactive bone surrounds the femur (*short arrow*). **B:** Coronal T2-weighted MRI shows high signal within the lesion (*long arrow*), periosteal reactive bone (*short arrow*), and extensive surrounding soft-tissue edema. Soft-tissue extension of the infection is present.

bone. Blood cultures are almost always negative, and cultures of the lesion are often negative as well. A rare complication of longstanding, chronic, and draining osteomyelitis is development of malignancy—mostly squamous carcinomas—along the sinus tract. In chronic osteomyelitis, foci of bacteria persist within bone cavities that are filled with granulation tissue. Dense bone surrounds the site, and the cortex may be thickened as a result of long-term deposition of reactive medullary and periosteal bone (Fig. 16.7). Serpiginous sinus

tracts may extend to the skin surface. Abscesses, sinus tracts, and sequestra may be obscured by the dense reactive bone, so that CT or MRI may be required. The radionuclide bone scan shows areas of increased uptake. Scans with gallium or labeled leukocytes should also be positive.

A Brodie abscess is a local, subacute bone abscess that is a fairly common cause of a solitary bone lesion. Symptoms of recurrent pain and local tenderness with swelling and erythema

**FIGURE 16.4.** Osteomyelitis with layers of involucrum (*arrow*).

**FIGURE 16.5.** Osteomyelitis and septic arthritis involving the second and fourth MTP joints in an adult diabetic. The third toe and MTP joint were amputated previously.

**FIGURE 16.6.** Diabetic osteomyelitis in the finger (*arrow*).

**FIGURE 16.8.** Brodie abscess in the distal tibia.

may be present for months or years. Most cases occur in adolescents and young adults, but the reported age range is from 6 to 61 years. Men are affected more often than women (by 2:1). The typical location is the metaphysis or diaphysis of the femur or tibia. A Brodie abscess may begin de novo, develop in the same site as a preceding episode of acute osteomyelitis, or follow an acute episode of osteomyelitis at another site. *S. aureus* appears to be the offending organism.

Radiographically, a Brodie abscess appears as a well-defined lucent area in cancellous bone with smooth, rounded geographic margins and a thick sclerotic rind that may merge imperceptibly with the surrounding bone (Figs. 16.8 and 16.9). The lesion may appear lobulated with lucent, serpentine tracts extending along the bone. CT is valuable for defining the reactive sclerosis and can permit

identification of tracts in the bone. The corresponding pathology is an avascular cavity, typically 1 to 4 cm in size, lined with granulation tissue and filled with fluid but not frank pus. Thickening of trabeculae adjacent to the lesion by reactive endosteal bone formation may form the sclerotic rind around the cavity.

Although Brodie abscesses have a characteristic appearance, they may be confused with other focal bone lesions, including tumors. The key radiologic feature of a Brodie abscess is the extensive reactive bone formation that has a sharp interface with the lesion but merges gradually with surrounding normal bone.

## ■ SPINE INFECTIONS

Pyogenic vertebral osteomyelitis occurs in elderly adults with genitourinary tract infections, patients who are immunocompromised, and intravenous drug abusers. Organisms from genitourinary tract infections ascend the vertebral column by way of the vertebral plexus of Batson, a valveless, venous bed that allows retrograde blood flow. The initial site of infection is the subcortial bone of the vertebral body adjacent to the intervertebral disk. The infection typically extends through the endplate, involving the disk and the adjacent vertebral body. Multiple levels of involvement are not uncommon, and the levels may be contiguous or noncontiguous. Lateral extension causes a paraspinal abscess; posterior extension can result in epidural abscess, cord compression, and meningitis.

The radiographic finding is disk space narrowing with destruction of the facing vertebral endplates. As the process evolves, increasing reactive bone production and sclerosis occur in the affected vertebral bodies on both sides of the involved disk space, often making it appear widened (Figs. 16.10–16.12). Bony ankylosis is one eventual outcome of this process. Paravertebral soft-tissue swelling may indicate extension into the soft tissues. CT and MRI can delineate the anatomic extent of involvement.

**FIGURE 16.7.** CT scan of chronic sclerosing osteomyelitis of the clavicle.

**A**                                                                **B**

**FIGURE 16.9.** Brodie abscess in the proximal tibia. **A:** Coronal T1-weighted MRI shows central lesion (*arrow*) with surrounding sclerosis. **B:** Coronal T1-weighted gadolinium-enhanced MRI shows enhancement of the periphery of the lesion (*arrow*), but not the center.

The clinical presentation is fever, back pain, and stiffness. Diagnosis is often delayed; radiographic findings may not be apparent until 2 to 8 weeks after onset. In 60% of cases, the recovered organisms are *S. aureus*; in 30% of cases, the organisms are species of *Enterobacteriaceae*. In 40% of cases, a remote source of infection is known (usually genitourinary tract, skin, or respiratory tract).

# ■ MISCELLANEOUS INFECTIONS
## Tuberculosis

Tuberculosis is becoming more common in North America but is usually associated with immunocompromised patients or immigrant populations. Musculoskeletal disease is the result of hematogenous spread, typically from the lungs. Perhaps half of all cases of musculoskeletal tuberculosis affect the spine. The body of L1 is the site most commonly affected, but involvement of multiple contiguous levels is frequent, and involvement of the cervical and thoracic region, posterior elements, and SI joints is known to occur. The infection usually begins in the anterior aspect of the vertebral body at an endplate. Infection may spread by extending into the disk space, along the subligamentous space, or into the paraspinal soft tissues (Fig. 16.13). Paravertebral psoas abscesses may burrow into the groin or thigh.

Tuberculosis may spread to the joints, resulting in a granulomatous synovial infection that requires synovial biopsy or joint aspiration for diagnosis. In the usual situation, the process is monoarticular and there is osteomyelitis adjacent to the involved joint. The classic radiographic appearance is juxta-articular osteoporosis, peripherally located erosions, and gradual joint space narrowing. However, multifocal disease, periostitis, sclerosis, and large soft-tissue abscesses may occur.

Tuberculous osteomyelitis may result from contiguous spread from an adjacent joint or from hematogenous spread. The ends of long bones are typically involved, and there may be multiple sites of involvement within the same bone or dispersed throughout the

**FIGURE 16.10.** Vertebral discitis and osteomyelitis with destruction of the adjacent inferior and superior endplates (*arrow*).

**FIGURE 16.11.** Lumbar vertebral discitis. **A:** Sagittal inversion recovery MRI shows fluid at the L4–5 disk space (*arrow*) and edema of adjacent vertebral body endplates. **B:** Sagittal T1-weighted fat-suppressed post-gadolinium MRI shows enhancement (*arrow*) around the L4–5 disk space.

**FIGURE 16.12.** Vertebral discitis, osteomyelitis, and epidural abscess. **A:** Sagittal T1-weighted MRI shows infection of the C6–7 level with epidural mass (*arrow*). **B:** Sagittal T1-weighted gadolinium-enhanced MRI shows an enhancing inflammatory mass with a low signal in the center. **C:** Axial CT scan at C6 shows vertebral body destruction.

**FIGURE 16.13.** TB spondylitis. **A:** Radiograph at presentation shows loss of height at the L3–4 disk level and early inferior endplate destruction at L3 (*arrow*). **B:** CT shows bone destruction and paraspinal inflammation. **C:** Axial T2-weighted MRI shows paraspinal inflammatory mass (*short arrow*) with left psoas muscle abscess (*long arrow*). **D:** Radiograph after 1 month shows further destruction of L3.

skeleton. On radiographs, osteolysis, erosions, and osteoporosis are the dominant features (Fig. 16.14). Soft-tissue extension with burrowing abscesses may be present, but reactive bone formation is sparse or absent. On MRI, the region of involvement has low signal on T1-weighted images and high signal on T2-weighted images, with enhancement after gadolinium injection. Periosteal reactive bone and subperiosteal involvement tend to be absent, unlike acute pyogenic osteomyelitis.

## Fungal Infections

Fungal infections are caused by dimorphic pathogenetic organisms. The mycelial form of the organism produces infectious spores that may be inhaled and converted to yeastlike pathogens in the host. The entire range of fungal infections that occur in the lungs may also involve the musculoskeletal system, especially coccidioidomycosis, histoplasmosis, and blastomycosis. The infections are often

**FIGURE 16.14.** Tuberculosis osteomyelitis. **A:** Coronal CT reformation of the knee shows focal lucency with sclerotic center (*arrow*) at the medial tibial metaphysis with overlying soft-tissue swelling. There is no reactive bone formation. **B:** Coronal T1 MRI shows focal bone lesion with sequestrum, cortical penetration, and soft-tissue swelling. **C:** Coronal T2 MRI shows high signal within the lesion and adjacent soft tissues. There is a joint effusion.

low grade and chronic but may become virulent when host defenses are compromised. Opportunistic infections such as candidiasis may also occur in immunocompromised individuals. Radiologic features of fungal osteomyelitis include osteolysis with discrete or permeated margins, surrounding sclerosis that is less florid than in bacterial infections, and variable amounts of periosteal reaction (Fig. 16.15). Extensive bone sclerosis and formation of sequestra are unusual. Fungal septic arthritis has a nonspecific appearance with soft-tissue swelling, diffuse joint space loss, and central and marginal erosions of bone. The progression of disease is slower and the host bone reaction milder than pyogenic infections.

**FIGURE 16.15.** Candidal osteomyelitis of the humerus. CT shows focal bone destruction and minimal reactive change.

## Cellulitis

Cellulitis is diffuse purulent inflammation of the loose subcutaneous soft tissues. The process may disseminate along anatomic planes. The early clinical presentation of cellulitis— particularly in children—is virtually identical to that of early osteomyelitis, but direct extension of cellulitis through the cortex of adjacent bone into the marrow space to cause osteomyelitis occurs only occasionally. On radiographs, cellulitis is evident as soft-tissue swelling and obliteration of normal tissue planes, the same early radiographic features of osteomyelitis. If a gas-forming organism is involved, soft tissue gas may be present. The three-phase bone scan can distinguish between cellulitis and osteomyelitis. On immediate postinjection flow images (radionuclide angiogram) and on blood pool images (obtained 5 min after injection, reflecting distribution of radionuclide in the extra-vascular space), both cellulitis and osteomyelitis show diffusely increased soft-tissue uptake. However, on delayed images (obtained 2 hours after injection), cellulitis shows no focal abnormality, but osteomyelitis shows focal tracer uptake in bone at the site of infection. MRI and CT are also highly accurate in delineating soft-tissue infections. On MRI, cellulitis is evident as reticular subcutaneous edema and enhancement after gadolinium injection (Fig. 16.16). Edema and enhancement of the underlying fascia, muscle, and bone are indicative of fasciitis, myositis, and osteomyelitis, respectively. If present, soft-tissue abscesses show rim enhancement after gadolinium injection. Soft-tissue gas is more difficult to identify on MRI than CT.

Noninfectious subcutaneous edema—as might occur after a bite from a spider or snake or after an allergic reaction to a bee sting—results in soft-tissue edema. The radiologic appearance is similar to infectious cellulitis except that gas formation and abscess formation do not occur. Osteomyelitis of the underlying bone does not occur.

## Necrotizing Fasciitis

Necrotizing fasciitis is an uncommon, deep soft-tissue infection caused by group A streptococci. Known in the lay literature as the

**FIGURE 16.16.** Cellulitis of the foot in a diabetic shown by axial MRI. **A:** T1-weighted images shows low signal in the lateral subcutaneous tissues (*arrow*). **B:** inversion recovery image shows edema (*arrow*). **C:** Following gadolinium-based contrast injection, T1-weighted fat-suppressed image shows enhancement (*arrow*).

disease caused by "flesh-eating bacteria," necrotizing fasciitis has a mortality rate of approximately 25%. Although it occurs more frequently in diabetics, intravenous drug abusers, immunosuppressed patients, and patients at risk for other infections, it may also occur in young and previously healthy patients, including athletes. The abdominal wall, extremities, and perineum are the most common sites of involvement, and necrotizing fasciitis may occur with streptococcal toxic shock syndrome. Both direct implantation of bacteria through a break in the skin and hematogenous spread may occur. Patients present with severe local pain, skin changes, and systemic toxicity. Radiographs of necrotizing fasciitis in the extremities may show extensive subcutaneous edema and gas (Fig. 16.17). The gas may track along fascial planes. On CT, gas in the soft tissues is more easily identified than on radiographs (Fig. 16.18). Diffuse thickening of the skin, edema of the subcutaneous tissues, thickening of the fascia, and fluid collections are other features of CT. On MRI, involved fascial planes have low signal on T1-weighted images and high signal on T2-weighted images. Enhancement of the fascia after gadolinium injection is indicative of inflammation, whereas lack of enhancement is indicative of tissue necrosis.

**FIGURE 16.17.** Necrotizing fasciitis of upper right arm in a patient with acute promyelocytic leukemia, showing gas (*arrow*) in the subcutaneous tissues and muscles.

**FIGURE 16.18.** Necrotizing fasciitis in the deep posterior compartment of the leg. Axial CT slice shows muscle edema and bubbles of gas (*arrow*).

**FIGURE 16.19.** Pyomyositis with abscess in the soleus muscle of the leg of an immunosuppressed patient. **A:** Axial T2-weighted MRI shows heterogeneous high signal in a lesion (*arrow*) in the soleus, with extensive subcutaneous edema and obliteration of the normal fat between the muscle fascicles. **B:** Axial T1-weighted fat-suppressed post-gadolinium MRI shows enhancement of the superficial posterior compartment and the rim of the abscess (*arrow*).

## Pyomyositis

Pyomyositis is caused by *S. aureus* in approximately 90% of cases; most of the remaining cases are caused by *Streptococcus*. Because healthy muscle is resistant to hematogenous infections, pyomyositis usually is found in the presence of predisposing conditions such as local trauma, nutritional deficiency, immunocompromise, or concurrent infections elsewhere. Pyomyositis is relatively unusual outside the tropics. Imaging by sonography, CT, or MRI shows extensive inflammation and abscess formation (Fig. 16.19). Direct extension to bone may occur. The definitive diagnosis is made by aspiration and culture.

## Gas Gangrene

Clostridial contamination of traumatic wounds may produce extensive tissue damage and gas formation in devitalized tissues (gas gangrene). The causative agent, *Clostridium perfringens*, is widely

**FIGURE 16.20.** Clostridia myonecrosis with widespread dissection of gas along muscle fibers, resulting in a feathery appearance.

**FIGURE 16.21.** Cysticercosis with calcified larvae in the posterior musculature.

distributed in nature. Unlike deep group A streptococcal infections, clostridial infections spare the fascia but cause rapid necrosis of muscle. Clostridial myositis is an acute, rapidly progressive, invasive infection of muscle that often results in myonecrosis and systemic toxicity. Exotoxins elaborated by the bacteria promote the rapid spread of infection by destroying healthy tissue and interfering with normal host responses. Clostridial myonecrosis has a classic radiographic appearance of extensive featherlike linear collections of gas that are widely dispersed throughout the affected muscles (Fig. 16.20). Therapy for clostridial myonecrosis includes surgery, antibiotics, and hyperbaric oxygen, with reported mortality rates of 5% to nearly 30%.

## Parasitic Infestation

Cysticercosis—infestation by the larval form of the pork tapeworm—may cause dense, widespread calcifications in the muscular tissues. Calcification is a late finding that is seen years after infestation. Larval death evokes a foreign body reaction that causes localized tissue necrosis with caseation. The calcifications may be up to 3 cm in size and tend to be oriented with the muscle fibers (Fig. 16.21). Parasitic infestation with other worms is unusual in the United States except among immigrants from endemic tropical regions of the world.

## Leprosy

Leprosy is a chronic granulomatous infection of the skin, peripheral nerves, mucous membranes, and other organs. It becomes evident after a lengthy incubation. Caused by *Mycobacterium leprae*, the disease is virtually unknown in the United States except among immigrants from Africa, South America, and parts of Asia. The most common radiographic abnormalities in leprosy are related to involvement of the peripheral nerves. Atrophic neuropathic osteoarthropathy may result from denervation and repetitive minor injury. On radiographs, findings may include atrophy, resorption, and tapering of the ends of the bones, particularly of the digits of the hands and feet. Involvement is generally asymmetric. Leprous periostitis, osteitis, and osteomyelitis occur, but they do so infrequently. There is a propensity for the development of squamous cell carcinoma at sites of cutaneous ulcerations. There is an increased risk of developing lymphoma and leukemia.

## HIV Infection and AIDS

Infection with HIV devastates cellular-mediated immunity, leading at a variable rate to AIDS and death. Musculoskeletal manifestations are less common than manifestations in the central nervous system, the gastrointestinal tract, and the lungs. These include infections, neoplasms, and rheumatologic conditions. Osteomyelitis may be caused by common and opportunistic organisms, including *S. aureus*, *Salmonella*, tuberculosis, fungus, and *Rochalimaea henselae* (the rickettsial species that causes bacillary angiomatosis). Bacterial myositis and septic arthritis may also be caused by common and opportunistic organisms. Non-Hodgkin lymphoma has an incidence 60 times greater in AIDS patients than in the general population. Primary and secondary involvement of the marrow is common. Kaposi sarcoma also may metastasize to bone. Anemia is common in HIV-positive patients and leads to reconversion of fatty (yellow) marrow to hematopoietic (red) marrow. Polymyositis and inflammatory arthritis have been reported in AIDS patients.

## ■ MARROW AND STORAGE DISEASES

The bone marrow is one of the largest organs of the body. Confined to the intramedullary space of bone, it consists of a meshwork of trabecular bone with fat cells, myeloid cells, reticulum cells, and supporting structures. At birth, the marrow cavities of tubular bones, flat bones, and vertebrae have a predominance of hematopoietic cells. With advancing age, the hematopoietic marrow regresses and is replaced by fatty marrow, beginning distally in the extremities and progressing to encompass incompletely the pelvis, spine, and cranium. The process may reverse (marrow reconversion) when there is an increased demand for hematopoiesis, as may occur in anemia or replacement of normal hematopoietic marrow by a pathologic process.

Radiographic findings of marrow disorders are indirect and nonspecific. When chronic marrow space expansion occurs in the growing skeleton, adaptive bone changes may occur during the development of the bone. Actual enlargement of the marrow space alters the normal bony contours; such changes do not occur acutely nor do they occur in the adult. The best method for direct imaging of the bone marrow is MRI. Because marrow is a conglomeration of different tissues, the appearance on MRI may vary, with the composition of the marrow as well as with the particular technical parameters. In general, fatty marrow has the predominant signal characteristics of fat, and hematopoietic marrow has signal characteristics more similar to muscle. Nuclear scans with technetium-99m (99mTc) sulfur colloid and 99mTc-methylene diphosphonate can provide physiologic assessments of the reticuloendothelial marrow elements and the surrounding bone, respectively.

## Mucopolysaccharidoses

The mucopolysaccharidoses are a spectrum of hereditary diseases resulting from various enzyme deficiencies in the metabolism of mucopolysaccharides. The individual diseases are differentiated by clinical features, inheritance, and specific biochemical defect, but all of them result in deposits of abnormal metabolites in the central nervous system, marrow space, and other sites. Dwarfism is common to all, and they have similar radiographic features that are collectively referred to as *dysostosis multiplex*. These features include macrocephaly with premature closure of the sagittal suture, hypoplastic paranasal and mastoid sinuses, a J-shaped sella, canoe paddle–shaped ribs, focal thoracolumbar kyphosis, and a distinctive hypoplastic "spinnaker sail" vertebra in the upper lumbar region with an inferior beak (Fig. 16.22). The diaphyseal and metaphyseal regions of the long bones are expanded, there is delayed epiphyseal ossification and cortical thinning, the iliac wings are flared with narrow supra-acetabular portions, and the metacarpals are short and wide with tapered ends.

## Gaucher Disease

The prototype for the lipid storage diseases is Gaucher disease (glucocerebroside lipidosis). In this autosomal-recessive condition, deficiency of glucocerebrosidase results in the progressive accumulation of histiocytes laden with glucocerebroside lipids in the bone marrow and other organs and tissues. Secondary changes in bone are observed. The classic radiographic finding is the Erlenmeyer flask deformity, which is undermodeling of the metaphysis due to marrow space packing (Fig. 16.23). Cortical thinning by endosteal erosion and osteopenia are additional radiographic abnormalities that may be evident. Osteonecrosis of the femoral head is a common association; this event is usually bilateral. After prolonged

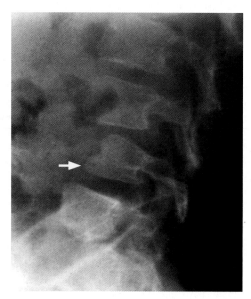

**FIGURE 16.22.** Hunter syndrome (MPS II). Lateral lumbar spine radiograph at age 11 shows hypoplastic "spinnaker sail" vertebra with inferior beak (*arrow*).

enzyme replacement therapy with macrophage-targeted glucocerebrosidase (glucosylceramidase), marrow composition, bone mass, and bone morphology revert toward normal.

# ■ OSTEONECROSIS (AVASCULAR NECROSIS, ASEPTIC NECROSIS)

Most bones have a dual blood supply. The periosteum has a rich network of vessels that supplies the periosteal portion of the cortex. The endosteal blood supply enters through one or more nutrient arteries and supplies the marrow, the trabecular bone, and the endosteal portion of the cortex. Portions of bone that are covered with articular cartilage or enclosed within joint capsules have no periosteum and therefore have only an endosteal blood supply, leaving them more vulnerable to ischemic infarction.

## Femoral Head

The femoral head is the most important clinical site of osteonecrosis. Men are affected more often than women (by 4:1), and the usual age range of patients is 30 to 70 years. The typical presentation is abrupt onset of hip pain without trauma. In 50% of cases, bilateral involvement is present; bilateral disease is usually asymmetric.

Osteonecrosis begins with interruption of the blood supply to the femoral head. The precise event that initiates the loss of circulation may be unknown, although a large number of clinical conditions appear to be associated with it (Table 16.1). One possible event is an increase in intraosseous pressure within the femoral head; when this pressure exceeds the perfusion pressure, blood flow stops. Ischemic necrosis of the marrow and bone follows with the onset of pain, but radiographs are normal. Intramedullary pressure measurements of the proximal femur are elevated. The typical distribution of infarction is a wedge-shaped region under the weight-bearing surface of the femoral head. The articular cartilage itself remains viable because its nutrition is derived from the synovial fluid. After infarction, the avascular area becomes revascularized from the periphery, and creeping substitution of devitalized bone occurs. When repair begins, plain films may show an increase in bony density around the periphery of the infarction. This increased peripheral density may slowly progress centrally as repair proceeds. Sometimes, the dead bone is incompletely resorbed, and a sclerotic zone remains indefinitely (Fig. 16.24). Because this repair process involves both resorption and replacement of bone, the mechanical strength may decrease transiently, and subchondral insufficiency fractures may result. Insufficiency fractures of the subchondral bone may be recognized by a crescentic lucent zone that separates the fragment. This late segmental collapse of the femoral head may lead rapidly to deformity and secondary osteoarthritis of the hip.

**FIGURE 16.23.** Gaucher disease. **A:** AP radiograph of both knees shows Erlenmeyer flask deformities of the femurs and tibias. **B:** Coronal T1-weighted MRI shows uniform replacement of the fatty marrow.

| TABLE 16.1 | Clinical Conditions Associated with Osteonecrosis of the Femoral Head in Adults |
|---|---|
| **Unilateral** | **Bilateral** |
| *Commonly associated conditions* | |
| Idiopathic | Alcoholism |
| Trauma | Corticosteroids |
| Surgery | Idiopathic |
| *Uncommonly associated conditions* | |
| Gout | Arteriosclerosis |
| Hemophilia | Caisson disease |
| Infection | Cushing disease |
| | Gaucher disease |
| | Hemoglobinopathy |
| | Systemic lupus erythematosus |
| | Pancreatitis |
| | Pheochromocytoma |
| | Rheumatoid arthritis |

**FIGURE 16.24.** Osteonecrosis of the right femoral head with collapse of the articular surface. The left femoral head is also osteonecrotic.

Early osteonecrosis is best demonstrated by MRI. The region of osteonecrosis is evident as a loss of the normal bright marrow signal on T1-weighted MRI (Fig. 16.25). Characteristically, the region of involvement is the superior weight-bearing quadrant of the femoral head. If marrow edema is present in the femoral head and sometimes, femoral neck, then the osteonecrosis is acute or subacute. Hip effusion is commonly present. As the osteonecrosis begins to remodel, edema and revascularization result in the "double line" sign. On T2-weighted MRI, the region of osteonecrosis is circumscribed by a peripheral zone of high signal and an adjacent outer zone of low signal. MRI can also depict late osteonecrosis and subchondral collapse of the femoral head. The radionuclide bone scan may initially show loss of radionuclide accumulation in the avascular stage with subsequent variable increases in accumulation in the reparative stage. The nuclear scan is less sensitive than MRI and gives poor anatomic detail. The common asymmetric bilaterality of osteonecrosis of the femoral head may complicate interpretation of the bone scan. The most sensitive test for early osteonecrosis of the femoral head is intramedullary pressure measurement.

Osteonecrosis may be treated by decompression of the femoral head, usually by drilling a hole in the lateral cortex through the neck and into the head. Sometimes a tantalum insert or vascularized bone graft is placed to encourage bone growth. Hemiarthroplasty and total joint replacement are options for end-stage disease.

A

B

**FIGURE 16.25.** Osteonecrosis of the femoral head. **A:** Coronal T1-weighted MRI shows serpentine low signal (*arrow*) surrounding the region of osteonecrosis. **B:** Axial T2-weighted fat-suppressed MRI shows subchondral collapse (*arrow*).

## Spontaneous Osteonecrosis of the Knee

Spontaneous osteonecrosis of the knee is typically found in adult women older than 50 years of age who present with persistent knee pain and tenderness. The medial femoral condyle is most commonly involved, but the lateral femoral condyle or even the tibial plateau may be affected. There is some controversy whether the lesion actually represents an insufficiency fracture. In any event, the condition appears to be self-limited, with resolution within a few months, but subchondral collapse may lead to secondary osteoarthritis. Radiographs may be normal, but if subchondral collapse occurs, then sclerosis, subchondral lucency, flattening of the condyle, and eventual secondary degenerative joint disease may be seen. On MRI, the affected region initially shows a geographic area of signal abnormality, with decreased signal on T1-weighted images and increased signal on T2-weighted images (Fig. 16.26). As the area becomes revascularized and remodels, the region of osteonecrosis becomes better defined by low signal around the periphery. If the lesion progresses to subchondral collapse, the condyle may become flattened, and overlying articular cartilage may be lost.

## Other Sites

Osteonecrosis has been described at various sites in the skeleton. The pathophysiology is the same regardless of site and follows the stages described above: ischemia, revascularization, repair, deformity, and osteoarthrosis. Examples include osteonecrosis of the humeral head (Fig. 16.27), osteonecrosis of the lunate (Kienböck disease) (Figs. 16.28 and 16.29). On MRI, medullary infarcts are usually multiple and have a diagnostic appearance. They have an irregular, serpiginous, sharply defined low signal border on T1-weighted and proton density (PD) images (Fig. 16.30). If there is a surrounding zone of high signal on T2-weighted MRI, then the infarcts are

**FIGURE 16.27.** Osteonecrosis of the humeral head. Coronal T1-weighted MRI shows subchondral collapse (*arrow*) of the humeral head.

acute or subacute. This zone of high signal on T2-weighted images corresponds to the margin of revascularization and remodeling. Contemporaneous radiographs are often normal, but the infarcted marrow may eventually calcify (Fig. 16.31). This dystrophic calcification in infarcts may resemble the mineralized matrix of an endosteal cartilage tumor.

**FIGURE 16.26.** Spontaneous osteonecrosis of the knee. Coronal inversion recovery MRI shows high signal (*arrow*) in the medial femoral condyle.

**FIGURE 16.28.** Osteonecrosis of the lunate (Kienböck disease) (*arrow*).

**FIGURE 16.29.** Osteonecrosis of the lunate (Kienböck disease). Coronal T1-weighted MRI shows sclerosis and deformity of the lunate (*arrow*).

## Osteochondroses

The osteochondroses are a group of heterogeneous conditions in which there is osteonecrosis of a growing epiphysis or apophysis. These are described in Chapter 14.

## ■ HEMATOLOGIC DISEASES
### Sickle Cell Anemia

Sickle cell disease is caused by an inherited structural defect in hemoglobin that leads to red cell dysfunction. The radiologic features of sickle cell disease in bone are the result of bone marrow hyperplasia, vascular occlusion, and osteomyelitis. Hyperplasia

**FIGURE 16.31.** Calcified marrow infarcts in the femur and tibia.

of the bone marrow expands the marrow space. Vascular occlusion results in osteonecrosis. Any portion of any bone may be involved; frequent sites include the medullary space of long bones, growing epiphyses, and the hands. Multiple small infarcts sustained over a period of years may result in sclerotic bones (Fig. 16.32). New periosteal bone apposed to necrotic cortex may result in a double layer of cortex that has been likened to tram tracks. Involvement of growing epiphyses leads to growth disturbances; if the femoral head is involved, the pathophysiologic events and sequelae are indistinguishable from those of Legg-Calvé-Perthes disease. A growth disturbance in the vertebral body leads to development of H-shaped

**FIGURE 16.30.** Medullary bone infarcts. Coronal T1-weighted MRI shows infarcts in the femur and tibia.

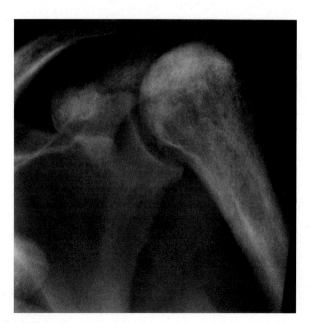

**FIGURE 16.32.** Sickle cell disease with diffuse sclerosis of the humerus from multiple infarcts.

**FIGURE 16.33.** Sickle cell disease with H-shaped vertebral bodies from infarctions during development.

vertebrae (Fig. 16.33). Localized infarctions of bone with repair or dystrophic calcification result in focal areas of bony sclerosis scattered about the skeleton. Hemosiderosis may follow repeated transfusions of blood (Fig. 16.34).

Patients with sickle cell disease have a high incidence of osteomyelitis. Unlike hematogenous osteomyelitis in other situations, the infection in sickle cell disease is most frequent at the diaphysis of the long bones, where the oxygen tension is lowest. In approximately

50% of cases, *Salmonella* species or mixed flora are the causative organisms (their presence is exceedingly unusual under any other circumstance); the remaining cases are usually caused by *Staphylococcus* species. Chronicity and recurrence are common. Osteomyelitis may be difficult to differentiate from infarction on both clinical and radiologic grounds; either one can be a complication of the other. The radiographic signs of osteomyelitis are superimposed on whatever preexisting bone changes are present from the sickle cell disease.

## Thalassemia

Thalassemia comprises a group of disorders caused by inherited abnormalities of globin production that lead to ineffective hematopoiesis and anemia. The defect is in the synthesis of one of the globin chains. There are many types of thalassemia that are distinguished on the basis of the specific globin chain affected and the particular molecular defect present. The radiologic findings of thalassemia in bone result from marrow hyperplasia and marrow space expansion. These lead to growth disturbances, modeling deformities from marrow space packing (Fig. 16.35), and premature closure of the growth plate. Localized bone infarcts and insufficiency fractures occur occasionally. Secondary hemochromatosis may follow repeated transfusions of blood. Bone marrow transplant may be curative and should lead to regression of the skeletal abnormalities.

## Hemophilia

Classic hemophilia is a bleeding diathesis caused by a sex-linked hereditary deficiency of coagulation factor VIII. Hemophilia B (Christmas disease) is a hereditary deficiency of factor IX, and hemophilia C is a hereditary deficiency of factor XI. The clinical features are similar, and the radiologic manifestations are

**FIGURE 16.34.** Sickle cell hemosiderosis. Coronal T1-weighted MRI of the pelvis shows marrow replacement.

**FIGURE 16.35.** Thalassemia with manifestation in the foot. The marrow spaces are packed with hematopoietic elements, causing the bones to have thin, scalloped cortices without much medullary structure.

**FIGURE 16.36.** Hemophiliac knee. **A:** Lateral radiograph shows marked synovial hypertrophy and effusion (*arrows*), with epiphyseal overgrowth. **B:** AP radiograph shows squaring of the condyles and degenerative changes.

indistinguishable. Approximately 90% of hemophiliac patients have spontaneous or traumatic hemarthrosis involving the large joints, often in repeated episodes. The hemarthroses are monoarticular in 70% of cases. The knee is most commonly affected, followed in frequency by the elbow or ankle (Fig. 16.36). Different joints may become involved in succession, leading to polyarticular involvement. During an acute bleed, joint effusion and osteoporosis may be seen. Chronic or repeated hemorrhage leads to synovial hypertrophy and chronic inflammation. As the abnormal synovium extends across the articular surface, the cartilage is dissolved, leading to degenerative changes. Subchondral cyst formation is common,

and overgrowth of the epiphyses results from chronic hyperemia; the younger the age at which these events begin, the more severe the changes. Secondary degenerative joint disease follows the destruction of the articular cartilage. Intraosseous bleeding and the subsequent inflammatory reaction that clears the hemorrhage may create radiolucent defects in bone called *pseudotumors*. Repeated bleeding into a pseudotumor may cause it to recur and enlarge, simulating malignancy (Fig. 16.37). When such a pseudotumor is large enough to contain several units of blood, life-threatening hemorrhage is possible. Many hemophiliacs have been infected with HIV during transfusions with contaminated blood products.

**FIGURE 16.37.** Hemophilia with pseudotumor in the pelvis. **A:** AP radiograph of the pelvis shows a large, expansile, lucent lesion involving the left iliac wing. **B:** CT scan shows heterogeneous attenuation within the mass without calcification.

## SOURCES AND READINGS

Berquist TH, ed. *MRI of the Musculoskeletal System.* 5th Ed. Philadelphia, PA: Lippincott Williams & Wilkins; 2005.

eMedicine. http://emedicine.medscape.com.

Fontes RA Jr, Ogilvie CM, Miclau T. Necrotizing soft-tissue infections. *J Am Acad Orthop Surg.* 2000;8:151–158

Griffin LY. *Essentials of Musculoskeletal Care.* 3rd Ed. Rosemont, IL: American Academy of Orthopedics; 2005.

Heitmann C, Patzakis MJ, Tetsworth KD, Levin LS. Musculoskeletal sepsis: Principles of treatment. *Instr Course Lect.* 2003;52:733–743.

Hirsch R, Miller SM, Kazi S, et al. Human immunodeficiency virus-associated atypical mycobacterial skeletal infections. *Semin Arthritis Rheum.* 1996;25:347–356.

Lew DP, Waldvogel FA. Osteomyelitis. *N Engl J Med.* 1997;336:999–1007.

Morton KA, Clark PB, Christensen CR, et al. *Diagnostic Imaging: Nuclear Medicine.* Salt Lake City: Amirsys; 2007

Resnick DL, Kransdorf MJ. *Bone and Joint Imaging.* 3rd Ed. Philadelphia, PA: WB Saunders; 2004

Steinbach LS, Tehranzadeh J, Fleckenstein JL, et al. Human immunodeficiency virus infection: Musculoskeletal manifestations. *Radiology.* 1993;186:833–838.

Tehranzadeh J, Wong E, Wang F, et al. Imaging of osteomyelitis in the mature skeleton. *Radiol Clin North Am.* 2001;39:223–250.

Trueta J. *Studies in the Development and Decay of the Human Frame.* Philadelphia, PA: WB Saunders; 1968.

Wheelees CR III, ed. *Wheeless' Textbook of Orthopaedics.* http://www.wheelessonline.com.

Wong CH, Chang HC, Pasupathy S, Khin LW, Tan JL, Low CO. Necrotizing fasciitis: Clinical presentation, microbiology, and determinants of mortality. *J Bone Joint Surg Am.* 2003;85:1454–1460.

# Postsurgical Imaging

## ■ IMAGING TECHNIQUES

Viewing images of postsurgical orthopedic patients can be mind-numbing if one does not understand the surgery that was performed. This chapter describes the imaging of the musculoskeletal system after a variety of orthopedic operations. Imaging after fracture treatment is described in Chapter 6.

The standard diagnostic imaging techniques for the musculoskeletal system can be applied to postsurgical patients. Many operations are guided by the use of intraoperative fluoroscopy or radiographs. Standard radiographs are generally obtained immediately after the surgery to document the postoperative results. At follow-up visits, radiographs are obtained to monitor healing and to screen for complications. When extensive hardware has been implanted, nonstandard, obliquely positioned radiographs—or even radiographs positioned under fluoroscopy—may be necessary to project the hardware away from the bone, allowing it to be visualized. More specialized techniques are generally reserved for problem solving. CT can be used to evaluate the progress of healing when radiographs are equivocal, especially in the presence of complex anatomy and hardware. Streak artifacts on CT result from the high X-ray attenuation by metal (Fig. 17.1). Improvements in CT scanners and reconstruction algorithms and in orthopedic hardware materials have reduced the impact of these artifacts. On MRI, extensive artifacts may be caused by metallic implants (Fig. 17.2). Large implants may affect the surrounding magnetic field and cause the computer to distort the anatomy around the implants. Even when no hardware has been left behind, artifacts may be present from microscopic metallic particles introduced by instruments. These artifacts tend to be minimized on T1-weighted images but become more extensive ("bloom") on T2-weighted or inversion recovery images (Fig. 17.3). However, previous surgery and orthopedic implants are not contraindications to MRI, and MRI may provide useful information in many situations. Arthrography should be considered when there is a question of joint infection or other postsurgical joint abnormalities. Stress views or examination under fluoroscopy may document motion at sites where none was intended. Radionuclide bone scan is useless in the immediate postoperative period because of tracer uptake at the surgical site. However, tracer accumulation returns toward normal after approximately 6 months, after which time the bone scan may be helpful (Fig. 17.4). Imaging with labeled leukocytes or gallium-67 may be indicated when there is a question of infection.

## ■ OSTEOTOMY

An osteotomy is any operation that involves a surgical cut through the bone. Osteotomies are commonly performed to change the alignment, length, or shape of a bone. For example, a fracture malunion with angular deformity may be revised by an osteotomy that realigns the fragments. Osteotomies may be described by their site and the direction of change in the distal fragment. A valgus osteotomy of a long bone realigns the distal fragment into the valgus relative to its original alignment. A lateral displacement osteotomy repositions the distal fragment laterally. Changes in the rotational alignment may also be made; these are called *rotational osteotomies*. Shortening is accomplished by the removal of a bone. Lengthening may be accomplished by displacement of overlapping fragments by the insertion of a bone graft or by bone distraction using an external fixator. The fixation and healing of osteotomies are similar to that of fractures, and the hardware devices used to treat fractures are applicable (see Chapter 6). Complications of healing are rare.

Osteotomies are also used to alter the alignment and biomechanics of joints. A high tibial valgus osteotomy is a common treatment for severe medial compartment osteoarthritis with varus deformity (Fig. 17.5). By realigning the tibial shaft, the varus deformity is corrected, and the mechanical axis of the knee is restored. This has the effect of reducing the weight-bearing stress on the diseased medial compartment and redistributing some of it to the lateral compartment. Distal femoral varus osteotomies can correct valgus deformities at the knee from the lateral compartment osteoarthritis. Similarly, angular or rotational osteotomies of the proximal femur alter the major weight-bearing portion of the femoral head in the treatment of hip dysplasia, early osteoarthritis, or similar conditions. An innominate osteotomy may be used to deepen the acetabulum.

A bunion is a symptomatic protrusion at the medial aspect of the head of the first metatarsal that is the result of a valgus deformity of the great toe and a varus deformity of the first metatarsal

**FIGURE 17.1.** Coronal reconstruction of CT scan through TKR shows severe artifact from the presence of metal, yet the metal-bone interface (*arrow*) of the tibial component is clearly visible.

**FIGURE 17.3.** MR with metal artifact from metal surgical instruments. T1-weighted axial spine MRI shows very dark areas (*arrow*) overlying the skin and the left posterolateral spinal canal in this patient with laminectomy. There were no actual metal clips or other implants present.

(also called *hallux valgus primus varus*). Tension along the flexors and extensors of the great toe acts like bowstrings to increase the angular deformities. The condition may be painful and is often compounded by the difficulty of fitting shoes. Surgical correction involves not only removing the bony prominence but also—more important—realigning the great toe with its flexors and extensors. Commonly, the first metatarsal is shortened, and the head is displaced laterally (Fig. 17.6).

**FIGURE 17.2.** Coronal T2-weighted MRI of the pelvis with major metal artifact on the left side due to the presence of a total hip replacement. The artifact (*arrow*) extends well above the actual location of the replacement.

**FIGURE 17.4.** Anterior view of the radionuclide bone scan of the patient with bilateral total hip replacements. A stress fracture was present in the lateral femoral cortex on the left (*arrow*).

**FIGURE 17.5.** High tibial valgus osteotomy with external fixator.

## ■ ARTHRODESIS

An arthrodesis is a surgical fusion of a joint. An intra-articular arthrodesis is accomplished by resecting the joint and fixing the ends of the articulating bones together. Internal or external fixa-

**FIGURE 17.7.** Ankle arthrodesis with locked IM rod fixation.

tion may be used as well as bone graft. A healed and remodeled arthrodesis has a continuous cortex and trabecular structure across the site. Adaptive changes may occur in adjacent joints in response to the loss of motion. Joint pain in arthritis can be eliminated by synovectomy and arthrodesis. Common sites for arthrodesis include the fingers, for treatment of arthritis; the wrist, for treatment of arthritis or posttraumatic instability; and the subtalar joint, for treatment of posttraumatic arthritis. One of the more common arthrodeses involving the foot is the triple arthrodesis, in which the subtalar joints, calcaneocuboid joints, and talonavicular joints are arthrodesed (Fig. 17.7). In the setting of arthritis, it may sometimes be difficult to distinguish an arthrodesis from a bony ankylosis (joint fusion caused by a disease). An extra-articular arthrodesis is accomplished by establishing a bony bridge across a joint that prevents motion without actually resecting the joint itself. Some spine fusions involve an extra-articular arthrodesis. An epiphysiodesis, a surgical fusion of an open growth plate, may be performed for correction of growth discrepancy.

## ■ ARTHROPLASTY

An arthroplasty is a surgical repair of a joint. Resection arthroplasty involves excision of one or both of the articular surfaces, leaving the ends of the bone to articulate with each other. Because the joint is not fixed, a pseudoarthrosis develops, preserving motion. Common sites for resection arthroplasty include the toes and hip. Many toe deformities result from soft-tissue contractures. Reducing the length of the bone through resection arthroplasty eliminates the effect of contractures (Fig. 17.8). Resection arthroplasty may be performed with resection of a small bone at a painful joint such as the trapezium from the first carpometacarpal (CMC) joint (Fig. 17.9). At the hip, a resection arthroplasty is called a *Girdlestone procedure*. Replacement arthroplasty involves replacing one or more articular surfaces with a prosthesis (discussed in "Joint Replacement").

**FIGURE 17.6.** Bunion repair with shortening and displacement osteotomy of the first metatarsal, fixed by K-wire. Also note osteotomy of the proximal phalanx of the great toe (*arrow*).

**FIGURE 17.8.** Resection arthroplasty of the IP joint (*arrow*) of the fifth toe.

**FIGURE 17.9.** Resection arthroplasty of the first CMC joint (*arrow*).

## ▪ JOINT REPLACEMENT

Prosthetic joint replacements are the most common elective orthopedic operations performed in the United States. A total joint replacement arthroplasty replaces both sides of the joint with prosthetic components. A hemiarthroplasty replaces one side of the joint with a prosthesis.

### Materials and Techniques

Metal, polyethylene, and cement are commonly used in manufacturing joint replacements. Metal components—usually titanium or a cobalt-chromium alloy—are used for strength and stiffness. The fatigue strength of these metals under cyclic loading is such that *in vivo* failure is rare. Ultrahigh-molecular-weight polyethylene is used for concave articular surfaces such as the acetabulum, tibial plateau, and glenoid fossa. This material is denser and stiffer than the polyethylene used in common kitchenware and is manufactured to have high resistance to abrasive wear. A metal back is often used to provide mechanical support. Polyethylene is radiolucent—like other plastics—but the presence of a metal back, especially at the acetabulum, may obscure the polyethylene on radiographs. Many polyethylene components have embedded metal markers that indicate their position on radiographs. Bone cement (polymethyl methacrylate or methyl methacrylate) is a rapidly polymerizing acrylic plastic that is used as an adhesive to fix metallic or polyethylene components to the bone. Cement is rendered radiopaque during manufacture by the addition of barium sulfate. Ceramics have become more popular for use as articular surfaces. For the small joints of the hands and feet, silicone rubber prostheses may be used. Recently, pyrolytic carbon components have been introduced for use in the hand.

Implanted metal components are often fixed into the bone with cement. Bubbles in the cement that might act as stress risers are removed before use by centrifugation or vacuum chamber, and the cement is injected into the medullary space under high pressure. A polyethylene plug at the bottom of the prepared cavity creates a closed space and prevents flow of cement down the medullary canal. Metal prostheses that are implanted without cement may have a mechanical press fit that provides immediate stability and a specially textured surface (porous coat) that allows ingrowth of the bone or fibrous tissue, providing eventual long-term fixation. A high degree of precision is ensured at surgery through the use of jigs, cutting guides, and mock-ups that allow the surgeon to achieve a perfect geometric fit between the bone and the prosthetic component. Screws temporarily secure some cementless components until bone ingrowth occurs. Hydroxyapatite crystals applied to the surfaces of cementless metal components during manufacturing may improve biologic fixation in the bone. The crystalline coating of the prosthesis is directly incorporated into the molecular structure of the host bone.

Because different materials deform to different degrees under mechanical loading (their stiffness is different), shear stresses develop at the interfaces, particularly between the bone and metal or the bone and cement. A layer of fibrous tissue that grows into these interfaces helps dissipate the forces by redistributing them over a greater surface area. This layer is similar to the periodontal ligament that cushions the teeth in the softer cancellous bone of the jaws. The fibrous layer may be visible on radiographs as a fine lucency (less than 2 mm thick) between the bone and cement or the bone and metal. An additional area of increased stress is the interface between the cement and metal; microscopic motion may occur at this interface, but no gap should be seen.

### Hip Replacement

There are several general types of hip replacements. A cup arthroplasty resurfaces the articular surface of the femoral head with a metal cup (Fig. 17.10). Hemiarthroplasties of the hip replace the

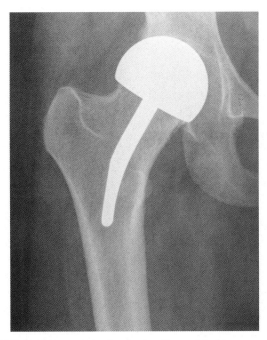

**FIGURE 17.10.** Resurfacing hemiarthroplasty of the hip.

**FIGURE 17.11.** Bilateral femoral endoprostheses, unipolar on the **right** and bipolar on the **left**.

femoral head and neck (Fig. 17.11). Simple femoral prostheses compose a single metal component with a stem that is fitted into the medullary canal and a head that articulates with the native acetabulum. Bipolar femoral prostheses have a metal femoral component comprising a stem and a head and an acetabular component comprising a metal socket with a polyethylene liner. The metal socket articulates with the native acetabulum, and the head of the femoral component articulates with the polyethylene liner. Although the acetabular component is not fixed, most of the motion takes place between the head and liner, preserving the native acetabular cartilage. Hemiarthroplasties are used for the disease of the proximal femur in which the acetabulum is relatively normal. For example, a femoral neck fracture complicated by osteonecrosis might be managed with a bipolar femoral prosthesis. A bipolar prosthesis may be converted to a total hip replacement (THR) with interchangeable components. A THR has both femoral and acetabular components that replace the native articular surfaces (Fig. 17.12). Most currently implanted prostheses have a metal acetabular component

A      B

**FIGURE 17.12.** Total hip replacements (different patients). **A:** Noncemented THR. **B:** Cemented THR.

**A**

**B**

**FIGURE 17.13.** Total hip replacements (different patients). **A:** Noncemented THR with metal-on-metal bearing surface. **B:** Noncemented THR with ceramic head (*arrow*).

with a polyethylene liner that forms the articular surface, so that the bearing surface is metal-on-polyethylene. Some newer implants have metal-on-metal, ceramic-on-polyethylene, or ceramic-on-ceramic bearing surfaces (Fig. 17.13). The components may be fixed to the bone with or without cement. Some surgical approaches require an osteotomy of the greater trochanter for exposure; it is usually reattached with wires or cables. If a nonunion develops, a lurching gait disturbance results. If a gluteal soft-tissue release is used for

surgical exposure, the gluteal musculature may be reattached to the greater trochanter with sutures, screws with washers, or soft-tissue anchors. Bone graft and specialized hardware may be inserted to buttress a deficient proximal femur or acetabulum.

The most common early complication of THR is dislocation. Typically, the femoral head rotates externally out of the acetabulum (Fig. 17.14). Loss of fixation of the acetabular cup may allow it to dislocate from the acetabular bed (Fig. 17.15).

**FIGURE 17.14.** Dislocated THR. The head has moved laterally and superiorly.

**FIGURE 17.15.** Dislocation of the acetabular cup from the acetabular bed, with dislocation of the femoral head from the cup.

**FIGURE 17.16.** Heterotopic ossification in bilateral THRs.

Heterotopic bone formation after THR is common; it may occasionally interfere with motion (Fig. 17.16).

Osteolysis in total joint replacements is usually caused by foreign body granulomatous reaction. The mechanical friction of metal on polyethylene abrades microscopic particles of polyethylene, which incite an osteolytic granulomatous foreign body reaction. Migration of polyethylene debris and its accompanying reaction along cement-bone or metal-bone interfaces—often in the form of a thin membrane—may eventually cause gross loosening. Massive localized osteolysis may also occur; these lesions are filled with the same polyethylene foreign body reaction that caused component loosening. Polyethylene osteolysis usually progresses slowly over many years. Debris may pass through lymphatics to regional lymph nodes. Because the radiolucent polyethylene liners of total joint replacements are responsible for the joint space on

**FIGURE 17.18.** Loose cemented total hip replacement with failure of the cement-metal bond of the femoral component (*arrows*).

radiographs, thinning or gross failure of the polyethylene is evident on radiographs as narrowing of the joint space (Fig. 17.17). Some newer prostheses have eliminated the polyethylene acetabular liner from their designs, replacing it with metal or ceramic liners. Their prostheses therefore have ceramic-on-ceramic or metal-on-metal bearing surfaces.

Radiographic findings that suggest loosening of prosthetic components include widening of the lucent zone at the cement-bone or metal-bone interfaces to greater than 2 mm, migration of components from their original positions, development of a lucent gap between the metal and cement, cement fracture, periosteal reactive bone, and osteolysis. Any gap between the metal and cement is abnormal (Fig. 17.18). A gap of more than 2 mm between the bone and metal or the bone and cement is abnormal. However, a component may not be clinically loose or symptomatic until the gap surrounds the component completely. With radiography, only the interface that is in tangent to the X-ray beam can be confidently assessed. Fragmentation of cement appears to be the result of mechanical failure rather than a biologic process.

## Knee Replacement

The most common total knee replacement (TKR) has a bicondylar femoral component, a tibial component, and a patellar component (Fig. 17.19). The tibial and patellar components have polyethylene articular surfaces. Some designs incorporate meniscal bearings that move with flexion and extension, attempting to duplicate more closely the normal kinematics of the knee (Fig. 17.20).Unconstrained TKRs depend on the muscles and ligaments of the knee for stability. A semi-constrained or intercondylar-stabilized TKR has a post that extends vertically from the tibial component into a slot in the bicondylar component (Fig. 17.21). This mechanism partially constrains the allowable motion of the prosthesis. If the soft-tissue supports of the knee are poor or have been sacrificed, a fully

**FIGURE 17.17.** THR with osteolysis (*white arrow*) around the acetabular cup and proximal lateral femoral stem. The head is asymmetrically positioned (*black arrow*) within the acetabular cup indicating polyethylene failure.

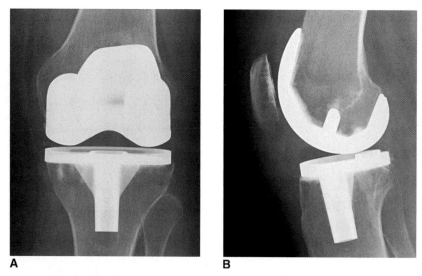

**FIGURE 17.19.** Bicondylar TKR. **A:** Lateral radiograph. **B:** AP radiograph.

**FIGURE 17.20.** Bicondylar TKR with meniscal bearings. **A:** Lateral radiograph. **B:** AP radiograph.

**FIGURE 17.21.** Intercondylar stabilized TKR. **A:** Lateral radiograph. **B:** AP radiograph.

A

B

**FIGURE 17.22.** Rotating hinge TKR. **A:** Lateral radiograph. **B:** AP radiograph.

constrained (rotating hinge) prosthesis may be used (Fig. 17.22). Because the normal knee rotates as it flexes, rotating hinge TKRs have a second articulation comprising a metal post that inserts into a polyethylene socket that allows rotation. The bone stock of the tibia is sometimes deficient because of previous high tibial osteotomy; bone graft may be used to supplement it. Cement is typically used as a surface adhesive to fix the components to the bone. The

ideal alignment of the tibial articular surface is parallel to the floor; this is best demonstrated on standing radiographs.

A unicondylar TKR is used when there is significant, symptomatic disease of either the medial or the lateral compartment but relative preservation of the other compartments. Both sides of the joint of the involved compartment are replaced (Fig. 17.23). The components are typically cemented in place. The bearing surface

A

B

**FIGURE 17.23.** Unicompartmental TKR with cemented polyethylene tibial component. **A:** Lateral radiograph. **B:** AP radiograph.

**A**

**B**

**FIGURE 17.24.**  TKR with loosening of the patellar component. **A:** Postoperative radiograph. **B:** Follow-up radiograph several months later shows resorption of the bone at cement-bone interface of the patellar component (*arrow*).

is polyethylene. The stability of these prostheses depends on the inherent stability of the host knee; the surgery can be accomplished with preservation of both the ACL and PCL. The cost is lower than a bicondylar TKR, and the rehabilitation is typically easier. The long-term results are less predictable, because intervening disease of the remaining compartments often leads to revision to a bicondylar TKR.

Most complications of knee replacements involve the patellar component (Fig. 17.24). Major trauma to limbs with prosthetic joints may result in fractures and dislocations. When fractures occur, they usually begin at a bone-metal interface that acts as a stress riser (Fig. 17.25).

Polyethylene wear and gross fragmentation of the polyethylene bearing surface of the tibia may occur (Fig. 17.26). Polyethylene

**FIGURE 17.25.**  Fracture of the femur through stress riser at the superior edge of the femoral component.

**FIGURE 17.26.**  TKR with polyethylene thinning in the medial compartment (*arrow*).

A    B

**FIGURE 17.27.** TKR with metal synovitis. **A:** Lateral radiograph shows increased radiodensity in the suprapatellar recess (*arrows*) and posterior capsule (*arrowheads*) from deposition of metal in the synovium. **B:** Axial CT scan shows metallic deposition within the synovium of the suprapatellar recess.
*Source:* From Chew FS, Ramsdell MG, Keel SB. Metallosis after total knee replacement. AJR. 1998;170:1556, with permission.

wear can be recognized on radiographs as a loss of joint space on weight-bearing views. Some polyethylene inserts have metal wires embedded within them, and displacement of these wires signifies displacement of the polyethylene. Polyethylene loss from the

patellar component is difficult to recognize without axial (sunrise) patellar radiographs.

Metal particles are also found around joint implants and may be carried to regional lymph nodes. Synovial discoloration is common around prostheses (seen at revision arthroplasty, not on imaging), and the deposition of metal particles has been associated with synovitis (Fig. 17.27). Other biologic effects of metallosis are suspected but not proved. Osteolysis may occur around TKRs, similar to the situation at the hip. Infection is an uncommon complication that often requires arthrocentesis for diagnosis. Soft-tissue swelling with a new effusion is a typical but nonspecific radiographic sign of infection. If organisms are not cultured from the joint fluid at arthrocentesis, an open synovial biopsy may be necessary. Infection of a prosthesis typically leads to its removal.

**FIGURE 17.28.** Total shoulder replacement with cemented polyethylene glenoid component.

**FIGURE 17.29.** Reverse total shoulder replacement.

**A**     **B**

**FIGURE 17.30.**  Total elbow replacement. **A:** Lateral radiograph. **B:** AP radiograph.

## Shoulder Replacement

Shoulder replacement may be used to treat incapacitating arthritic pain (Fig. 17.28). A typical shoulder replacement has a metal humeral component with a head and an intramedullary (IM) stem, as well as a polyethylene glenoid component. Simple humeral head replacements may be used after resection of the native humeral head for problems such as tumors, osteonecrosis, or severe fracture dislocations. Conventional shoulder prostheses are unconstrained, depending on the stability provided by the native soft tissues. When the soft tissues are deficient, reverse shoulder replacement may improve function by placing the prosthetic socket on the humerus and the articulating ball on the glenoid (Fig. 17.29), allowing the deltoid to assume the function of the rotator cuff.

## Elbow Replacement

Elbow replacement is sometimes performed in patients with advanced arthritis, typically rheumatoid arthritis (Fig. 17.30). Total elbow prostheses are linked and replace the hinge articulation between the distal humerus and ulna. The proximal radioulnar joint is sacrificed. Radial head replacements may be used when there is isolated radial head disease, such as severely comminuted fractures.

## Wrist Replacement

Arthroplasties of the wrist are usually reserved for patients with deformities from inflammatory arthritis. Total wrist prostheses with metal components and polyethylene articular surfaces are available; placement of these devices requires resection of the proximal carpal

**A**     **B**

**FIGURE 17.31.**  Total wrist replacement. **A:** PA radiograph. **B:** Lateral radiograph.

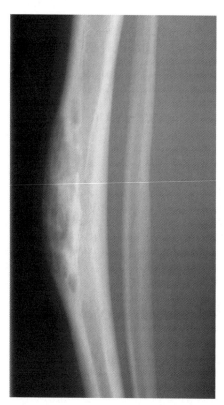

# INDEX

Page numbers in "*italics*" denote figures; those followed by a "t" denote tables.